P023046

D0284839

Taking Charge of the Change

A Holistic Approach to the Three Phases of Menopause

Taking Charge of the Change

A Holistic Approach to the Three Phases of Menopause

LENNIE MARTIN

PAM JUNG

DELMAR

THOMSON LEARNING

Australia   Canada   Mexico   Singapore   Spain   United Kingdom   United States

DELMAR

THOMSON LEARNING

Taking Charge of the Change: A Holistic Approach to the Three Phases of Menopause
by Lennie Martin and Pam Jung

Health Care Publishing Director:
William Brottmiller

Product Development Manager:
Marion S. Waldman

Product Development Editor:
Jill Rembetski

Editorial Assistant:
Robin Irons

Executive Marketing Manager:
Dawn F. Gerrain

Channel Manager:
Gretta Oliver

Production Editor:
Mary Colleen Liburdi

Cover Design:
Mary Colleen Liburdi

COPYRIGHT © 2002 by Delmar, a division of Thomson Learning, Inc. Thomson Learning™ is a trademark used herein under license.

Printed in Canada
1 2 3 4 5 XXX 05 04 03 02 01

For more information, contact Delmar, 3 Columbia Circle, PO Box 15015, Albany, NY 12212-0515

Or you can visit our Internet site at http://www.delmar.com

ALL RIGHTS RESERVED. No part of this work covered by the copyright hereon may be reproduced or used in any form or by any means—graphics, electronic, or mechanical, including photocopying, recording, taping, Web distribution, or information storage and retrieval system—without permission of the publisher.

For permission to use material from this text or product, contact us by
Tel   (800) 730-2214
Fax   (800) 730-2215
www.thomsonrights.com

Library of Congress Cataloging-in-Publication Data
Martin, Lennie, RN.
    Taking charge of the change : a holistic approach to the three phases of menopause / Lennie Martin & Pam Jung.
        p. cm.
    Includes bibliographical references and index.
        ISBN 0-7668-3276-7 (alk. paper)
        1. Menopause.   2. Menopause—Psychological aspects.   3. Self-care, Health.   4. Middle aged women—Health and hygiene.   I. Jung, Pam. II. Title.
    RG186 .M326 2001
    618.1'75—dc21   2001047318

NOTICE TO THE READER

Publisher does not warrant or guarantee any of the products described herein or perform any independent analysis in connection with any of the product information contained herein. Publisher does not assume, and expressly disclaims, any obligation to obtain and include information other than that provided to it by the manufacturer.

The reader is expressly warned to consider and adopt all safety precautions that might be indicated by the activities herein and to avoid all potential hazards. By following the instructions contained herein, the reader willingly assumes all risks in connection with such instructions.

The Publisher makes no representation or warranties of any kind, including but not limited to, the warranties of fitness for particular purpose or merchantability, nor are any such representations implied with respect to the material set forth herein, and the publisher takes no responsibility with respect to such material. The publisher shall not be liable for any special, consequential, or exemplary damages resulting, in whole or part, from the readers' use of, or reliance upon, this material.

CONTENTS

PREFACE

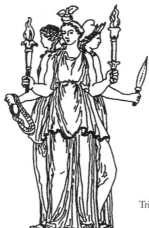

Triple Hecate (the Triple Goddess).
Reproduced with permission.
Copyright © Kate Cartwright.

Menopause is a body-mind-spirit experience that can revolutionize women's lives. This event signals moving from the first half of life to the second half. It is a developmental transition of major importance. The physical and emotional symptoms that begin in perimenopause act as harbingers of this transition, and are catalysts for body-mind changes. These often propel women into new relationships with self and others. Frequently, what women are interested in, committed to, and willing to invest their energy in undergoes a shift. Values and priorities change. Women begin to relate differently to themselves, as earlier aspects fade and new self-expressions emerge. What gives a woman "juice"—what energizes and activates the imagination, what fascinates and attracts interest—may come from surprising sources.

As an event of life-changing significance, menopause has been receiving wide coverage in articles, books, and other media. In part this is caused by the large number of baby-boomer women entering menopause. This book draws upon many excellent sources, and adds a fresh dimension through its holistic, integrative approach. We take a definite path in our presentation of levels of health and well-being, moving from the outward, in the form of the physical aspects, to the inward in the form of mental-emotional aspects, and finally to the deepest level of the spiritual and archetypal dimensions. We feel that it is only through integrating all these levels that a woman can truly feel whole.

Menopause is a gateway into a new phase of life. The symbol of passing through a gate signifies crossing a boundary, going from one reality to another, or moving from one terrain to another. Once the boundary is crossed, you cannot remain the same person as before. Many aspects of women's lives change around menopause. Although facing uncertainty in this new terrain, most women now approach the transition with confidence and anticipation. Many sense that they are moving into greater freedom to be their authentic self. Fresh forms of self-expression begin to take shape, and avenues for creativity may open up that were not possible while fulfilling the demands of family and professional life. For most women, this is a spiritually expansive phase.

If you are a woman between 30 and 60 years of age, you will find much of interest in these pages. Because perimenopause can start a decade before actual menopause, it actually is not too early to begin learning about it in your mid-30s. For women in their 50s and beyond who have achieved menopause, this book gives information on how to maintain physical and mental health and vitality well into the later years.

The population of menopausal women is growing rapidly. By the year 2000 more than 50 million women had achieved 50-plus years of age. It is becoming more apparent that mature women are a force that is actively shaping society and its priorities. One of those priorities is health, broadly defined in the body-mind-spirit literature of today. More women are taking charge of their well-being rather than leaving it to society, doctors, or the media to define. They are searching for new models, and rejecting the old model in which menopause is seen as a deficiency disease curable by artificial estrogen. Women want to learn all they can about this change in their lives, find out what their options are, then make decisions with the help of their therapists and health-care providers. Women today want to:

- understand what is actually happening in their bodies, in user-friendly terms.
- know what options exist to relieve symptoms (both Western medicine and alternative).
- get reliable, up-to-date information.
- know that they are not alone during these challenging times.
- be assured that they will have many more productive, sexy, and vital years.

> The number of women now entering midlife is an unprecedented historic event that I firmly believe is sowing the seeds for a cultural reawakening of feminine value.
>
> —Joan Borysenko, *A Woman's Book of Life*

> Today, millions of us are moving into our fruitfulness and our wisdom
> with potential undreamed of in other generations. I have often said
> that the hope for the future may well rest with the truthfulness and
> wisdom of postmenopausal women.
>
> —Christiane Northrup, *Health Wisdom for Women*, February, 1996

Menopause is also about what is happening on a woman's soul or spirit level. Women are searching for archetypes that foster qualities of the mature woman with which they can identify. Transcultural images of powerful, compassionate, wise elders who are continually co-creating a reality that is healing and inclusive are coming more clearly into view. Not only are individual women in need of this enlightened feminine energy, so too is the world. We share a vision of what this could look like in the chapters on spirituality and archetypes.

AN INTEGRATED APPROACH TO HOLISTIC MENOPAUSE

Our primary motivation for writing this book came through our personal journeys through menopause. In our professional practice, teaching, research, and personal lives we came to realize that menopause is much more than hormone changes, coping with physical or mental symptoms, and adjusting to changes in family or career configurations. Indeed, the menopause experience encompasses the whole woman. Patterns of thinking shift. Priorities are readjusted. Yearnings from deep within reveal themselves, and women feel drawn to creative self-expression and spiritual exploration. A need surfaces for feeling complete, integrated, and anchored in our core being, the authentic self. We wanted to find ways to share these processes with other women, and to communicate what we have learned so that others can find validation and support in their menopause transitions.

A great deal has been written about the physical aspects of menopause. Much also has been written about the mental-emotional aspects. Some has been written about the spiritual and archetypal aspects. However, it is not easy to find a book that includes all these aspects and integrates them into a comprehensive view of the whole-woman menopause experience. In this book, we provide just such an integrated approach; it is both inclusive and holistic in its philosophy and its practical suggestions for dealing with symptoms.

Some writers seem to equate a holistic approach with alternative therapies. We believe the holistic approach includes the whole range of options, spanning western allopathic medicine as well as herbal therapy, nutrition, and yoga. Many practitioners are now envisioning health care as a continuum, from which therapies are selected that are best suited to the person and the condition. This is called integrative medicine. Women are provided with options ranging from pharmaceutical drugs or surgery to control symptoms, to nutraceutical or energy-body-mind therapies to restore balance, to a meditation retreat for gaining clarity and peace about their lives.

In this process, there is acceptance of the woman's individual choices. The health practitioner's responsibility is to offer the woman information, to review a range of options, and to discuss possible consequences of decisions. Medications, herbal and nutraceutical therapies, and lifestyle choices such as diet, exercise, service, stress reduction, and mind-calming practices may all be considered. Then, support is given to each woman in making the decisions that affect her life. Emphasis usually is placed on preventive and health-promoting actions. This is the partnership paradigm that we adhere to in our book.

Women today often must be their own health advocates. Given the limited time for visits in most managed-care health settings, we urge women to be well-prepared when they see their health practitioner. We suggest that a woman does some research first and makes a list of questions, goals, and preferences. If appropriate, fax the list in advance of your visit so that the professional may prepare for your appointment. This sets the tone for partnership, and provides a basis for discussing options. This book can be helpful to both you and your health practitioner by offering:

- current research on pharmaceutical, herbal, and nutraceutical therapies.
- inclusive view of how this major life transition impacts women.
- review of contemporary thinking of leaders in menopausal women's health.
- discussion of areas of controversy in diagnosing and treating problems.
- description of the natural, human-identical hormone therapy that women are now requesting.
- emphasis on lifestyle choices, which have profound implications for health in midlife and beyond.

Our philosophy supports women having a choice in all aspects of their lives, including health. To have informed choices, a woman needs to educate herself, establish partnerships with experts, and cultivate the ability to follow her own inner guidance.

Blending Science, Philosophy, and Spirituality

Women experience their lives as an integrated whole, although the focus from moment to moment shifts from one aspect to another. We have constantly been intrigued by the flow in women's experiences from physical and social realities, to their inner emotional and conceptual perceptions, to wrapping their minds around scientific explanations offered by physics and brain research, to having mystical or intuitive episodes that provide flashes of sudden insight. In this book, we blend a good deal of science with philosophies of living and spiritual or archetypal frameworks. We hope to help women find wholeness through acknowledging and supporting these interwoven processes. In our fragmented, fast-paced, technological society, it is easy for women to feel they are not in control of their destinies. They may find little time to contemplate the deeper meanings of life. There may be little sense of the connection of womankind through time and various cultures, through our "herstory" and feminine traditions. By including these in our book, we hope to lend strength, comfort, and healing to contemporary women.

Spirituality, in the context of this book, does not mean any particular religious perspective. We draw examples from a number of religious traditions to provide insight into women's spiritual processes. Our purpose is not to cover every religious viewpoint, but to offer perspectives we, or other women, have found meaningful. Our discussions with many women going through menopause support the idea that it is a major spiritual transition. We encourage women to pay attention to the ineffable aspects of their lives. Being aware of the spiritual dimensions, and realizing that more is happening during menopause than meets the eye, might provide an opening for the Spirit or the Divine to come more consciously into a woman's life.

CONCEPTUAL APPROACH AND ORGANIZATION

Our conceptual framework moves from a broad overview of an integrated, holistic approach to menopause, into the details of women's physical and mental-emotional experiences, and then to an exploration of the characteristics of women's spiritual journeys and the archetypal patterns that often find expression during midlife and menopause.

Chapter 1: Holistic Menopause describes our philosophy of holistic menopause and self-care, and what is needed to take charge of this major life transition. Thereafter, the book is organized by three broad aspects of menopause: the physical (Chapters 2 and 3), the mental/emotional (Chapter 4), and the spiritual/archetypal (Chapters 5 and 6).

Chapter 2: The Physical Experience: Symptoms, Risks, and Testing describes perimenopausal and menopausal symptoms, hormone patterns, risk factors for health problems, and diagnostic tests and health screening appropriate at midlife and later.

Chapter 3: The Physical Experience: Hormones, Herbs, and Lifestyle provides an in-depth discussion of prescription hormone replacement therapy (HRT) and considerations in using these hormones (both synthetic and human-identical hormones), and approaches to managing menopause naturally, including nutrition, supplements, herbs, lifestyle, and other alternative therapies. It contains a health matrix giving a concise overview of most therapy options for symptoms and health problems.

Chapter 4: The Mental-Emotional Experience examines the phases of midlife women's psychological development, and describes recent research and information about brain and mental functions, depression and mood disorders, and other related symptoms. It addresses the impact of stress and adrenal fatigue, and reviews a wide range of therapies for managing symptoms and problems.

Chapter 5: Women's Spiritual Journey explores menopause as a spiritual passage and presents a model of energy fields and centers that connect spirit and body-mind. It reviews possible relationships between quantum physics and neurotheology, and the experience of expanded states of consciousness. Unique characteristics of women's spiritual path are proposed, with suggestions for enhancing spiritual growth. Traditions, rituals, and ceremonies for spiritual expression are included, with examples of women mentoring others and transforming their own lives. The purpose of the wise woman in contemporary society is addressed.

Chapter 6: Archetypes of Midlife and Menopausal Women ventures into the realm of archetypal thought forms and their importance during this major transition. The roots of the sacred feminine are traced in newly revealed information about ancient goddess-centered peoples and early gnostic Christians. Archetypes are explored as a bridge between the world of mind and that of spirit, connecting women to universal patterns. Several examples are given of archetypes that find expression during this time in women's lives, and a new Creatrix archetype, forming a fourth face of the traditional triple goddess, is described. Processes for healing ourselves and future generations, and the new world vision of wise women are examined.

FEATURES AND BENEFITS

Several features make this book unique. As a holistic approach to midlife and menopause, it provides a balanced view of the benefits and side effects of Western medical and alternative therapies for the entire range of menopausal concerns. Body-mind and spirit are equally honored for their functions in women's lives, for it is the health of all these that makes us whole. Comprehensive information is provided in a user-friendly way with numerous graphs, illustrations, charts, and worksheets to enhance learning and allow women to individualize the material.

Special focus is placed on art that represents expansive, powerful, and symbolic aspects of women, including a wide array of goddess and mythic images. The path of women's spiritual unfolding is described, with special features connected with the feminine divine. Women are brought in touch with the long heritage of feminine archetypes in history and myth, and offered guidance in drawing upon the energies of archetypes to bring deeper aspects of the self into expression.

Some specific features and their respective benefits include:

Feature: The matrix
Benefit: This summary of several therapies for each symptom or aspect of menopausal health provides a clear, quick reference.

Feature: Holistic coverage
Benefit: A woman can see the range of choices available to her, on a continuum from Western medicine to alternative therapies to lifestyle.

Feature: Body-mind and spirit are included in one book.
Benefit: By viewing menopause in its entirety—and working on all levels simultaneously—this transition, and the changes it requires, may be navigated in greater depth, and made easier to understand and accept.

Feature: Expressive art and insightful quotes from women's experiences
Benefit: Meaningful illustrations and quotes add to the enjoyment of the book and help anchor concepts in the mind.

Feature: Boxed material, Appendices
Benefit: Examples, stories, and related information are presented in a way that enriches the material while not interrupting the flow of the narrative.

Feature: The science of a symptom is correlated with a possible spiritual or energetic explanation for that symptom. An example is hot flashes, which are defined scientifically as hormonally mediated vascular instability causing destabilization of the brain's temperature regulating mechanism. On the level of energy fields and spiritual forces, however, it has been explained as kundalini (life force) rising in a woman's spine to open her awareness and expand her consciousness.
Benefit: Considering a "symptom" in this new context can add to a woman's sense of well-being and lead to a much deeper understanding and acceptance of self.

Feature: Extensive references are included at the end of each chapter.
Benefit: Readers who wish to study the subject further will find a wealth of both up-to-date and classic resources from which to draw.

Feature: Worksheets and exercises.
Benefit: Through exercises and activities, a reader personalizes the material, makes valuable self-assessments, and practices her skills.

Sheer numbers, if nothing else, are forcing a re-examination of negative stereotypes of the older woman. We are also witnessing a renaissance of self-help groups. . . . Menopause support groups are now found all around the country. . . . Working as a unit, women have the chance to explore every aspect of their changing, developing lives . . . it is not enough to merely reject the negative concepts of the menopausal and postmenopausal woman. We need positive, strong role models to take their place.

—Jane L. Mickelson, "Changing Woman," in *Women of the 14th Moon*

REFERENCES

Borysenko, J. (1996). *A woman's book of life: The biology, psychology, and spirituality of the feminine life cycle.* New York: Riverhead Books.

Mickelson, J.L. (1991). Changing woman. In Taylor, D., & Sumrall, A.C. (Eds.). *Women of the 14th moon.* Freedom, CA: The Crossing Press.

Northrup, C. (1996). Listening to your body's wisdom: The wisdom of menopause. *Dr. Christiane Northrup's Health Wisdom for Women, 3:*6–7.

ABOUT THE AUTHORS

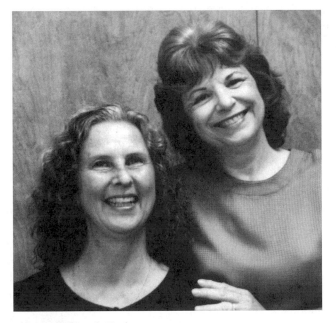

Pam Jung and Lennie Martin
Co-founders, Women at the Gateway
Website: *www.women-at-the-gateway.bigstep.com*

LEONIDE (LENNIE) MARTIN, RN, MSN, FNP, DrPH

Lennie retired early from her university nursing position to live in a spiritual community and work as a family nurse practitioner in a rural clinic. She is an emeritus professor, has held many leadership positions, received academic and professional honors, and published and presented at conferences and workshops. Currently Lennie practices as an FNP at Sierra Family Medical Clinic, Nevada City, California. Certified in Intuitive Healing by Holos Institute, Springfield,

Missouri, she also provides health and intuition consulting and co-founded Women at the Gateway, an organization that educates women about holistic menopause.

Lennie describes her menopause journey:

> My menopause transition at age 55 was relatively smooth. The last 5 years before menses stopped were the most difficult with a lot of pelvic congestion symptoms. Herbal teas (PMS tea) and vitamin B_6 really helped relieve this. As my periods dwindled off, I coped with hot flashes by using wild yam cream and vitex tincture (prepared by my co-author, Pam Jung). Although familiar with hormone-replacement therapy, I never felt that my symptoms or risk assessment were severe enough to need this assistance.
>
> My professional background includes graduate nursing and public health degrees, with a long academic career and many years specializing in women's health. In my current work as a family nurse practitioner, I assist women in managing their menopause transitions. My patients have shared a wide variety of journeys during this life-change phase. I believe in offering women a full range of choices, from prescription hormones, to herbals and nutraceuticals, to nothing more than a healthy lifestyle. My goal is to help empower women to gain knowledge of their menopausal transition process. By better understanding their inner self, women can make the choices that most enhance their personal-spiritual growth and body-mind health.
>
> It is, however, the symbolic, archetypal meanings of symptoms and illness that hold special fascination for me. The body is a "true messenger," giving us important communications in code language. Using intuition and energy-body analysis (drawing from the works of Caroline Myss, Jean Shinoda Bolen, Mona Lisa Schultz, and others), I provide consulting to assist people to understand the messages of their body-mind. In this work, I use many techniques from my spiritual studies that are powerful ways to accomplish change.
>
> In addition to a passion for the wise-woman archetype, and my many professional interests, my life includes the wonderful companionship of my husband, David, the delight of our children and grandchildren, and the joy of our horses and cats, and the wild creatures and trees with which we share our home in the Sierra Nevada Mountains of California.

PAMELA JUNG, BA

After a career in public relations and advertising, Pam studied herbalism and nutrition, and now wildcrafts local herbs and consults on women's groups, ritual, and ceremony. She co-founded Women at the Gateway and offers experiential workshops symbolizing women's midlife and menopause transitions. Currently Pam is a freelance writer, contributing a series of articles to *The Union,* among other projects. Pam lives in Nevada City, California.

Pam describes her menopause journey:

> My menopause was an early one, completed by age 48. My physical symptoms were relatively minor, with only mild-to-moderate hot flashes disrupting my life for a

while. I did, however, find the mental/emotional symptoms troubling, ranging from feeling moody on a regular basis to feeling occasionally depressed. As I had no successful menopausal role models in my life at the time, I turned to research to learn all I could about "the change."

Being a bit of a rebel at heart, I did not take any advanced degrees but rather set out on my own to study alternative therapies. I became a backyard herbalist (someone who makes her own tinctures and teas from what she grows or wildcrafts locally) in the process. After reading book after book and article after article in the burgeoning field of menopausal studies, I realized how confusing it must be to someone just beginning to learn. My organizational nature connected with my skills as a writer to produce a matrix that summarized the nutritional, herbal, and lifestyle therapies that both the researchers and my own personal experience showed were effective for relieving symptoms associated with menopause. Later, with Lennie's pharmaceutical contributions, this matrix became a seminal part of this book.

The more I shared this information with the women I knew, the more I found that it was becoming a primary interest of mine. The word "menopause" can produce fear and anxiety in people who don't know what to expect. Our cultural stereotypes certainly exacerbate this fear with their underlying denial of aging. Thus, in this book I am teaching and writing honestly about the ups and downs of menopause, and touting its promises.

In addition to being a principal in Women at the Gateway—the business Lennie and I founded to do educational research in menopause—I am involved in death and dying through my volunteer work with hospice and in my elder-care work. As a postmenopausal single woman, I am also helping, along with many sisters, to bring a new archetype into being.

HOW TO GET IN TOUCH WITH US

We appreciate your feedback and ideas. Women enjoy telling their stories. It is wonderful to be listened to and heard. We all learn from hearing how others manage and grow from their experiences. You may contact us at:

Women at the Gateway
P.O. Box 2196
Nevada City, CA 95959
Website: *www.women-at-the-gateway.bigstep.com*

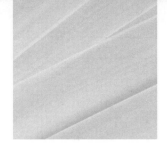

ACKNOWLEDGMENTS

Thanks are due to all the researchers, health providers, authors, and scientists whose works have given the foundation upon which we have built.

Our special appreciation to the artists, whose imaginations have captured visually the essence of women's midlife journeys down through the ages. Artists Kate Cartwright, Alta Wertz, Sharyn McDonald, Sandra Stanton, and Margo Gal have helped us present the incredible richness of feminine symbolism, across cultures and time.

Much gratitude to all the women who have participated in our classes and retreats, sharing their life stories, difficulties, and wisdom with us; to these sisters we owe a special debt and we honor them ever in our hearts.

David Gortner, Lennie's husband, deserves special thanks as our "computer angel"—he is a great electronic trouble-shooter and a patient sage for teaching computer relations.

The publisher, editors, and staff at Delmar Thomson Learning have provided invaluable assistance in bringing this book into form. Bill Brottmiller, publisher, Marion Waldman, project development manager, Jill Rembetski, product development editor, Robin Irons, editorial assistant, and Mary Colleen Liburdi, production editor offered support essential for successful completion of this project. Thank you, too, to Nancy Crompton for her expert help in editing. Special thanks to Lynn Keegan, series editor, for her continuous encouragement and enthusiasm, which kept our energy flowing toward the goal. We would also like to thank Roberta B. Hollander, PhD, MPH, Kathleen Palladino, RN, Lynn Rew, EdD, RNC, HNC, FAAN, Joann Venes, MSN, CRNP, and Wendy Wetzel, RN, for reviewing the manuscript and offering valuable suggestions toward its improvement.

CHAPTER 1

Holistic Menopause

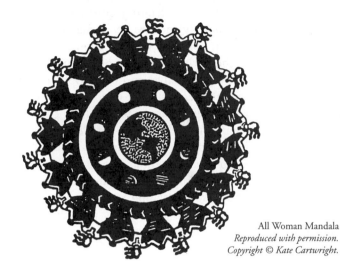

All Woman Mandala
Reproduced with permission.
Copyright © Kate Cartwright.

A lovely Spanish women came to our class on menopause as a major life transformation. At age 62, she was vibrantly alive with curly brown hair cascading to her shoulders and sparkling bright black eyes. Her menopause had occurred several years before with minimal symptoms, which she had managed with herbs including black cohosh and vitex. Her interest in coming to the class was spurred by a feeling that there was something much bigger about menopause than the end of periods and a few years' worth of symptoms. She sensed there was a deep and profound transition happening within her in psychological and spiritual ways. This process seemed to have connections with other women around the world, and with changes happening in the consciousness of our whole planet. She wanted to become a more conscious participant in this process.

This is exactly what happens for women during midlife and menopause: a transition of profound proportions, a change from one phase of life to another. It is a time of many endings, of completions, of coming to terms with our shadow, looking at what is and is not working in our lives, facing the specter of our fears, and breaking through limiting beliefs and thought patterns. Simultaneously it is a time of beginnings, discoveries, awakenings to our deepest self, and the expansion of boundaries. Typical of such great changes, this time is often fraught with challenges and difficulties.

The current generation of midlife women is taking a whole new approach to these challenges. The "baby boomers" born after World War II are now in the perimenopause years, with some having completed menopause already. This group's experiences of menopause are changing cultural definitions and expectations. Always proactive, this generation of menopausal women is now bringing an explosion of awareness to society and individuals about this phase of women's lives. Breaking the silence of their mothers' generation, when "the change" was barely acknowledged, they are accelerating cultural evolution by energetically embracing these changes in body and psyche, and actively seeking ways to bring balance to their lives during this time. Going beyond even that, they are plumbing inner depths to find the spiritual meaning of the menopause transition.

This chapter presents the perspectives and philosophy of the authors on taking a whole-woman approach to menopause. It introduces themes that run throughout this book: the three phases of menopause, taking charge of one's life as the core of self-care, understanding the scientific basis of menopause physiology and therapies, blending the practical with the inspirational, respecting a range of choices to meet individual needs, listening to and honoring inner guidance, the personal and transpersonal importance of menopause, and exploring the metaphysical aspects of menopause by relating to symbolic and archetypal patterns. Later chapters develop these ideas more fully, providing references for further study and activities for applying them to your own life.

40 MILLION MENOPAUSAL WOMEN

As the 21st century begins, the world is seeing a dramatic rise in the numbers of women entering menopause. About 40 million American women are presently experiencing menopause, with another 20 million women expected to reach it in the next 10 years (Finkel, Cohen, & Mahoney, 2001). More women than at any time in history are now perimenopausal or menopausal. Nearly one-half of the female adult population in the United States is in this age range (Jacobowitz, 1996). In the United States and Canada, more than 4,000 women achieve

> Ultimately, I've found this journey bracing, exciting, and health-enhancing. . . . So please join me—and the millions of others who have come before and will come after—as we transform and improve our lives, and ultimately our culture, through understanding, applying, and living the wisdom of menopause.
>
> —Christiane Northrup, *The Wisdom of Menopause*

menopause every day. Worldwide, 24.5 million women reach menopause each year (North American Menopause Society, 2000).

The average woman's life expectancy has increased significantly. Until quite recently, few women lived beyond menopause. In 1900, women lived on average 50 years, but by 1997 this rose to nearly 80 years. By the year 2020, a baby girl born in a developed country will have an average life expectancy of 90 years (Doctor's Guide, 1997). An American woman who was 60 years old in the 1990s has a life expectancy of 83.1 years (National Center for Health Statistics, 1996). By 2030, more than 70 million Americans will be over 65 years old, the majority of whom will be women. The present group of menopausal women may expect to live 30 years or more after menopause—about one-third of their lives (Amerongen, 2000).

Could the phenomenon of millions of menopausal women around the world have a deep significance? As these millions of women enter their wisdom years, and change the thinking of their societies about midlife and older women, this may serve to bring a powerful feminine consciousness into the world. Feminine energy is intuitive and supportive. It is concerned with connectedness, nurturance, and acceptance. It encourages diversity and is life-sustaining for all forms of life and the earth itself. Feminine energy seeks to harmonize with the cycles of living systems, and resonates with the greater cycles of earth, the moon, the sun and planets. The masculine consciousness that has dominated the world for centuries has advanced science and technology, but has also brought serious imbalance to the environment, social systems, and relations among nations. The earth needs the expanding feminine consciousness brought by menopausal women to ensure its survival and well-being.

Cycles of a Woman's Life

Women's lives have rhythms that put them in phase with earth and moon cycles. In traditional cultures, women's menstrual patterns followed moon phases. The processes of childbearing and caretaking connected women with the cycles of human life. Their roles in providing food and nourishment traditionally connected women with the cycles of nature and growing things. Being close to nature

> The midlife woman has the power and the voice to bring the message of respect, care, and interdependence to all people and help rekindle a reawakening to these core feminine values throughout society. It's no mistake that the current movement of psychospiritual healing is composed largely of women in their thirties, forties, and fifties. We are awakening en masse and beginning to deliver a much-needed message of health, hope, and healing to the world.
>
> —Joan Borysenko, *A Woman's Book of Life*

brought women into harmony with the seasons of the year, which are symbolically connected with the four directions. The phases of the moon are associated with the seasons, directions, and qualities of being that are brought into expression through the energies created in this merging. These processes relate to the unfolding of women's spirituality, and to the archetypal patterns that represent complementary states of consciousness.

The menopause transition is associated with the third phase in this system. This is the time of the waning moon, of autumn with its richness and abundance, and of the West as the sun begins to set beyond the vast waters. The energy needed is that of flowing with change, with processes that lead to the unknown. The state of consciousness evoked in the mature, midlife woman is one of being complete, fulfilled, and at the height of creative expression. From this fullness, she blesses others and the world with her gifts of love, compassion, generosity, and wisdom. This phase of the Creatrix archetype may last for many years, and lays the

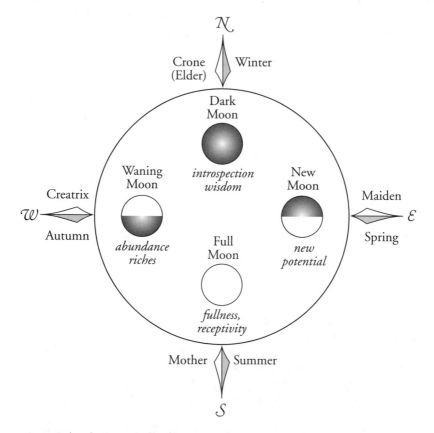

Figure 1–1 Cycles of a Woman's Life. The greater cycle of a woman's life is associated with moon phases, seasons of the year, the four directions, the four major archetypes, and qualities associated with each phase.

> So we are connected to the moon. That gives us a power, a connec-
> tion to the earth and the moon, men don't know about.
>
> —Cecilia Mitchell, Mohawk, in *Wisdom's Daughters:*
> *Conversations with Women Elders of Native America*

foundation for moving into the last phase of life. This closing of the cycle as an elder wise woman, at the dark moon phase, brings the great transformation into spirit. (See Figure 1–1. These ideas are described more fully in Chapters 4 and 5.)

WHAT IS HOLISTIC MENOPAUSE?

In our view, holistic menopause means engaging with all aspects of a woman's being during this time of transition: the physical, the mental-emotional, and the spiritual. Holistic means to be whole, a unity, complete, oneness with no part left out. It also recognizes that the whole is more than the sum of its parts, having a transcendent quality that defies definition. Holism involves understanding the individual as an integrated whole, interacting with both the internal and external environments (Keegan & Dossey, 1998). This integrated body-mind-spirit approach is the inspiration and guiding force for our approach to menopause.

Menopause is certainly an intense physical experience with a wide array of symptoms. Some women feel overwhelmed by these compelling body sensations, such as hot flashes, insomnia, fatigue, and menstrual problems. Others have milder symptoms but still are very aware of their body changing. The mind often seems to malfunction, with symptoms of forgetfulness and poor concentration. There also is a sense of the brain firing up, activating intense connections that bring novel perceptions and understandings, and enhancing intuition (Northrup, 2001). Emotionally, women may feel fragile or explosive, with wildly fluctuating moods and bouts of depression or anxiety. Profound moments of unimagined compassion and radiant universal love may also manifest. The range of experiences is great, but virtually every woman senses that she is going through transitions that will make her different in some very important ways.

The spiritual aspect of the menopause journey is deeply felt by most women, who experience the need to get their lives in order. Menopause prompts a developmental stage that says, "Bring unfinished business in your life to completion, learn the lessons of adversity, integrate all life's experiences, heal and release the past." There is urgency around resolving issues and getting in touch with inner, core values. No longer can women put things off because they are too busy tending their family, running a household, or building a career. This great push for resolution is a springboard for the phase of accelerated spiritual growth that follows midlife. As human beings, we are biologically programmed for this move

> With our child-rearing years behind us, our creative energies are freed. Our search for life's meaning begins to take on new urgency, and we begin to experience ourselves as potential vessels for Spirit.
>
> —Christiane Northrup, *The Wisdom of Menopause*

into fuller spiritual expression. Perimenopause is the messenger and menopause the initiator of this spiritual unfolding.

Menopause has profound significance in women's lives. It offers opportunity for vast expansion and fulfillment. The more informed women are about the experiences and processes involved, the greater their ability to flow with events, transform challenges into valuable knowledge, and gather to themselves the mantle of wisdom.

In keeping with this holistic philosophy, this book is structured to cover all aspects of menopause: physical, mental-emotional, and spiritual. While all three happen simultaneously in the menopause experience, these aspects are discussed in separate chapters. The divisions in this book are merely a tool of communication, and we hope that the chapters will flow together smoothly as an undivided web of inner understanding to guide your menopause transition.

Alaina: Menopause Mysteries

At around age 48, Alaina began noticing changes in her menstrual cycles, with heavier flow, more intense premenstrual pelvic pressure and bloating, and increased emotional sensitivity. Her cycles had always been mild, and these new symptoms were tolerable. During this time she was also initiating a new phase of psychological and spiritual exploration. Having participated in several religious traditions, including Christian and Eastern, she was now drawn to study earth religions with foundations in goddess traditions. This exploration was gradually moving her away from her current church, into a wide network of associations with women's spiritual groups. This was an exciting but unsettling time of participating in ritual and personal spiritual practices that in many ways contradicted her former belief systems.

A professional woman with a successful career, Alaina was in her second marriage and had grown children. She faced some challenges on all fronts. Well-established patterns of honest communication, and respecting each other's viewpoints, supported family relationships through this time.

(Continued on next page)

However, she was increasingly dissatisfied with work, feeling a strong drive inside to move into her own "mission," though that was ill-defined. Alaina had always been a free-thinking person who defied many social and cultural dictates during her adolescence and younger adulthood. Now the hormonal changes of perimenopause were fueling her journey toward another level of seeking inner truth and guidance.

Hot flashes began to add their urgency a couple of years later, although Alaina was still having periods. She related to these "power surges," as signals of the rising inner fire of transformation (called "kundalini rising" in Eastern traditions). Pressure was building, and Alaina knew she needed to make some real-world changes in her life. She reduced her time at work and began to develop her own business, which provided channels for creativity and self-expression. She challenged some rules and practices of her church that she found constraining. When little change occurred, she became more involved with other groups that supported her need for spiritual expansion. For the physical symptoms of menopause, Alaina used herbs and soy isoflavones with good results.

Holistic Approach to Taking Charge of the Change

Holistic therapies are often regarded as the same as alternative therapies (also called complementary medicine). However, in a truly holistic approach the entire range of therapies is considered. This includes Western (allopathic) medical treatments as well as alternative therapies, nutrition, lifestyle modifications, and self-care methods. Each woman's needs and preferences are unique. Presenting a broad spectrum of therapies and methods provides women with information about various options for managing perimenopause and menopause.

The field of alternative therapies has exploded in recent years, and it is not feasible here to discuss every method available. Our focus is upon therapies that are specific to women during midlife and menopause, and are widely used or well documented for relief of menopausal symptoms. These include herbal therapies, nutrition and diet, lifestyle (habits, stress, exercise), yoga, and methods for working with the mind (beliefs, attitudes, and values).

Inherent in this approach is a deep honoring of each woman's right to choose her own methods of managing her menopause. Health practitioners, friends, experts, family members, and organizations often have strong opinions about how to manage symptoms and stay healthy during this time. The huge amount of information on menopause, much of it conflicting, leaves many women feeling confused and overwhelmed. At first it may seem easiest to leave decisions to someone else, particularly an expert or health practitioner. If you do not feel comfortable with a therapy, however, or have deep misgivings, even if they are vague, this may be the voice of inner wisdom giving you guidance. The most important thing is to listen to your body and its messages, whether they manifest as "gut feelings" or in a more subtle manner. Seek the advice of respected experts, learn as much as possible about your options, and then look within for confirmation of your choices.

Any therapy works for some women some of the time. Certain approaches have more risks than others, some work faster, some are more gentle and natural. Some choices for therapies have social consequences or impacts on other creatures or cultures. Use as wide a framework as you wish in considering your choices. Realize that others may disagree or think another way is better. The more your choices are drawn from deep self-knowledge and resonate with your core values, the better they will work in your life.

Blending Science and Inspiration

You will find more science here than in most books written for the layperson. Research related to midlife and menopause is rapidly expanding. It is amazing how many studies are being conducted about various aspects of menopause, especially in the areas of hormone-replacement therapy, cardiovascular (heart) health, osteoporosis and bone health, cognition and brain functioning, and female cancers (breast, uterine, and ovarian). There are controversies in a number of these areas that bear directly on women's health and choices during menopause. Key research studies are reviewed in this book in clear and understandable terms. You deserve to know what scientific evidence is revealing, so that you can make the most informed decisions.

Scientific research can be tricky to read and understand. Most studies have some limiting factors, such as the sample size and characteristics or how well the study results can be applied to a wider population of women. The statistical methods used in research cannot "prove" something is true, but can say only that there is a very small probability that the results occurred from chance (thereby implying that the results were caused by the factors being studied). Thus, one has to be careful of the interpretation of research results, especially by the popular media. For example, results showing a decrease in breast cell proliferation (growth) when progesterone cream is applied to breasts are many steps removed from concluding that this approach will curtail growth of breast cancer cells or prevent breast cancer.

Still, research offers important information for our decision making. The medical world relies heavily on research results to guide recommendations for treatment, especially for use of drugs and diagnostic tests. Some health practitioners do not keep up with the latest research in women's health, or disregard study results that do not agree with their preformed ideas. Particularly controversial are studies about mammography and the risk of breast cancer, and hormone-replacement therapy (HRT) for preventing heart disease. The relationship of HRT and breast cancer is still not completely clear, with conflicting research results. The use of bone-density testing to predict fracture risk from thinning bones raises issues around technology reliability and the natural history of bone aging and susceptibility to fractures. Research has recently questioned how often women should have Pap smears when prior results are normal. There are also issues around screening tests for ovarian cancer.

While keeping informed about the research related to menopause is important, of equal or greater value is the inspiration this life transition brings to women. It is a time of coming fully into one's own true self. In coming to realize how beautiful and precious our inner core being truly is, we cannot help but be inspired and uplifted. We are continually reminded of the wholeness of our being when seeing the intricate connections between consciousness and biochemistry, attitudes and experiences, nutrition and vitality, and symptoms and symbolic meanings. The bodily and emotional-mental experiences of menopause provide the vehicle for psychological and spiritual growth. Our journey into spiritual unfolding is the pathway to inner self-discovery, metamorphosis, and transformation.

TAKING CHARGE IS THE CORE OF SELF-CARE

The essential energy arising in women at midlife is being "at choice" about our lives. From childhood, forces in family and society mold women toward being caretakers, whether of children, husbands, parents, or friends. We learn to keep our antennae up and sense the feelings of others, to be alert to situations and to how we could be supportive. We learn to suppress our inner reactions if these are in conflict or disagreement with keeping harmony in the situation. Over many years, these deeply ingrained patterns place veils over our inner awareness and outer vision. The effects of reproductive hormones reinforce this role by keeping women focused on meeting the needs of others, nurturing and supporting their families (Northrup, 2001). These dynamics often keep women from making choices and taking actions that express their own deepest values related to self-integrity. And sometimes, if this social and neurochemical conditioning is strong enough, women are out of touch with the values that must be honored in order to bring them to integrity.

During perimenopause, the hormone changes affecting our bodies also have profound effects on the brain and nervous system. The brain chemistry and neural network change, and the nervous system is "re-wired" for different types of thoughts, ideas, and connections. More neural circuits develop to the intuitive centers in the temporal lobes and midbrain structures (Schultz, 1998). Women have more psychic and mental energy available than at any time since adolescence. Sometimes it feels like a volcano erupting, a fiery core needing to burst outward into expression.

This group (midlife women) is no longer invisible and silent, but a force to be reckoned with: educated, vocal, sophisticated in our knowledge of medical science, and determined to take control of our own health.

—Christiane Northrup, *The Wisdom of Menopause*

These surges of expressive, creative energy can be both exhilarating and intimidating. The way that we see our world changes. In situations where before we compromised and held back to maintain peace, we now have a sharper awareness of injustice and inequality. Where we have been silent in order to avoid disagreement, we now experience the necessity to voice our truth (Borysenko, 1996).

There is almost no escaping the upheaval of change at midlife. Like the caterpillar, we are transforming within the chrysalis, losing our prior form and reshaping our very molecules into a new form. Through the struggle of our own efforts, we break through the chrysalis's hard shell to emerge as the multi-jeweled butterfly. This process calls for a deep level of self-nurturing, of focusing our loving feelings upon ourselves. For most women, imbued with the virtue of placing others first, this is an uncomfortable idea. But the intensity of physical and emotional events puts a mandatory quality on self-care. It is not a luxury or indulgence now, but a necessity. Without self-care, it feels as though we may fall apart.

Donna: Menopause Metamorphosis

Donna's experience of life had been dramatic and intense, and perimenopause was no exception. Vivacious and outgoing, she was emotionally expressive and physically attractive at age 50. Her partner in a traditional marriage for 24 years, Donna's husband had recently retired and her youngest child was finishing college. During her reproductive years, Donna had severe PMS with headaches, cramps, and crying episodes that kept her in bed about two days per month. During this time, the family had to get their own dinner, tend to each others' needs, and keep quiet around Donna. The rest of the time, she carried out the family caretaker role. Donna's husband made all the decisions, kept his emotional distance, and was often critical of her.

Through the years, Donna had coped by creating a world of her own filled with women friends, volunteer work, and her children's activities. Whenever she was at cross-purposes with her husband, she became

(Continued on next page)

submissive and compliant. This kept the relationship stable for years, until perimenopause starting at age 45 began upsetting Donna's coping patterns. Her PMS symptoms not only were worse, but seemed to occur two or three times a month at erratic intervals. She could not count on more than a week of feeling good during each cycle. Her irritability led to arguments with her husband, as she felt less able to suppress her thoughts and feelings. She saw him drawing farther away emotionally, and spending less time at home.

As her periods became irregular, Donna began having intense hot flashes. She was drenched with sweat up to 15 times daily, and continually pulled off sweaters or blouses, only to don them again as chills set in. At night, she rarely slept more than one to two hours without awakening with a wet gown and sheets. Up and down all night changing linens, she felt exhausted in the morning, and fatigued all day. Her husband often slept in the spare bedroom so his night would not be disrupted. Donna obtained prescription hormones from her doctor, which reduced her symptoms but did not eliminate them.

Deep inside, Donna knew things were not right in her life. She felt a sadness underlying her irritability and a yearning for self-expression. She wondered who she really was, what her life was all about, and where it was going. Friends suggested counseling, which Donna did on her own, because her husband was not open to it. As Donna learned about the consequences of self-denial and dependence, she began to wonder about ending her marriage and striking out on her own. This was really frightening, but perhaps it was her intuition at work. Shortly after Donna reached age 50, her husband announced he was getting a divorce, as he had fallen in love with a younger woman and wanted to marry her. After several difficult months, with support from friends and therapist, Donna came to appreciate this opportunity to take control of her life and chart a creative future for herself. After 10 months without a period, her hot flashes became less frequent and her energy began to return. Donna began to feel a new zest for life as she expanded involvement with college classes, women's groups, and volunteer activities.

What Is Required to Take Charge

Taking charge of this change in our lives resonates on all levels. Hormone upheavals open the window to seeing what changes are needed in order to live our lives fully and honestly, in ways that support health and growth. Some requirements for taking charge, being at choice in this midlife transformation are:

- getting in touch with what you truly value.
- knowing yourself ever more deeply—exploring "Who am I?"
- taking full responsibility for your share in the problems in your life.
- becoming clear about what you are willing to accept, and what requires too much from your essential self.
- letting go of what no longer serves your growth.
- being willing to feel the pain of loss, and grieve for parts of the self left behind.
- learning to recognize, respect, and follow your inner authority.

The strands of each woman's life web flow together during menopause. Women are called to mend the frayed fibers and interweave each strand into a whole.

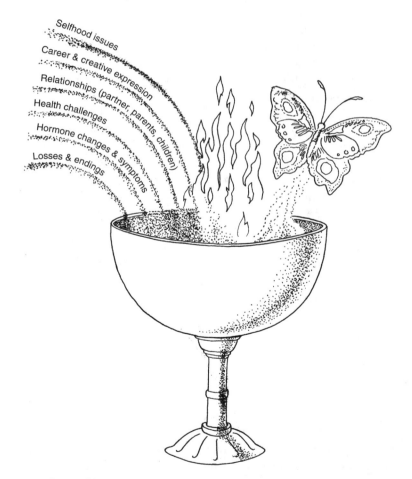

Figure 1–2 The Crucible of Menopause. The web of life is transformed through the fire of body-mind changes, until the radiant new self emerges, full of inner strength, vision, and new potential.

The Crucible of Menopause

In midlife, there is a convergence of life's channels into the crucible of menopause (see Figure 1–2). As if drawn by an unseen force, the strands of life's web flow together at this moment of truth. Like a pressure cooker with the fire turned high, the midlife woman's psyche faces:

- selfhood issues.
- career and creative expression needs.
- relationship issues.
- changing needs of teenage or young-adult children.
- growing dependence of elderly parents.
- health challenges.
- hormonal upheavals with multiple symptoms.
- losses of many kinds (deaths, divorces, dreams, identities).

Through this fire of transformation, the pure essence of being emerges, as all that is not needed, not serving the mandate of growth, is melted away. The profound changes occurring within the body-mind-spirit usher forth a woman of clarity, wisdom, creative energy, and integrity.

THE THREE PHASES OF MENOPAUSE

Menopause is usually divided into three phases: perimenopause, menopause, and postmenopause. While these are discussed thoroughly in Chapter 2, here we present brief descriptions of these phases. The average age for onset of symptoms and health conditions, and their usual duration, are discussed in relation to perimenopause, menopause, and postmenopause (see Figure 1–3).

Perimenopause

Perimenopause is the time leading up to actual menopause. It may last for a decade, usually beginning in a woman's 40s, but sometimes occurring as early as the mid-30s. During this time, women's hormones begin to act differently, often causing physical and emotional symptoms, many of which are grouped under the rubric of premenstrual syndrome (PMS). This time signals the beginning of major changes in self-concept, as women move from the young adult to the mature adult stage. Spiritually it is a time of going inward and experiencing the shadow side, as many issues surface for healing and resolution. Women experience the phenomenon of *enclosure,* feeling wrapped within a compelling field of change. One important

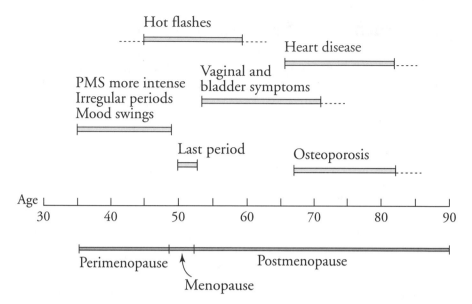

Figure 1–3 Timeline for Menopausal Symptoms. The average age for onset of symptoms and health conditions, and their usual duration, are shown in relation to perimenopause, menopause, and postmenopause.

archetype expressing the energies of perimenopause is the Alchemist, who taps into her inner sage to turn lead (adversity, suffering) into gold (valuable lessons, wisdom).

Early in perimenopause women often are dealing with some of the following symptoms.

- Not being able to count on the predictability of menses, experiencing flooding and spotting, and having long periods or very short ones at differing intervals. This is all caused by gyrating hormones.
- Moodiness, irritability, and depression.
- Discomfort: pelvic congestion, which may include bloating and cramps, pains during ovulation, breast tenderness, and heart palpitations.
- Erratic receptiveness to sex, with fluctuating sex drive.

Later in perimenopause these symptoms are more likely to occur, although hot flashes may occur quite early and be one of the first symptoms noticed.

- Hot flashes and night sweats, the hallmark symptoms of this time, occur to varying degrees. Most women have mild to moderate symptoms, but some

> Menopause is not just a single event or ceremony, it is really a long transition, a change on all levels of a woman's inner life.
>
> —Jean Mountaingrove, "Nature's Plan," in *Women of the 14th Moon*

suffer severely with repeated daily and nightly episodes interfering with sleep and functioning.

- Urinary tract changes, such as needing to void frequently, urgency, and feeling as though the bladder has not been completely emptied.
- Vaginal dryness and frequent vaginal infections.
- Skin changes, such as itching or crawling sensations; dryness, thinning.
- Changes in mental functioning, called fuzzy brain; feeling less sharp mentally and becoming more forgetful.

Menopause

Menopause, the permanent cessation of menstruation, is known only in retrospect. It is a point in time when you realize that you have not had a period for 13 months (some experts says 18 months). Some symptoms experienced in perimenopause continue during these months, but a woman no longer has periods. For some women, new symptoms appear or symptoms such as hot flashes intensify. It is clear that a new phase of life has occurred, and women are called upon to accept and embrace a new identity. Negotiating the previous physical and emotional upheavals brings forth inner strength, clarified values, and enhanced intuition. Spiritually this is a time of testing new powers, and finding their highest forms of expression. Women experience the phenomenon of *metamorphosis,* a radical change of form. The Guardian archetype often emerges, with a fierce directness that cuts to the heart of things. The Queen or Matriarch archetype expresses the energies of a noble, victorious spirit who can set examples for younger women.

The dominant symptoms during this 13–18 month phase are:

- hot flashes and night sweats.
- insomnia, sleep difficulties.
- mental function changes.
- fatigue, low energy.
- vaginal and urinary changes.
- low libido.

Postmenopause

Postmenopause is the time after menopause is completed, and lasts the rest of a woman's life. Having been transformed through the menopausal journey, women emanate a different consciousness. Often a sense of deep inner peace and harmony with life is expressed. This is usually a time of increased creativity, expanded consciousness, self integration, and spiritual adventures. Women experience the phenomenon of *emergence,* bringing forth their new self into the world.

> The most creative force in the world is the postmenopausal woman with zest.
>
> —Margaret Mead

The Wise Woman archetype manifests during this time, through which women integrate all of life's experiences and bring perspective, comfort, guidance, and inspiration to others. The Creatrix archetype enters women's lives during this phase as they express their expanded creativity, and give to the world through their inner abundance, fullness, and completeness.

Physical symptoms that are related to the long-term diminished hormone production may include:

- thinning vaginal and bladder walls.
- an increased risk of heart disease, starting around age 60.
- continuing skin and hair changes.
- usually reduction and ending of hot flashes.
- usually improved mental functions.
- osteoporosis (thinning of the bones).

A healthy body continues to produce hormones after menopause, although the levels are lower than before. Only a small percentage of women experience symptoms that are truly difficult. Most symptoms cease altogether at some point. Many natural, symptom-relieving choices are available. Achieving menopause is a relief to many women, as it acts as a launching pad into a fascinating next phase of life.

TAKING CHARGE OF THE CHANGE: TOOLS

The transition through perimenopause, menopause and into postmenopause can be exhilarating, empowering, and liberating. This experience is a passage through the gateway to the second half of our lives. In this book, we offer facts and information, philosophical perspectives, and practical self-help tools to assist you in negotiating the challenges as well as taking advantage of the opportunities that arise. These include the necessary ingredients for you to successfully take charge of your transition.

- Information about what happens in your body physiology, mental and emotional processes, and spiritual experiences.
- Discussion of tests on hormone levels, bone density and turnover, and cancer screening.

- Methods for understanding your unique personal profile of risk for health problems, including heart disease, osteoporosis, cancers, and brain disorders (such as Alzheimer's).

- Information on a wide range of therapies, from self-care with nutrition and lifestyle, herbs, supplements, and natural hormones, to consulting with your health practitioner about using prescription hormones and medications.

- Exploration of a larger perspective on the purpose of the menopause transition as a catalyst for psychological growth and spiritual initiation.

Welcome to menopause. May you find this passage an adventure into your authentic self, which brings integration of all aspects of your life journey, and supports you in healing into wholeness.

REFERENCES

Amerongen, D.V. (2000). Menopause in managed care. *Women's Health in Primary Care* (Suppl.), 3, 3.

Borysenko, J. (1996). *A woman's book of life: The biology, psychology, and spirituality of the feminine life cycle.* New York: Riverhead Books.

Doctor's Guide. (1997). Women's life expectancy to soar ahead of men's—smoking blamed. Accessed 4/01: *http://www.docguide.com/dg.nsf.*

Finkel, M.L., Cohen, M., & Mahoney, H. (2001). Treatment options for the menopausal woman. *The Nurse Practitioner, 26,* 5–15.

Jacobowitz, R.S. (1996). *150 most-asked questions about menopause: What women really want to know.* New York: William Morrow.

Keegan, L., & Dossey, B.M. (1998). *Profiles of nurse healers.* Albany: Delmar Publishers.

Mead, M. (2001). Post-menopausal zest. Accessed 8/01: *http://www.jeanshinodabolen.com/feat_mothersday.html.*

Mitchell, C. (1993). Mohawk. In S. Wall (Ed.). *Wisdom's daughters: Conversations with women elders of Native America.* New York: Harper Perennial.

Mountaingrove, J. (1991). Nature's plan. In D. Taylor & A. C. Sumrall (Eds.). *Women of the 14th moon: Writings on menopause.* Freedom, CA: The Crossing Press.

National Center for Health Statistics. (1996). *Vital statistics of the United States, 1992* (Vol. II). (Section 6, Life tables). Accessed 4/01: *http://www.lifeexpectancy.com/usle.html.*

North American Menopause Society. (2000). Accessed 3/00: *http//www.menopause.org.*

Northrup, C. (2001). *The wisdom of menopause: Creating physical and emotional health and healing during the change.* New York: Bantam Books.

Schultz, M.L. (1998). *Awakening intuition: Using your mind-body network for insight and healing.* New York: Harmony Books.

The Physical Experience:
Symptoms, Risks, and Testing

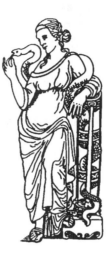

Hygieia, Greek goddess of
health and healing.
Reproduced with permission.
Copyright © Kate Cartwright.

Around 35 to 40 years of age, our bodies begin to change as we enter peri-menopause, an experience that may last several years, or even as long as a decade. There is a wide range in symptoms, from very mild to quite severe. A few women sail smoothly through these changes, but most have some symptoms. At first the changes are subtle, such as menstrual periods that are a few days closer together, or a day more of PMS. Then changes may become very noticeable; in fact, they may almost seem to shout out, "Things are *not* the same anymore!" The body often becomes unpredictable. Menstrual periods may be heavier, longer, and more painful. Pelvic congestion may start around ovulation (at midcycle) and last until menses begin. Crampy sensations, bloating, and fullness in the pelvic region may cause discomfort for up to three weeks out of four. Hot flashes may start during one's thirties, although they are more common later on. For some women, the main symptoms are mental or emotional, such as mood swings, depression, and changes in mental functioning.

> From the very beginning of my perimenopause, and for the next five years, it felt as though some strange and powerful force was relentlessly destabilizing and restructuring my body, mind and psyche. No dramatization, this!
>
> —Chris Karras, "Climacterium," in *Women of the 14th Moon*

SYMPTOMS OF MENOPAUSE

The symptoms of menopause may be divided into those that usually appear early in the process, and those most likely to appear later. However, women may have almost any symptom at any point in perimenopause.

Early Symptoms of Perimenopause

- Irregular menses, less predictable (cycles become shorter, sometimes more regular during the last few years, then begin occurring at longer time intervals)
- Heavy flow (or lighter at times)
- Intensification of PMS, ovulation symptoms
- Emotional changes (moodiness, irritability)
- Changes in mental functioning ("brain fog," less memory and concentration)
- Changes in sexuality (usually less libido, sometimes more)

Later Symptoms of Perimenopause

- Hot flashes ("power surges")
- Sleep disturbances (changed sleep patterns, such as waking every 3–4 hours, inability to get to sleep, or awakening early)
- Vaginal dryness
- Urinary tract changes (discomfort, frequency, leaking)
- Skin changes (dryness, itching, crawling skin sensation)

All these symptoms are caused by hormones, mainly the estrogens and progesterone in our bodies, but also some testosterone. Often the question is "If I'm feeling PMS-like much of the time, or having hot flashes, is it my estrogen or my progesterone that's the problem?" The following section discusses what most experts, such as Christiane Northrup M.D., John Lee, M.D., and others have to say about hormones and symptoms.

Hormones and Symptoms

The following symptoms are associated with too much (dominance, excess) or too little (deficiency, low) of the hormones listed.

ESTROGEN DOMINANCE

fibrocystic breasts
breast swelling and pain
PMS, bloating
pelvic congestion, pressure
heavy, irregular menses, cramps
depression, headaches
recurring vaginal yeast infections
leg cramps

ESTROGEN DEFICIENCY

hot flashes, night sweats
palpitations, anxiety
vaginal dryness
insomnia, headaches
moods, depression
memory loss, mental fuzziness
shortness of breath
bladder symptoms

EXCESS PROGESTERONE

sleepiness
drowsiness
depression

LOW PROGESTERONE

headaches
PMS, irritability
depression, moods
low libido and energy
anxiety, nervousness
food cravings
more facial and less head hair

EXCESS TESTOSTERONE

acne, especially on face and scalp
increased facial hair, deeper voice
mood disturbances

LOW TESTOSTERONE

low libido, slower arousal and
    orgasm
less sensitivity to sexual stimula-
    tion (nipples, clitoris, vagina)
lower vital energy
loss of muscle tone
thin, dry hair and skin
genital atrophy (shrinking)

TAKING INVENTORY OF YOUR SYMPTOMS

The first step in taking charge of your perimenopause and menopause involves keeping track of your personal set of symptoms. As you can see, menopausal symptoms cover a wide range with some overlap as to which hormones are

> . . . We are living longer than ever before. We must ensure that our long lives will be healthy and happy, we must stay abreast of medical developments and share our experiences. Most of all, we need to take responsibility for our own health, reading, taking advantage of medical expertise, but always listening to our own bodies and intuition and not being afraid to ask for help.
>
> —Vickie C. Posey, "What It Was, Was Menopause,"
> in *Women of the 14th Moon*

responsible. Your experience of any symptom may be mild, moderate, or severe. Symptoms may appear at different points during your transition, and some may come and go. The picture gets much clearer when you keep a record of what you experience and when symptoms occur. This personal symptom profile can guide you in self-care choices, and assist your health practitioner in deciding if diagnostic testing or prescription therapy is necessary.

See Worksheet 2–1 at the end of this chapter as a guide for keeping track of symptoms.

HORMONE HISTRIONICS: THE UPS AND DOWNS OF THINGS

What causes so many symptoms as women go through perimenopause? To understand why so many different things can happen, we need to visit the ups and downs of hormone activity. Women's menstrual cycles are regulated by hormones from the hypothalamus, pituitary, and ovary. The communication between these hormones and body organs (ovaries, uterus, breasts, brain) is harmonious and finely tuned. It causes girls to begin sexual development, regulates menstrual cycles, and supports pregnancy. When women reach their mid 30s changes often begin to happen in the female hormonal system. Over the next 15 years or so, these changes intensify and cause major shifts in menstrual cycles and symptoms. Finally, the ovaries stop responding to hormone stimulation, the phase of menstrual cycling ends, and menopause occurs. The players in the hormone cycle are:

FSH—follicle stimulating hormone

LH—luteinizing hormone

EST—estrogen (primarily estradiol)

PRO—progesterone

The Reproductive Years

The cycle is started by the hypothalamus, a structure located near the base of the brain with many nerves connecting it to other areas in the brain. These nerve connections in the brain make the hypothalamus responsive to whatever is going on emotionally and physically anywhere in the body. The hypothalamus sends out signals of "releasing factors" to the pituitary gland, an endocrine gland located somewhat lower in the brain. Then the pituitary releases follicle stimulating hormone (FSH) directly into the bloodstream. FSH travels through blood vessels to the ovaries, where it gives the signal to begin the development of an egg inside a small cyst in the ovary called a follicle. As the egg nears completed growth, the pituitary releases luteinizing hormone (LH) to complete the egg's growth and cause ovulation to occur. LH reaches a high peak in the blood just before ovulation, causing estrogen (EST) and progesterone (PRO) to rise in the blood and stimulate growth of the inner lining of the uterus. Estrogen drops when LH falls rapidly, but as progesterone increases to complete the development of the uterine lining in preparation for pregnancy, estrogen rises again. In the last part of the cycle, both estrogen and progesterone are quite high, which may contribute to PMS symptoms by causing swelling of tissues. If the egg is not fertilized, and pregnancy does not occur, estrogen and progesterone fall off rapidly over three to four days and soon menstrual bleeding begins. Even as the cycle is ending, however, FSH is starting to rise to prepare for the next cycle (see Figure 2–1).

During Perimenopause

Perimenopause usually starts with minor changes in menstrual cycles. Women's periods occur somewhat closer together, and sometimes more regularly. The amount of bleeding often increases, becoming heavier. Cramping before and during periods often becomes more severe. PMS symptoms may intensify, including irritability, moodiness, headaches, bloating, and breast/nipple tenderness. Ovulation often becomes noticeable. Before perimenopause most women do not know when they ovulate because the signs are quite subtle. Now, they feel pain in the lower abdomen on one side or the other. It may be just slight discomfort, or pain so intense they think it's appendicitis. The pain lasts one to three days, then disappears or lessens. Some women have pelvic congestion, which is fluid buildup in the pelvic tissues. It may begin around ovulation and last until into the next period. Sometimes women feel heaviness and pressure in the pelvic region right after their period, because hormones are already rising to get the next cycle underway. This congestion and pressure may be so intense that women describe it as feeling like "the bottom falling out" in their pelvic region.

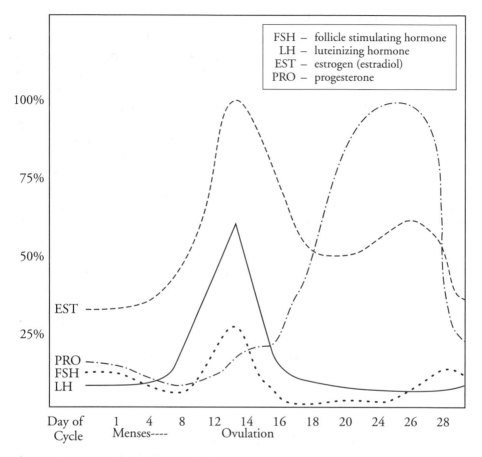

Figure 2–1 Menstrual Cycle: The Reproductive Years. FSH initiates the cycle by prompting the ovary to ripen an egg. Around days 8 to 12, LH rises sharply to complete egg ripening and cause ovulation. Estrogen (EST) rises as ovulation occurs, then drops afterward, making another, smaller rise shortly before menstruation begins. Progesterone (PRO) rises rapidly after ovulation, peaks, and drops precipitously if pregnancy does not occur. The sharp decline in progesterone signals the uterus to begin menstrual bleeding.

WHAT THE HORMONES ARE DOING

During the perimenopause phase, the body is flooded with hormones which are released erratically. FSH is trying to get the ovary to produce an egg, but the ovary is becoming more resistant. It has fewer eggs remaining, and these are more diffi-cult to ripen. The membrane around the ovary is getting tougher, so the egg follicle builds up more fluid before it ruptures to release the egg into the tube. This greater amount of fluid falls onto the inside abdominal wall, causing a "chemical" irrita-tion that adds to pain and swelling of surrounding tissues. As FSH fluctuates, it takes estrogen with it, causing congestive symptoms. LH also rises and falls, but

> So this was menopause! The first two to three years were the worst,
> given my . . . heavy periods, more severe migraines, hot flushes,
> abdominal bloat, stress-incontinence, heart palpitations, . . .
> irritability, free-floating anxiety, horrific nightmares, insomnia, and
> a rapidly eroding self-confidence and self-esteem. The combined
> pressures were immense: I still refer to this period in my life as
> my twilight zone.
>
> —Chris Karras, "Climacterium," in *Women of the 14th Moon*

progesterone does not do much until an egg finally ripens and erupts (causing ovulation). However, now progesterone is acting on tissues already swollen and irritated from the higher FSH and estrogen levels (see Figure 2–2). This situation can lead to overgrowth of the endometrium (uterine lining) because it is being overstimulated by estrogen. Heavy bleeding, clots, flooding, and PMS symptoms are common.

As Menopause Draws Near

As menopause approaches, bleeding and congestion symptoms lessen. However, a new group of symptoms begins. These include hot flashes, night sweats, sleep disturbances, foggy brain, fatigue, moodiness, depression, skin crawling, and a host of others. Periods become irregular and lighter when they do occur. Women may skip several months, only to have another period after as long as six to twelve months. Remember, you know you've completed menopause only in retrospect. Most authorities say a woman must be without periods for 13–18 months before she can be declared as having gone through menopause.

WHAT THE HORMONES ARE DOING

When menopause is complete, the hormones quiet down and become more steady. A woman's body is designed to continue producing hormones from places other than the ovaries. Women continue to make estrogen, now from fatty tissue and the adrenal glands in the forms of estriol and estrone. The ovaries, which produce mostly estradiol, play a much smaller role and estradiol remains at low levels. Much less progesterone is made, as it is mainly produced by the ovaries after ovulation. However, estrogen, progesterone, and testosterone are also produced in body fat, skin, adrenal glands, the brain, and some nerves, and these sources provide a lifetime supply. At times women feel premenstrual, when hormone levels rise, but this usually subsides without any bleeding (see Figure 2–3). Now that estrogen levels are lower, levels of testosterone, which women make in small amounts (primarily in the adrenal glands), become relatively higher. While this

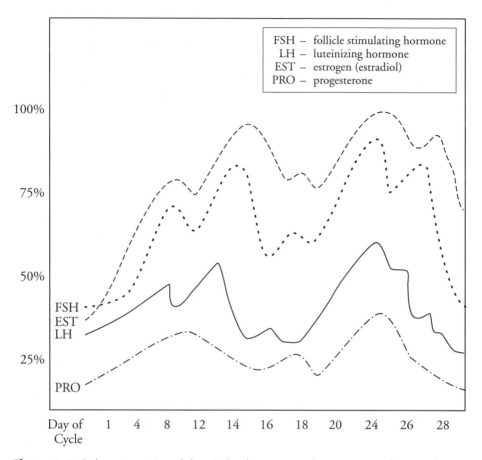

Figure 2–2 Perimenopause: Anovulation. During the years preceding menopause, the ovary does not ripen eggs efficiently. FSH rises and dips, attempting to stimulate egg ripening. LH follows the ups and downs of FSH but at lower levels. Estrogen (EST) soars upward, often higher than during reproductive years, causing many perimenopausal symptoms. Progesterone (PRO) remains at relatively low levels, as its release is triggered by ovulation.

may cause undesirable changes, such as hair on upper lips and chin, it may also provide a source of energy and stamina.

FSH and LH remain quite elevated during menopause and afterwards. Even many years after the ovaries have stopped responding, levels of these stimulating hormones are high. In addition, GnRH (gonadotropin releasing hormone), produced by the hypothalamus gland in the brain, which signals the pituitary to release FSH and LH, remains high. Why this is so has puzzled scientists, as the pituitary and hypothalamus should stop making these molecules after some months of no ovarian response. Some experts believe that one reason may be the neurotransmitter

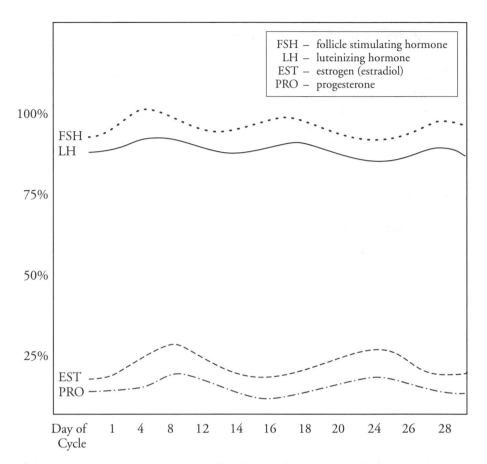

Figure 2–3 Postmenopause: Hormone Stability. After some time, the ovaries no longer respond to the signal of FSH to ripen an egg. FSH and LH remain very high for several years. Estrogen (EST) and progesterone (PRO) levels stabilize. Estrogen levels fluctuate somewhat, but remain around 25 percent of their highest level during the reproductive years. Progesterone continues at low levels, with minor fluctuations.

(messenger molecule) effect they have on the brain, which causes re-wiring of neural circuits and altered brain chemistry meant to produce changes in how women's minds work after menopause (Northrup, 2001; Pert, 1997; and Schultz, 1998). This concept is more fully explored in Chapter 4.

The Hormone Cascade

The sex-steroid hormones—estrogen, progesterone, testosterone, DHEA, and cortisol—are in a class by themselves. They work together like a cast of characters, supporting each other. The ovaries in women, testes in men, and the adrenal

Physiology of Hot Flashes

The "roller-coaster ride" of hormone levels during perimenopause results from very high to very low swings of FSH and LH . The hormones attempt to stimulate the ovary to produce an egg, but the ovary becomes less able to respond. Levels of estrogen rise and fall. When estrogen levels drop, norepinephrine is metabolized differently in the brain. This neurotransmitter is a messenger peptide carrying signals between brain, immune system, and body organs. The heat regulation center in the brain is affected, and it sends erratic signals to blood vessels making them suddenly dilate (open up). Sudden dilation makes skin surface temperature increase, causing a "flush" or flash of heat, usually in the upper body and face. Sweating occurs to reduce body surface heat. The body readjusts by causing blood vessels to constrict (close down), thus decreasing skin temperature and causing the chilly sense that follows hot flashes. The uncomfortable, edgy sensation deep inside the chest that many women feel probably relates to neurotransmitter effects on large internal blood vessels and the heart.

However, another way to think of hot flashes is as a burst of *internal energy* becoming available to us. This could relate to increased flow of prana/chi through the chakras, which seems to happen in women during their late 40s and early 50s. It may also be nature's way to kill abnormal precancerous cells, which become more common as we age, by raising body temperature to activate the immune system. Perhaps we can think of these as *power surges* given by Mother Nature for our growth and health. (See Chapter 5 for more energy and spiritual meanings.)

glands produce most of the sex-steroid hormones, but they can also be made by the brain, liver, skin, and fat. All these hormones are made from cholesterol, an essential building block. While having too much cholesterol in the bloodstream contributes to fatty plaque in arteries, we do need an adequate amount for making steroid hormones. Our bodies use cholesterol to make the precursor hormone pregnenolone, which can be converted into the other sex hormones, and each of these hormones may be transformed into one or more of the others. For example, DHEA can become testosterone and estrogen. Progesterone can turn into estrogen, testosterone, DHEA, or cortisol. Testosterone can become estrogen or progesterone. When this transformation happens, it is called a hormone cascade effect (Figure 2–4).

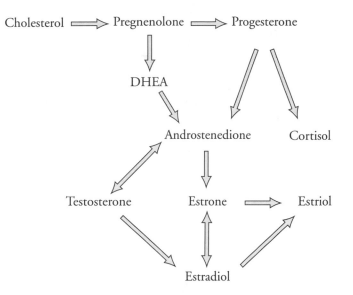

Figure 2–4 The Hormone Cascade. Each sex-steroid hormone has the ability to transform into one or more of the others. They are made from cholesterol, which becomes the precursor hormone, pregnenolone, which transforms into DHEA and progesterone. From there, the hormones cascade into androstenedione, which becomes testosterone or estrone. Testosterone can transform into estradiol, which can become estrone or estriol. This flexibility allows the body to maintain its hormonal stability.

Using the hormone cascade, your body exercises its innate wisdom. The body knows which hormones are needed, and by turning those it already has available into those that may be at lower levels, it maintains hormonal equilibrium. Before menopause, the ovaries make most of our estrogen (estradiol). However, after menopause the ovaries no longer make as much estradiol, so your body transforms DHEA or testosterone stored in fat cells into estrone or estriol. Progesterone is also transformed into estrogen when needed (Ahlgrimm & Kells, 1999).

Other Hormones Affecting Menopause

Two other endocrine glands play important roles in perimenopausal symptoms (see Figure 2–5). The interrelationships among the ovaries, thyroid, and adrenal glands help maintain balance and smooth coordination of our needs for energy and reproductive function. This interaction also affects moods and mental state. An imbalance or malfunction of one or more glands often leads to symptoms of fatigue, anxiety, or depression. If a woman feels chronically tired, depressed, and unable to deal with ordinary stresses, or if she starts her day feeling she has not had adequate rest, then she may have problems with her thyroid or adrenal glands.

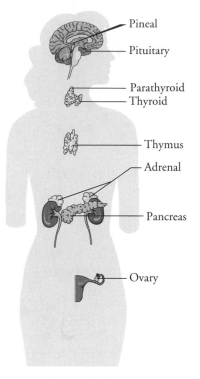

Pineal

Pituitary

Parathyroid
Thyroid

Thymus

Adrenal

Pancreas

Ovary

Endocrine glands

Figure 2–5 Glands that Produce Hormones. During the menstrual years, the ovaries produce most of a woman's estrogen and progesterone, under the direction of stimulating hormones from the pituitary glands. After menopause, the adrenal glands and body fat take over most of the estrogen and progesterone production. The thyroid, pancreas, and adrenal glands coordinate the body's needs for energy and regulate metabolism. The pineal gland keeps the other glands in harmonious relationship and secretes melatonin. The thymus gland communicates with the immune system and heart rhythms.

THYROID FUNCTION

Thyroid gland problems are quite common during perimenopause and menopause. The thyroid, located at the base of the neck, secretes two types of thyroid hormones and calcitonin. These regulate energy metabolism and calcium balance in the blood. About 26 percent of perimenopausal women are diagnosed with hypothyroidism (low thyroid) (Massoudi, Meilahn, & Orchard, 1995). The symptoms of deficient thyroid hormones include low energy, weight gain, depression, irritability, sleep disturbances, and mental confusion. You can see how these might get confused with symptoms of perimenopause.

According to Dr. John Lee, symptoms of hypothyroidism may be related to estrogen dominance. When estrogen is not balanced with an adequate amount of progesterone, it can block the action of the thyroid hormones. When this happens, a thyroid test may show normal levels in the blood, but the body cannot use the thyroid hormones properly because estrogen is blocking their use by the cells (Lee, Henley, & Hopkins, 1999). If an estrogen-dominant woman is prescribed estrogen therapy, this compounds the problem even more. Taking thyroid supplements will not correct the situation. What is needed to bring this hormone situation into balance is progesterone supplementation.

If thyroid testing does show low levels of hormones, then thyroid medication is indicated. As two thyroid hormones are needed for restoring balance, the current trend is to supplement with both T_3 (triiodothyronine) and T_4 (thyroxine).

ADRENAL FUNCTION

The two small adrenal glands, sitting on top of each kidney, secrete three important hormones, epinephrine, cortisol, and DHEA, that help us respond to the stresses and demands of life. Keeping these hormones at healthy levels is critical to preserving our health, energy levels, and vitality as we enter the second phase of life. If a woman's life has been full of chronic, unrelenting stress, she probably will have depleted her adrenal glands by the time she enters menopause. Adrenal depletion leads to a state of persistent exhaustion, lower resistance to disease, and decreased capacity to respond to ordinary life stresses.

Epinephrine (adrenalin)   The "fight-or-flight" hormone pours into the body when you sense danger. It causes rapid, pounding heartbeat, deeper breathing, pupil dilation, less saliva and tears, slower digestion, increased tendency for blood to clot, greater blood supply in muscles and less in internal organs, and alerts the brain to be on guard. This prepares the body for intense physical action to deal with danger. In daily life, however, our "dangers" consist of dealing with conflicts, time pressure, criticism, or pushing too hard when we are fatigued. Only occasionally do we get to use these epinephrine surges to react quickly in physical ways, such as avoiding a fall or traffic accident. Over many years, chronic stresses overactivate the alarm part of the nervous system, and we lose the ability to relax fully. In addition, continued demands on the adrenal glands without adequate restoration by frequent times of peacefulness and harmony reduce the gland's ability to produce hormones.

Cortisol   Affects the storage and availability of energy in the cells, increases appetite, and dampens allergic and inflammatory responses of the immune system. The body uses cortisol to counteract the effects of infections, trauma, and temperature extremes. It helps maintain stable emotions and makes us feel perky. Under healthy conditions, cortisol is secreted only when the body needs it. After a jolt of epinephrine, released because of an accident that causes cuts and bruises, cortisol helps the tissues recover and heal. When people have severe allergic reactions, such as severe poison oak eruptions or prolonged asthma, the synthetic versions of cortisol (prednisone, cortisone) are used to stop the body's out-of-control reactions. In situations of chronic stress, cortisol levels remain too high for too long. This may lead to bone demineralization, muscle wasting, kidney damage, fluid retention, high blood sugar, weight gain, and vulnerability to infections, allergies and cancer.

DHEA (dehydroepiandrosterone)   Made by both the adrenal glands and ovaries, DHEA is an androgenic (masculine acting) hormone. It appears in inverse relation to cortisol; when DHEA is up, cortisol is down, and vice versa. DHEA counteracts the effects cortisol has in suppressing the immune system response, thus improving resistance to disease and infections. Other effects of DHEA are increasing bone density, keeping LDL cholesterol levels normal ("bad" cholesterol that builds plaque in arteries), maintaining normal sleep patterns, keeping the mind sharp and focused, and aiding recovery from episodes of trauma and other stresses. Healthy DHEA levels provide a sense of vitality and energy. As DHEA is the main ingredient used by the body to make testosterone, low levels often cause lack of libido. DHEA is highest in our 20s, and declines slowly as we age. This decline is thought to be one factor which causes the aging process.

TAKING CHARGE OF YOUR SYMPTOMS

At this point you might be asking "My hormones may be going crazy, but how do I know what estrogen, progesterone, testosterone, DHEA, or cortisol are actually doing in my body? Also, what about the condition of my bones? Am I at more risk for getting heart disease or cancer?" You can get answers to these and other questions by looking at your personal risk factors, and by taking diagnostic tests that are commonly recommended for screening during the menopausal years.

RISK FACTORS FOR HEALTH PROBLEMS

For many women, menopause signifies entering one of the healthiest and most balanced phases of their lives. They are no longer coping with the swings of menstrual cycles. Their home and work responsibilities often become less demanding. They have learned much from their experiences, and feel more comfortable with themselves. Increased awareness of healthy living leads to lifestyle and dietary changes that support health and longevity. Getting older has previously been connected with more health problems, but the current generation of menopausal women is doing a lot to change the statistics. The following review of risk factors for problems that may appear around menopause is intended to help you be more aware of the areas where you may be "at risk," so that you can make changes to support health. The media emphasize these problems, driven by advertising for drugs and products. When we respect and care for our bodies and selves, these problems need not develop.

Osteoporosis

Loss of mineral (primarily calcium) from the bones occurs in about 20–25 percent of women after menopause. The most rapid loss happens during the first five years after menses stop. Some loss begins during the last few menstrual years. A woman's greatest bone density is established by age 30. How dense bones are at their maximum is a major factor in later osteoporosis.

FACTORS THAT INCREASE RISK OF OSTEOPOROSIS

- Smoking cigarettes
- Lack of exercise, or overly-vigorous exercise (causes calcium loss)
- Thin, fair complexion, less than 18 percent body fat
- Mother or grandmother with osteoporosis (hip, wrist, or humerus fracture, "Dowager's hump," or vertebral compression fractures)
- Early menopause, before 40 years of age
- Taking steroids (cortisone) or thyroid hormone
- Anorexia, bulimia, and amenorrhea (not having periods, which often occurs in female athletes), causes of low estrogen levels

DIETARY FACTORS IN OSTEOPOROSIS

- Diet low in calcium, magnesium, vitamins C and D, and trace minerals
- Diet high in protein, especially animal protein (40–60 grams of protein daily is healthy, but the average adult American consumes over 100 grams of protein daily)
- More than two alcoholic drinks per day
- More than four cups of coffee or colas per day
- Excess phosphorus intake (sodas, junk foods). The proper phosphorus-calcium ratio is one-to-one; but the average American consumes two to four times more phosphorus than calcium
- Excess dairy products (negative calcium balance), which causes accelerated calcium excretion to maintain serum balance; too much protein
- Excess sugar leaches calcium out of the bones

Heart Disease

After menopause, women often have increased risk of heart disease. Estrogen is protective during the menstrual years by its effects on vascular walls, cholesterol, and blood-clotting factors. Heart disease is the leading cause of death for women after age 50, which is also when estrogen levels fall. However, the relationship between heart disease and estrogen is complex (see pages 64–65). Nutrition and lifestyle appear to be more important for heart health than do hormones (Stampfer, Hu, Manson, et al., 2000).

FACTORS THAT INCREASE RISK OF HEART DISEASE

- Smoking cigarettes
- Obesity (more than 20 percent over normal weight for height and age)
- High blood pressure (above 140/90, although less than 130/80 is healthier)
- Cholesterol: LDL (low density lipoprotein) above 120–129 mg/dl, and HDL (high density lipoprotein) less than 35 mg/dl; 50–60 mg/dl is healthy
- Family history of heart disease (high blood pressure, heart attacks, angina, and strokes, especially if these occur before age 50)
- Lack of exercise
- High fat diet (more than 35 precent calories from fat, 10 percent saturated fat)
- High animal protein diet (source of saturated fats)

The Physiology of Palpitations

Heartbeat is regulated by the electrical signals "fired" by two nodes, the sinoatrial, which signals the upper two heart chambers (atria), and the atrioventricular, which signals the lower two chambers (ventricles). Abnormalities of electrical impulses can happen at either node, or in the conduction system between ventricles. After nodes fire, a rest period is needed for "depolarization" (time for the electrical signal to die away) so tissues can respond to the next electrical impulse firing. During perimenopause, the heart's electrical rhythm system becomes more sensitive, probably because of hormone fluctuations. Many women have *palpitations*—becoming more aware of heartbeat, fluttering sensations, or skipped beats. Sometimes dizziness, blurry vision, and faintness accompany palpitations.

Most of the time this does not indicate heart disease. It is caused by disturbances in electrical firing or conduction resulting from changing hormones. The atria or ventricles are signaled to contract too frequently, or out of rhythm. Usually this only lasts a few seconds, and corrects itself spontaneously. However, women's risk of developing heart disease does

(Continued on next page)

increase around menopause. Having high blood pressure and cholesterol increases the risk. Women with persistent palpitations should get a medical checkup, including ECG, blood pressure, and measurement of blood cholesterol.

Palpitations may represent the need to follow the heart's wisdom. Stresses that we tolerated before become less bearable at midlife. Unresolved issues and unsatisfying aspects of our lives present themselves more insistently. Stress affects blood flow to heart vessels (coronary arteries), causes hormone fluctuations, and alters electrical impulses in the heart. We need to honor the heart's increased sensitivity, by reducing stimulants (caffeine, MSG, aspartame, scary or violent entertainment), and listen to its message that it is time to resolve issues.

Breast Cancer

One of every eight women who live to be 85 will develop breast cancer. There are about 175,000 cases of breast cancer diagnosed each year (Olopade & Cummings, 2000). Risk increases steadily with age. Breast cancer before age 50 is more dangerous than if it occurs when older. While the relationship between breast cancer and estrogen is complex and not entirely clear, it appears that both length of exposure and type of estrogen are important factors (see pages 73–75).

FACTORS THAT INCREASE RISK OF BREAST CANCER

- Menstruating for over 40 years (menarche before age 15, menopause after age 55)
- No children, or first child born after age 30
- High fat and animal protein diet. This connection, found in early studies, is now in question, as the Nurses Health Study found no increased risk with more than 20 percent fat calories, regardless of the type of fat (Northrup, May, 1999).
- More than 2 alcoholic drinks per day. This possible connection was found in early studies; however, in 1999, the Framingham study found no increased risk (*UCB Wellness Letter,* May, 1999).
- Low fiber and antioxidants in diet. Studies link low fiber to colon cancer and low antioxidants to overall cancer risk.
- Smoking cigarettes
- ERT/HRT (estrogen/hormone replacement therapy) for more than 5 years. Most studies used equine conjugated estrogens, and combined estrogen

and progestin showed the greatest increased risk. Human identical hormones (made from plants, biologically identical to hormones made by the human body) (see pages 58, 61) have recently been included in studies, although results are not yet available.

- Family history of breast cancer in two first-degree relatives (mother, sister) under age 60, and family history of ovarian cancer

How to Reduce Your Risks

When you have identified risk factors for yourself, there is much you can do to take charge of your health to reduce or eliminate risks. At the end of this chapter and in Chapter 3, you will find worksheet exercises and advice for each area. You may rate your risks for osteoporosis, heart disease, and cancer, and then learn about your choices to change factors in your life to reduce these risks. Of course, some factors cannot be changed, such as family history, ethnic background, and age when menstrual periods began. But most of the risk factors can be changed, because they relate to choices you make about diet and lifestyle.

Worksheet 2–2; *Determining your risks,* at the end of this chapter, provides a checklist for you to complete, which lets you see at a glance what factors may be increasing your risk. You may want to copy this worksheet to fill out in four to six months, after you complete your self-care program to support bone and heart health and to reduce cancer risks. You may be surprised by how your number of risk factors has decreased.

DIAGNOSTIC TESTING

Gathering information about the status of your hormones, bones, breasts, cervix, and ovaries is important for self-care and informed decision-making. Most women choose to take action in order to relieve menopausal symptoms that are interfering with their quality of life. In assessing your options, it's helpful to know whether you have increased risk for other health problems that might be affected by the type of therapy you select. If you have thinning bones, high blood pressure or cholesterols, or cancer risks, this information may guide you in selecting the most appropriate therapy to manage menopause symptoms. The following diagnostic tests are usually recommended during the menopausal years.

Menopause is preparing us for independent strength, friendship with death, wisdom.

—Sandy Boucher, "Meeting the Tiger," in *Women of the 14th Moon*

Saliva Hormone Tests

Saliva hormone tests are often recommended for the steroid hormones (such as estrogen, progesterone, testosterone, cortisol, DHEA, and melatonin) (Northrup, July, 1997). Numerous research studies carried out over 30 years validate the use of saliva to measure the biologically active part of steroid hormones. Saliva tests are more accurate than blood (serum) tests because steroid hormones are not bound by carrier proteins when they enter saliva, while 90–99 percent of these hormones are bound to proteins while in the bloodstream. After centrifuging blood samples to remove the cells, the carrier proteins also are largely removed, so the amount of hormone left in the serum (upon which "blood" tests are based) is a poor representation of the true steroid hormone levels.

The steroid hormones, when not bound to carrier proteins, diffuse freely from the bloodstream into tissues and saliva because their molecules are quite small. Saliva reflects the biologically active (free or non-bound) part of steroid hormones, which is what produces effects in our tissues and organs (Ahlgrimm & Kells, 1999). Saliva hormone normal ranges have been standardized for collection in the early morning (6–8 A.M.). As women take the saliva kits home, it is easy to take the specimen at the right time. This allows a more accurate comparison of your values with the normal ranges.

Where to get this test   You can have saliva testing done on your own (see Resources). However, it may be easier to go to your health care provider, as you might want help understanding test results. She or he can deal directly with a laboratory providing this testing. Not all clinical laboratories provide saliva hormone testing.

Blood Tests

Hormone levels may be checked using blood (serum) tests. An "ovarian panel" includes estrogen (estradiol), progesterone, FSH, and LH. When health practitioners test to see if you are menopausal, they usually order serum FSH, alone or with LH. Once FSH and LH levels both go above 30 MIU/ml and remain high, menopause may be diagnosed. Serum levels of hormones may fluctuate, however. Women have tested in the menopause range, only to begin having regular periods again with return of FSH and LH to premenopause levels. Similarly, estrogen and progesterone levels vary during different phases of the menstrual cycle, and may be quite low when women in perimenopause are not ovulating, only to rise again as the body produces more hormones and ovulation resumes. Once menopause has been completed, FSH and LH levels remain high for about eight years, then slowly decline. Both progesterone and estrogen (estradiol) are usually in the low range in serum after menopause.

Several other blood (serum) tests are commonly done to check for conditions that may produce symptoms often confused with menopause. To obtain more accurate results, free (unbound) hormone levels may be ordered. Hormone levels vary throughout the day, and each woman's daily variations may be unique. This makes it harder to compare your values with the normal range. Examples of common serum tests are:

- A thyroid panel checks levels of the thyroid hormones T_3 and T_4, and TSH (thyroid stimulating hormone). A deficiency of thyroid hormones may cause fatigue, weight gain, memory changes, and skin and hair changes. Thyroid hormone excess causes anxiety, palpitations, insomnia, and hot flashes.

- Diabetes is tested by a fasting blood glucose or 2-hour glucose test. Diabetes causes weight gain, fatigue, and dizziness.

- Anemia is tested by a red blood count. It causes fatigue, dizziness, difficulty concentrating, irregular periods, and shortness of breath.

- A cholesterol panel is used to assess risk for heart disease. High cholesterol may lead to angina (heart pain) and palpitations if coronary arteries are partly blocked. Total cholesterol level is a combination of low density (LDL) and high density (HDL) lipoproteins. LDL causes fatty deposits in arteries, while HDL indicates healthy metabolism of fats. It is important to know all the cholesterol levels. For women, having inadequate HDL increases risk for heart disease more than having a slightly elevated LDL.

Where to take these tests   Your health practitioner usually needs to order these tests. Health screening offered at health fairs or by special insurance programs is often available, although you may not be able to have all these tests performed.

Table 2–1 shows saliva hormone values for estrogens, progesterone, and cortisol. This reflects the normal range of saliva hormones (estrogens, progesterone) from an early morning sample in women not taking hormone replacement therapy. Cortisol values are shown for both morning and evening.

Table 2–2 shows saliva hormone values for DHEA and testosterone, reflecting the normal range for these hormones from an early morning sample, in women not taking supplements.

Bone Density Tests

The mineral content of bones, primarily calcium and magnesium, is measured by an X-ray technique called dual-energy X-ray absorptiometry (DEXA). It is the most precise X-ray measurement, and has a low level of radiation exposure (*The Medical Letter,* 1996). Most often, DEXA tests are done on bones in the lumbar spine and hip (neck of the femur). Heel and wrist tests are less accurate, but if bone density is low these can alert women to have a full DEXA. Women with risk factors for osteoporosis are advised to start getting bone density tests around age 35–40. It is recommended for all women by age 50.

TABLE 2–1	Saliva Hormone Values for Estrogens, Progesterone, and Cortisol

HORMONE	PHASE OF MENSTRUAL CYCLE/MENOPAUSE	NORMAL RANGE
Estradiol	Premenopause:	
	First half of cycle (follicular)	0.5–5.0 pg/ml
	Midcycle (ovulation)	3.0–8.0 pg/ml
	Second half of cycle (luteal)	0.5–5.0 pg/ml
	Postmenopause	<1.5 pg/ml
Estriol	Premenopause	4.4–8.3 pg/ml
	Postmenopause	3.0–11.8 pg/ml
Estrone	Premenopause	2.6–5.4 pg/ml
	Postmenopause	2.6–5.4 pg/m
Progesterone	Premenopause:	
	First half of cycle (follicular)	<0.1 ng/ml
	Second half of cycle (luteal)	0.1–0.5 ng/ml
	Postmenopause	<0.5 ng/ml
Cortisol	Morning	1.0–8.0 ng/ml
	Evening	0.1–1.0 ng/ml

TABLE 2–2	Saliva Hormone Values for DHEA and Testosterone

AGE RANGE	TESTOSTERONE (pg/ml)	DHEA (pg/ml)
20–29	17–54	106–300
30–39	15–44	77–217
40–49	13–37	47–200
50–59	12–34	38–136
60–69	12–35	36–107
70–79	11–34	32–99

Three Perimenopausal Women

Patty, now 42, was diagnosed with endometriosis three years ago and had surgical treatment to reduce the amount of endometrial implants. She has severe menstrual cramps with premenstrual bloating, pelvic pressure, irritability, moodiness, and depression. After skipping periods for three months, her symptoms improved. Now, after six months of having regular periods again, her symptoms are getting worse. She is wondering if perimenopausal hormone changes may be a factor. A serum (blood) hormone test shows that Patty has normal levels of estradiol, progesterone, FSH, and LH. She is not yet showing changes in her hormone levels that could indicate the end of her menstrual cycles. Patty has chosen to use supplements plus an antidepressant medication to help her symptoms.

Marianne is still having periods at age 54. She is moderately overweight despite being active: gardening, walking, and swimming three times a week at the gym. In the past year she has noticed more mood swings, bloating, and hot flashes, with occasional night sweats. Her energy fluctuates but is generally good. She has been using wild yam cream for six months, but her symptoms are not changing. Saliva hormone tests show her estradiol in the high-normal range with low progesterone. The ratio between estrogen and progesterone is out of balance, making Marianne estrogen dominant. She has decided to use prescription-grade progesterone cream to bring her hormones into balance.

Lisa has skipped a couple of periods at age 47, but returns to cycling. Her main symptom is insomnia, a long-standing problem made worse by perimenopause. The week before her period starts, the insomnia becomes more pronounced and sleeping aids are less effective. She wonders if hormone imbalances are contributing to this, although she does not have any other symptoms of perimenopause. Lisa's serum (blood) hormone test shows normal estradiol, low progesterone, high LH and moderately high FSH. This is a typical perimenopause hormone pattern. Lisa has chosen to take oral natural progesterone to support hormone balance during the premenstrual week.

These women's stories are continued in Chapter 3, including details about their choices for therapy and results. Table 2–3 shows their hormone test values.

TABLE 2–3	Hormone Values for Patty, Marianne, and Lisa				
	AGE/TEST	ESTRADIOL	PROGESTERONE	FSH	LH
Patty	42/serum	52 pg/ml	9.0 mg/ml	5.6 miu/ml	2.3 miu/ml
Marianne	54/saliva	10 pg/ml*	0.5 ng/ml	–	–
Lisa	47/serum	120 pg/ml	0.9 mg/ml	41 miu/ml	90 miu/ml

*Saliva estradiol levels are much lower than blood (serum) levels. Progesterone is measured by different values in saliva and blood. The range of values in blood is much greater than in saliva, making comparisons unreliable.

Interpreting the results of bone density tests calls for a good understanding of both the process of bone turnover and technical factors in taking the DEXA test. Bone cells are constantly in the process of breaking down and building up, a process called bone remodeling. It takes almost two years for each individual bone cell to finish its life cycle, die, and be replaced. Of course, the millions of bone cells in the body are on different start and finish times. By age 20, girls have built up most of their bone structure, and maximum bone density is set by around age 30. This is one reason why good nutrition is so important during adolescence. After menopause, the bone breakdown process speeds up, caused by declining estrogens. About 25 percent of menopausal women in the United States are at risk for osteoporosis (severe thinning of bones). As women become elderly, about half are vulnerable to osteoporosis (Lindsay, Marcus, & Recker, 1996). At a very old age, the process of building up new bone becomes less effective, and bones thin even more. When bone density is decreased, but not severe enough to be osteoporosis, the condition is called osteopenia (see Figures 2–6 and 2–7).

One bone density test does not give the full picture. A woman taking a DEXA test in her 40s may have had that level of bone density for years. The key is to see in what direction bone density is moving—is it going down, up, or staying the same? Bone changes slowly, so at least two tests should be done, one to two years apart. Also, there is "test variation" with a tendency for results to average out over time (Cummings et al., 2000), and the unavoidable statistical variance in measurement (see page 43, Interpreting Bone Mineral Density Tests). Women with risk factors for osteoporosis should get a baseline bone density before menopause occurs.

Where to take this test: Most hospitals with a radiology department do DEXA testing, and there are special bone density screening centers. Your health care provider needs to order the test for you. You may take a heel or wrist test on your own, when available at such places as a local pharmacy or health fair.

URINE DPD (DEOXYPYRIDINOLINE)

Urine Dpd is not a test for osteoporosis, but is useful to monitor the process of bone turnover. It measures the urinary excretion of cross-linked substances to

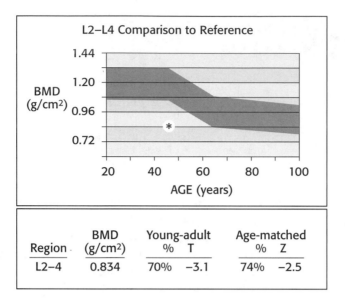

Figure 2–6 Bone Densitometry: Osteoporosis. The lumbar spine density of this 46-year-old woman has a T score –3.1, and Z score –2.5, both well below range for both young women and women her age. She has 70 percent of the BMD of young women, and 74 percent of the BMD of women her age. She has significant osteoporosis, and is at increased risk for fractures.

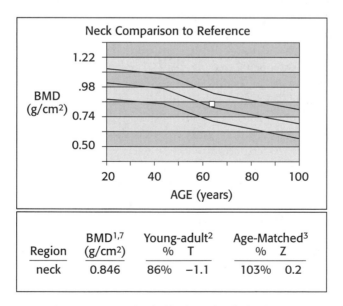

Figure 2–7 Bone Densitometry: Osteopenia. The hip (femoral neck) density of this 65-year-old woman has a T score –1.1, slightly below range for young women, and Z score 0.2, within range for women her age. She has minimal osteopenia, compared to a 35-year-old woman. Compared to women her age, she has average bone density.

Interpreting Bone Mineral Density (BMD) Tests

DEXA tests shoot two beams of photons from an X-ray tube through bone, and measure how much of the beams are absorbed by the bone. Bone density values are reported in terms of standard deviations (SD) removed from mean values in young adults and in age-matched controls. The test uses the bell-shaped curve, in which about 90 percent of values cluster near the average, within one SD above or below the mean. These statistical calculations take into account normal variation in bone denseness among women. To conclude that *any* difference from mean (average) values really exists, the BMD score must be more than 1 SD in either direction from the mean, either +1 SD above the mean, or –1 SD below the mean. Two values are given: **T score**, which compares your BMD to that of a 35-year old woman, and **Z score**, which compares your BMD to that of women your own age. For example:

- +1 SD (or more): Excellent bone density
- 0.0 to –1.0 SD: Normal bone density (within expected variation)
- –1.0 to –2.5 SD: Osteopenia (mild decreased density)
- –2.5 SD (or more): Osteoporosis (moderate to severe decreased density)

Sources: National Osteoporosis Foundation. (1998). *Physician's guide to prevention and treatment of osteoporosis.* Belle Meade, NJ: Excerpta Medica, Inc.
Licaca, A. A. (1999). Update on osteoporosis: Strategies for prevention and treatment. *Women's Health in Primary Care, 2,* 229–244.

type I collagen, which makes up 90 percent of bone matrix. Dpd is formed by enzyme action and released into urine during the bone breakdown process. Dpd is not affected by diet or calcium supplements. When Dpd levels are above the range of normal, then bone turnover is being accelerated. If this continues long enough, bones will thin and women may develop osteopenia or osteoporosis.

As urine Dpd is a simple test and can be done at home, women may want to start with this test before a DEXA. Collection materials are supplied by laboratories or health providers. You take the sample from your first morning urination, then send it to the laboratory. If your Dpd level is high, your bone turnover is more rapid than normal. You may need to review factors in your diet and lifestyle that might be causing this. After discussions with your health provider, you might consider a DEXA test.

Where to get this test: Dpd testing is provided by many clinical laboratories, and must be ordered by your health provider. Pyrilinks-D is a quantitative test of Dpd excretion, which you may have done on your own (see Resources, Aeron Lifecycles Laboratory).

Three Menopausal Women

Janice, now 52, stopped having periods three years ago. She has up to 10 hot flashes daily, is not sleeping well, partly because of night sweats, and tires more easily. She began using progesterone cream from the health food store, but it did not change her symptoms noticeably. In the past year, she has experienced vaginal dryness, discomfort with sexual intercourse, and pressure sensations with mild discomfort when urinating. A saliva hormone test shows that Janice has low-normal levels of estradiol, low progesterone, and low-normal testosterone and DHEA. She has chosen to use prescription dermal progesterone cream and vaginal estrogen cream to help her symptoms.

Arlene had an early menopause at age 45. Now 46, she has minimal symptoms with only a moderate decrease in energy. A health-conscious single woman, Arlene wanted a thorough checkup with Pap smear, blood tests, and hormone and bone density testing. Saliva hormone tests show low-normal estradiol, very low progesterone, low-normal testosterone, and normal DHEA. Other tests are normal, except her bone density, which shows significant osteoporosis in both the lumbar spine (T score: −3.1) and hip (T score: −3.2). Always one to take action for problems, Arlene has decided to use prescription oral estrogen and progesterone, testosterone gel, and the drug biphosphonate to increase her bone mineral.

Rosalyn is one year past menopause at age 51. She is having hot flashes and night sweats, disturbed sleep, and less energy than before. After trying black cohosh and vitex for several months, she did not find much relief of her symptoms. A saliva hormone test shows low estradiol, progesterone, and testosterone, with normal DHEA. Rosalyn initially asked to take oral estriol, the most popular form of estrogen in her native country, Germany. She has also agreed to take natural oral progesterone to support hormone balance and protect her uterine lining.

In Chapter 3, these women's stories continue, including details about their experiences with therapy. Table 2–4 shows their hormone test values.

TABLE 2–4	Hormone Values for Janice, Arlene, and Rosalyn				
	AGE/ TEST	ESTRADIOL	PROGESTERONE	TESTOSTERONE	DHEA
Janice	53 /saliva	0.5 pg/ml	0.01 ng/ml	23.4 pg/ml	68.4 pg/ml
Arlene	46 /saliva	1.4 pg/ml	0.01 ng/ml	19.0 pg/ml	185.5 pg/ml
Rosalyn	51 /saliva	0.6 pg/ml	0.02 ng/ml	17.9 pg/ml	167.5 pg/ml

Mammograms

A monthly self–breast exam is still the most frequent way that women detect abnormal growths. Low dose, focused X-ray mammography is a common screening test for early breast cancer. It often can detect very small tumors, or micro-calcifications that might indicate a malignant growth. In combination with clinical breast exams done by a health provider, mammograms aid in early detection of breast cancer. However, it is not 100 percent accurate, and having a normal mammogram is not a guarantee that your breasts will stay healthy. Radiation exposure is relatively low. Regular mammograms are considered the standard of care for women over 40. The American Cancer Association and many medical groups recommend yearly or biennial mammograms after age 40. If you are concerned about yearly radiation exposure to your breasts, you will need to carefully weigh your risk factors for breast cancer against the advantage of earlier detection.

Breast cancers identified in earlier stages are more curable than those found at later stages. Women who get regular mammograms are more likely to have breast cancer diagnosed at an earlier stage, resulting in better survival rates (McCarthy, Burns, Freund, et al., 2000). The five-year survival rate for women with localized (early) breast cancer is 97 percent, for those with regional spread of cancer it is 72 percent, and for those with distant metastases it is only 22 percent (Olopade & Cummings, 2000).

Although mammography is considered routine in current medical practice, some issues exist about widescale screening. The balance between beneficial and harmful effects seems very delicate. The recommendation for regular mammograms is

Get annual or biennial mammograms . . . or other screening if you have a positive family history for breast cancer or if you find that this screening puts your mind at ease. (Peace of mind produces very positive biochemical changes in the body.)

—Christiane Northrup, *The Wisdom of Menopause*

based on five large Swedish clinical trials showing that mammography screening lowered deaths from breast cancer by 29 percent in women ages 50–69. (Nystrom et al., 1993). Later Swedish studies have called these results into question. A meta-analysis of eight large clinical trials of half a million women in the United States, Scotland, Canada, and Sweden found that six of the trials had flaws in their research methods. These six reported the best results for regular mammography in reducing breast cancer deaths. The two well-designed trials did not find significant reduction in breast cancer deaths with mammography (Gotzsche & Olsen, 2000).

Regular mammography often leads to additional testing and surgery. Studies found breast biopsies and lumpectomies were much more common among women having regular mammography compared to control groups who did not. Benign biopsies were two to four times higher in mammography screening groups (Miller et al., 1992). This means that women who get regular mammograms will end up having more surgeries for benign breast conditions. Women undergoing surgery have increased risks from anesthesia and complications, such as infections and cardiovascular problems.

Psychological stress is another factor, but studies rarely take it into account. About half the women having regular mammograms will have at least one false positive result over a period of ten years (Gotzsche & Olsen, 2000). This means that women will be told there is something suspicious in their breast, will need further diagnostic tests, and may need to undergo surgery, only to find out that they do not have anything wrong or their breast lesion is benign—and they will go through the emotional trauma this entails. Data from these studies suggest that for each breast cancer death avoided using regular mammography, there are six other deaths from complications of procedures and surgery.

Thus the question still remains: Does having regular mammography reduce the risk of dying from breast cancer enough to justify the increased health dangers from more surgery, complications, and emotional distress?

In addition, mammograms are less accurate in detecting abnormal growths in women with dense breast tissue. During their 30s and 40s, most women have denser breasts than in their 50s and 60s. Studies have found an association between dense breast tissue on mammogram, and increased risk of breast cancer (Yaffe, et al., 1998). However, technical factors involved in mammography techniques affect this association. Newer breast imaging techniques, such as ultrasound, thermography, and magnetic resonance imaging, which do not use ionizing radiation, are under exploration. As radiation exposure is known to damage DNA, it is considered a carcinogen (causing cancer). Regular screening mammography for women in their 40s, when dense breast tissue reduces the accuracy of the test, has been questioned given the risk of cell damage from radiation.

Menopausal women taking hormone replacement therapy (HRT) also face less accuracy in their mammograms. An Australian study (Kavanagh, Mitchell, & Giles, 2000) found the sensitivity of screening mammography over a 2-year interval was lower in HRT users than non-users. Among women who were diagnosed with breast cancer during the two-year screening interval, HRT users were more likely to have a false negative result. Also, among women who did not have cancer diagnosed in the interval, HRT users were more likely to have a false positive result.

Making decisions about screening mammograms can be challenging. Some women choose not to have them, or to wait several years between screenings. Others feel more comfortable knowing (to the extent possible) that they do not have breast cancer, and decide to have yearly screening mammograms. You should discuss these concerns with your health care provider and stay informed. If you or your provider detect a breast lump, however, then you should not hesitate in getting a mammogram. In this instance, you will receive a diagnostic (not screening) mammogram to help determine the characteristics of the lump so that the next steps in evaluation and treatment can be planned.

Where to take this test: Start by asking your health care provider for recommendations. You may call your local hospital or look in the phone book in the Yellow Pages under "Mammography." Sometimes your local newspaper will advertise a mobile unit's schedule in your area. You will need an order from your health care provider for a mammography, unless it is offered at special screenings and health fairs.

On the horizon: New technologies for detecting breast cancer without exposure to X rays are being explored. MRI (magnetic resonance imaging) uses electromagnetic waves to create layered images of tissues, and can clearly define tumor stage. Thermography detects increased skin temperature, caused by higher metabolism of underlying tumor cells. Ductal lavage (also called nipple aspirate) uses thin catheters to wash cells out of nipple ducts with saline solution (many breast cancers originate in these ducts). These techniques are not widely available, and require special technology that needs further study and standardization.

Pap Test and Pelvic Exam (Cervical Cancer Screening)

For over 30 years, annual pelvic exams and Pap smears have been recommended for women. The Pap test detects abnormal cervical cells, which can range from atypical to cancerous. Found early, cervical cancer is among the most curable. The widespread use of Pap smears has decreased deaths from cervical cancer by an estimated 70 percent (Northrup, 1998). Nevertheless, nearly 14,000 cases of cervical cancer are diagnosed each year in the United States, and about half of these have local invasion into surrounding tissue. The five-year survival rate for women with more advanced disease is 65 percent (Research Report, 2000).

Recent studies have addressed how often women should have Pap tests. Data from the National Breast and Cervical Cancer Early Detection Program show that it is uncommon to have serious abnormalities within three years of a normal Pap test (Sawaya, Kerlikowske, Gildengorin, & Washington, 2000). In postmenopausal women taking HRT, no significant abnormalities occurred on Pap tests within two years of a normal result (Sawaya, Grady, Kerlikowske et al., 2000). This led researchers to recommend a two to three year interval between Pap tests for women with normal results.

A Pap test is performed by taking a sample of cells from the place where inner cervical cells meet outer cervical cells (the squamocolumnar junction), because this is where abnormalities first develop. Sometimes this junction is deep inside the cervical canal, making it necessary to use a tiny brush to get the sample. The test is sent to a laboratory for interpretation; many use computerized readings that are checked by technicians if any abnormalities appear. About 10–13 percent of Pap smears give a false negative report, meaning they fail to detect abnormal cells. Failure of the practitioner to get a good sample causes two-thirds of false negatives, and one-third are caused by laboratory misreading (Northrup, 1998). Pap reports use a descriptive classification, as follows:

- Within normal limits, benign
- Atypia, cells that are not typical but are not clearly abnormal
- Dysplasia, cells that are abnormal but are not clearly cancerous
- Squamous intraepithelial lesion (SIL), abnormal cells that are not clearly cancerous, ranging from mild to severe
- Cervical intraepithelial neoplasia (CIN), which means the same as SIL
- Carcinoma in situ (CIS), an early form of cancer
- Invasive carcinoma, more advanced cancer rated according to how deeply the malignant cells penetrate into cervical or surrounding tissue

Most abnormal Pap smears do not mean a woman has cervical cancer. Often atypical cells revert back to normal, as do many cases of dysplasia and mild CIN/CIS. About 50 percent of mild cervical abnormalities resolve without treatment. Your practitioner will usually recommend re-testing in two to three months. A new Pap procedure called "ThinPrep" uses a liquid preservative rather than making a smear directly on a glass slide. More cells are collected in the liquid, which is filtered to remove debris and spread in an even, thin layer on a slide allowing better identification of cells. The same specimen can be used to test for human papilloma virus (HPV). This avoids the need for an additional office visit and repeat Pap smear. It also eliminates the stressful two to three month waiting period until retesting.

Regular Pap smears also detect human papilloma virus (HPV) infection of the cervix. HPV infections often cause cervical atypia and dysplasia. HPV also causes genital warts, which appear on the labia, buttocks, thighs, and perineal skin (between the vagina and rectum). If HPV infection, inflammation, or vaginal infection is present, these are treated, as they may be the cause of abnormal cells.

If abnormal cell growth continues it may lead to cervical cancer. Cells identified as dysplasia and SIL/CIN are considered "pre-cancerous." If cancer develops, the earlier it is found, the simpler the treatment. Some lesions progress rapidly, and prompt medical treatment is the standard for moderate-to-severe categories. Methods used to remove or destroy the abnormal cells include laser, cryotherapy, or LEEP (loop electrical excision procedure). These are done in the doctor's office. Surgical conization, the removal of a cone of tissue in the cervical opening, is performed in outpatient surgery centers or hospitals under anesthesia. The cure rate of these procedures is over 90 percent. Once cancer cells have become invasive, they penetrate deeper into cervical tissues and potentially can spread through the lymphatic system or blood stream. Invasive cervical cancer requires more extensive surgery, usually removal of cervix and uterus, and checking surrounding lymph nodes for cancerous spread.

Where to take this test: A physician; a family or women's health nurse practitioner.

Ovarian Cancer Screening

The pelvic exam can detect uterine or ovarian enlargements. These range from simple ovarian cysts and uterine fibroids to cancers. Ovarian cancer is a "silent" disease, producing almost no symptoms until the tumor is quite large, and by then it often has metastasized to other organs. An annual pelvic exam is used to detect early ovarian cancer, but only about 15 percent of ovarian cancers are actually found this way. The risk increases after menopause; each year 40 out of 100,000 women ages 50 to 75 years are diagnosed with ovarian cancer (Gemignani & Hoskins, 2000). Half of these women survive for five years, but for those diagnosed early, the survival rate is 95 percent (Olopade & Cummings, 2000). This highlights the importance of early diagnosis, so treatment (usually surgery and radiation) can be done immediately, thus giving better results for cure and life expectancy.

To date, there is no simple, reliable screening test for ovarian cancer. When ovarian enlargements are found, pelvic ultrasound is done to further assess the characteristics of the mass. However, pelvic ultrasound is not very accurate in distinguishing between benign and malignant masses. The only way to determine for certain whether ovarian masses are benign or cancerous is through biopsy or surgical removal of the ovary, with pathological examination of the tissues. This makes pelvic ultrasound impractical for screening the general population of women. It would result in many biopsies or surgeries, the vast majority done for benign cysts or tumors.

A blood test, CA 125, tests for glycoproteins associated with ovarian cancer, but it is not specific to that condition alone. CA 125 is elevated in 80 percent of women with ovarian cancer. Many other conditions including uterine fibroids, ovarian cysts, and endometriosis can cause CA 125 to be high. Its levels are normal in more than 50 percent of women with early (stage I) ovarian cancer. Thus, measuring CA 125 is not a reliable screening method for ovarian cancer

(Gemignani & Hoskins, 2000). Many women must be tested to detect very few cases. In one study of 22,000 women with elevated CA 125 on screening, when surgery was performed to determine if ovarian masses were benign or malignant, only 20 percent were found to have cancer (Jacobs et al., 1993). Common conditions which can cause elevated levels of CA 125 are:

Uterine fibroids

Benign ovarian cysts

Endometriosis

Pelvic inflammatory disease (infection)

Pregnancy

CA 125 is most useful to monitor for recurrence of ovarian cancer, once it has been diagnosed and treated. In postmenopausal women, elevated CA 125 is more likely to point toward ovarian cancer, because the other conditions causing increased levels are less common after menopause. Combining pelvic ultrasound with CA 125 appears to offer better accuracy. At present, routine screening for ovarian cancer is not recommended for the general population.

If you have certain risk factors, you should discuss these tests with your health provider. Having a mother or sister with ovarian or breast cancer is the biggest risk factor. Hereditary ovarian cancers account for about 10 percent of all ovarian cancer cases. Hereditary breast-ovarian cancers carried in the BRCA1 susceptibility gene account for 65–75 percent of cases, and those carried in the BRCA2 susceptibility gene are thought to account for the rest (Olopade & Cummings, 2000). However, 90 percent of ovarian cancers are not the hereditary type. These are believed to result from gene mutations and defects which leave the immune system unable to properly destroy abnormal cells, or which cause abnormal cells to continue growing into cancers.

Where to get this test: A physician or nurse practitioner should evaluate whether it would be appropriate to get a CA 125 test, or a pelvic ultrasound.

TAKING CHARGE OF SYMPTOMS, RISKS, AND TESTS

The first steps in self-care require that you become an expert on yourself. The more aware you are of your particular bodily changes and symptoms, the better you can make choices about how you want to handle them. Use the worksheets at the end of this chapter to track your symptoms and your risk factors. Some principles for taking charge:

• Be familiar with your body, symptoms, and risk factors.
• Get the tests that help you assess your hormones and risks.
• Create a partnership with a health practitioner who will respect your views.

- Learn about the physical, chemical, and hormonal changes you may expect.
- Remember that physical symptoms are closely related to your emotions, mental state, and satisfaction with your life.

REFERENCES

Ahlgrimm, M., & Kells, J.M. (1999). *The HRT solution: Optimizing your hormone potential.* Garden City Park, NY: Avery Publishing Group.

Boucher, S. (1991). Meeting the tiger. In D. Taylor & A. C. Sumrall (Eds.). *Women of the 14th moon.* Freedom, CA: The Crossing Press.

Cummings, S.R., Palermo, L., Browner, W., et al. (2000). Monitoring osteoporosis therapy with bone densitometry. *Journal of the American Medical Association, 283,* 1318–1321.

Gemignani, M.L., & Hoskins, W.J. (2000). Screening for ovarian cancer: Who, how, when? *Women's Health in Primary Care, 3,* 205–212.

Gotzsche, P.C., & Olsen, O. (2000). Is screening for breast cancer with mammography justifiable? *Lancet, 355,* 129–134.

Jacobs, I., Davies, A.P., Bridges, J., et al. (1993). Prevalence screening for ovarian cancer in postmenopausal women in CA 125 measurement and ultrasonography. *British Medical Journal, 306,* 1030–1034.

Karras, C. (1991). Climacterium. In D. Taylor & A. C. Sumrall (Eds.). *Women of the 14th moon.* Freedom, CA: The Crossing Press.

Kavanagh, A.M., Mitchell, H., & Giles, G.G. (2000). Hormone replacement therapy and accuracy of mammographic screening. *Lancet, 355,* 270–274.

Lee, J., Henley, J. & Hopkins, V. (1999). *What your doctor may not tell you about menopause: Balance your hormones and your life from thirty to fifty.* New York: Warner Books.

Lindsay, R., Marcus, R., & Recker, R. (1996). Osteoporosis: What's new in prevention and treatment. *Patient Care, 30,* 24–53.

Massoudi, M.S., Meilahn, E.N., & Orchard, T.J. (1995). Prevalence of thyroid antibodies among healthy middle-aged women. Findings from the thyroid study in healthy women. *Annals of Epidemiology, 5,* 229–233.

McCarthy, E.P., Burns, R.B., Freund, K.M., et al. (2000). Mammography use, breast cancer stage at diagnosis, and survival among older women. *Journal of the American Geriatric Society, 48,* 1226–1233.

The Medical Letter on Drugs and Therapeutics. (1996). Bone densitometry. *38:*1–2.

Miller, A.B., Baines, C.J., To, T., & Wall, C. (1992). Canadian National Breast Screening Study: 2-breast cancer detection and death rates among women aged 50 to 59 years. *Canadian Medical Association Journal, 147,* 1477–1488.

Northrup, C. (July, 1997). Welcome to the hormone revolution! *Dr. Christiane Northrup's health wisdom for women, 4,* 1–4.

Northrup, C. (1998). *Women's bodies, women's wisdom: Creating physical and emotional health and healing.* New York: Bantam Books.

Northrup, C. (May, 1999). Dear Reader. *Dr. Christiane Northrup's health wisdom for women, 6,* 1–2.

Northrup, C. (2001). *The wisdom of menopause: Creating physical and emotional health and healing during the change.* New York: Bantam Books.

Nystrom, L., Rutqvist, L.E., Walls, S., et al. (1993). Breast cancer screening with mammography: Overview of Swedish randomized trials. *Lancet, 341,* 973–978.

Olopade, O.I., & Cummings, S. (2000). Breast and ovarian cancer, part 1: What you need to know about inherited risks. *Consultant, 40,* 1809–1814.

Pert, C. (1997). *Molecules of emotion: Why you feel the way you feel.* New York: Scribner.

Posey, V.C. (1991). What it was, was menopause. In D. Taylor & A. C. Sumrall (Eds.). *Women of the 14th moon.* Freedom, CA: The Crossing Press.

Research Report. (2000). Combined therapy for cervical cancer. *Women's Health in Primary Care, 2,* 479–480.

Sawaya, G.F., Grady, D., Kerlikowske, K., et al. (2000). The positive predictive value of cervical smears in previously screened postmenopausal women. The Heart and Estrogen/Progestin Replacement Study (HERS). *Annals of Internal Medicine, 133,* 942–950.

Sawaya, G.F., Kerlikowske, K., Gildengoren, G., Washington, A.E. (2000). Incidence of Pap test abnormalities within 3 years of normal Pap test—United States, 1991–1998. *MMWR Morbidity and Mortality Weekly Report, 49,* 1001–1003.

Schultz, M.L. (1998). *Awakening intuition: Using your mind-body network for insight and healing.* New York: Harmony Books.

Stampfer, M.J., Hu, F.B., Manson, J.E., et al. (2000). Primary prevention of coronary heart disease in women through diet and lifestyle. *New England Journal of Medicine, 343,* 16–22.

UCB Wellness Letter. (May, 1999). Wellness facts. *15*:1.

Yaffe, M.J., Boyd, N.F., Byng, J.W., et al. (1998). Breast cancer risk and measured mammographic density. *European Journal of Cancer Prevention (Suppl)*, *1*:S47–55.

SUGGESTED READING

Bender, S.D. (1998). *The power of perimenopause: A woman's guide to physical and emotional health during the transitional decade.* New York: Three Rivers Press.

Checklist: My Perimenopause and Menopause Symptoms

Enter the dates on which you began having each symptom that applies, and check whether mild, moderate or severe. This gives you a summary of your symptoms to use in selecting remedies.

Symptom	Date(s)	Mild	Moderate	Severe
menstrual changes	_____	☐	☐	☐
heavy bleeding	_____	☐	☐	☐
worse PMS	_____	☐	☐	☐
worse cramps	_____	☐	☐	☐
pelvic pressure	_____	☐	☐	☐
irregular periods	_____	☐	☐	☐
breast tenderness	_____	☐	☐	☐
bloating	_____	☐	☐	☐
headaches	_____	☐	☐	☐
moods, irritability	_____	☐	☐	☐
depression	_____	☐	☐	☐
fatigue	_____	☐	☐	☐
sleep disturbances	_____	☐	☐	☐
food cravings	_____	☐	☐	☐
memory loss	_____	☐	☐	☐
less concentration	_____	☐	☐	☐
hot flashes	_____	☐	☐	☐
night sweats	_____	☐	☐	☐
palpitations	_____	☐	☐	☐
decreased libido	_____	☐	☐	☐
crawling skin	_____	☐	☐	☐
vaginal dryness	_____	☐	☐	☐
frequent urinating	_____	☐	☐	☐
dribbling urine	_____	☐	☐	☐
dry, itchy skin	_____	☐	☐	☐
more facial hair	_____	☐	☐	☐
thinner head hair	_____	☐	☐	☐
less muscle tone	_____	☐	☐	☐

Determining Your Risks

These general guidelines are to increase your awareness. If you check two or more boxes, you need to look more closely at your health risks.

Osteoporosis	*Previous*	*Present*
Small frame (low bone mass)	☐	☐
Lack of weight-bearing exercise	☐	☐
Over-vigorous exercise	☐	☐
High animal protein intake (> 60 gm/day)	☐	☐
Cigarette smoking	☐	☐
Excess alcohol (> 2 oz/day)	☐	☐
Diet low in calcium, magnesium, Vitamin D	☐	☐
Excess phosphorus (sodas, junk food)	☐	☐
Excess caffeine (> 2 cups/day)	☐	☐
Excess salt, sugar, or dairy products	☐	☐
Mother, grandmother with osteoporosis	☐	☐
Steroids (prednisone), thyroid hormone, benzodiazepines, anticonvulsants	☐	☐

Heart Disease		
Cigarette smoking	☐	☐
Obesity (> 20% overweight)	☐	☐
Lack of aerobic exercise	☐	☐
High fat, cholesterol diet (> 30% calories)	☐	☐
High LDL: low density cholesterol > 130mg/dl	☐	☐
Low HDL: high density cholesterol < 35mg/dl	☐	☐
Diabetes, Type I or II	☐	☐
High blood pressure > 130/85	☐	☐
Low intake of antioxidants	☐	☐
Family history of heart, blood pressure problems	☐	☐

Breast Cancer		
Cigarette smoking	☐	☐
Longer estrogen production in body (> 40 years menstruating)	☐	☐

Mother, sister (first-degree relative) with breast
   or ovarian cancer   ☐   ☐

ERT/HRT used for > 5 years (data based on progestins
   and conjugated equine estrogens)   ☐   ☐

Possible risk factors—not clearly proven:

Diet low in fruit, vegetables, fiber   ☐   ☐

Low intake of antioxidants   ☐   ☐

Excess alcohol (conflicting data)   ☐   ☐

CHAPTER
3

The Physical Experience: Hormones, Herbs, and Lifestyle

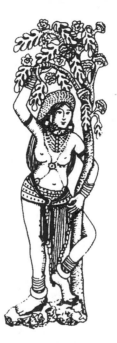

Tree goddess.
Reproduced with permission.
Copyright © Kate Cartwright.

Women have many choices for managing symptoms during perimenopause and menopause. From a holistic perspective, these choices range from prescription hormones to herbs, nutrition, and lifestyle. One choice is not inherently better than another, although using herbs may be gentler and more closely aligned with nature, while prescription hormones can act more quickly and provide stronger symptom relief. Each woman's body-mind is unique, and her experience of the menopause transition will reflect personal energy patterns. By using self-knowledge and information about personal characteristics, and developing a partnership with a health practitioner when needed, you can select the best therapy options for your own situation.

HORMONE REPLENISHMENT THERAPY

Why would a woman choose to take estrogen and progesterone therapy? Because taking hormones can help relieve symptoms, and may have health promoting effects such as reducing risk for osteoporosis, dental disease, and dementia (Alzheimer's disease). The benefits of hormone therapy for preventing heart disease are less clear. For some women, hormones make the difference between feeling like themselves and feeling physically miserable, emotionally distraught, or mentally dysfunctional. Hormones can be a tool for women to use to ease the menopause transition and as an aid to reduce risk of some diseases. Remember, using hormones is always your choice.

Most women want a "natural" choice for hormone therapy. We think of natural products as those that are closest to how the substance occurs in nature, made by Mother Nature herself. Products in the purely natural state, such as wild Asian yams, however, often do not have much effect in the body when taken in a natural way, such as eating. So it is necessary to refine natural sources of hormones (soy, wild yams) to some degree to get the desired effects on the tissues. That is what is done in natural hormone products.

The "natural" forms of estrogen and progesterone are made from plants, mainly soy and wild yams. Molecules are extracted from these phytochemicals and are used to make hormones that are identical in structure to human hormones, called human identical hormones (HIH) or bioidentical hormones. Their action in women's bodies appears to be the same as our own hormones (Wetzel, 1998). Using human identical hormones is called natural hormone-replacement therapy (NHRT). The HIH estrogens and progesterone are available in pill, dermal, and vaginal cream forms, mostly by prescription. These hormones do not appear to have the same risks as pharmaceutical synthetic hormones, which are made in laboratories from materials other than human sources. However, very little research has been done on bioidentical hormones, because they have not been in use very long. The huge, ongoing Women's Health Initiative studies have recently added groups of women using HIH. Those studies will provide the most comprehensive data on the effects of plant-derived hormones, but results will not be published until 2005 (Consumers Union, 2000).

Synthetic hormones are made in a chemistry laboratory. Most forms of estrogen and progestins produced by drug companies are made from a plant base (soy

I think if you get through the door of menopause and continue to face life as a fascinating, though frequently troubling, journey, and trust in that journey, your post-menopausal life will be extraordinary. . . . In a crazy way, it's something to look forward to. I feel more centered now, more so than at any time in my life.

—Elaine Goldman Gill, "Blowing the Fuse," in *Women of the 14th Moon*

or yams). The biologically active molecules are taken out, broken apart, and reconfigured so that they look chemically like human hormones. However, other byproducts and binders such as lactose and starch are present in the pills. Human identical hormones such as triestrogen, biestrogen, and micronized progesterone are also made from soy and yams, but the active molecules are simply extracted and concentrated—not synthesized. Their naturally occurring chemical form is not changed, as it is with synthetic hormones. The HIH micronized progesterone often is suspended in peanut oil. Women with peanut oil allergy can ask their pharmacist to customize the suspension with another type of oil.

Synthetic estrogens probably increase women's risks for hormone-related cancers, blood clots, gallbladder disease, and liver disease, although there are some conflicting studies (Bosarge, 2000). Synthetic combined hormones (estrogen plus progestins) reduce the beneficial effects of estrogen on high- and low-density cholesterols. The drugs made by pharmaceutical companies are very powerful synthetic compounds, purified and concentrated to have maximum effect on target areas of the body. This is both their advantage and their risk: The effect is predictable and noticeable in a short time, and the dosage can be carefully regulated—but side effects and complications are common. Hormone replacement therapy options, for both synthetic and human identical hormones, are reviewed in Table 3–1.

Steps for Figuring Out Your Hormone Needs

These guidelines can help you decide if hormone replacement therapy would fit with your needs. This is not an either/or decision, but a process guided by understanding your own symptoms and experiences. Taking or not taking hormones is your choice. There are many other options for easing symptoms and maintaining health during menopause, discussed later in this chapter.

- Determine what your goals are, what you would like to achieve.
- Have hormone tests done to determine your current hormone profile.
- Assess the impact of your symptoms, and how much relief hormones might provide.
- Assess your personal risk factors for osteoporosis, heart disease, and dementia, and how much benefit hormones are expected to provide.
- Assess your personal risk factors for breast cancer, and consider how you feel about hormone-replacement therapy possibly increasing that risk.

(Continued on next page)

- Think about what type of HRT fits best with your needs and beliefs, either human identical hormones or synthetic hormones.
- Consider what route of administration suits you best: oral, patches, dermal creams, vaginal creams, or sublingual tablets.
- Have an idea about how long you want to continue taking HRT, because risks and complication rates go up with longer duration of use.
- Review options for phasing off hormones, should you decide to use them.

Considerations in Using Hormone Replenishment Therapy

Making the decision to use hormones often is a big step for women. Most are aware that risks can be associated with taking hormones, in particular, estrogen. Some women, understanding that menopause is a natural process, are reluctant to tamper with nature's plans. They wonder if something deeper is happening that might be offset by keeping hormone levels artificially high. On the other hand, women may want to reduce the disruptions in their lives caused by hormonal changes. They also may seek to preserve their attractiveness and vitality, or decrease the risks of some diseases, by using hormone replenishment. Probably the main reason why women take hormones is for symptom relief.

Nature provides women with sources of hormones after menopause. The hormone shift that changes the balance between types of estrogen (less estradiol, more estriol), and alters the relative amounts of estrogen, progesterone, and androgens, supports different biochemistry in our brains and bodies. This is part of our life transformation, with its expanded vision and different modes of thinking. If we have not taken good care of ourselves, however, our body-mind may be depleted when we arrive at menopause. Our body may not be capable of providing adequate amounts of hormones to support healthy functions in the second half of life. In that case, hormone replenishment therapy may be an important support for weathering the upheavals of menopause.

You can check your hormone "bank account" to see whether your balance is sufficient for supporting you through menopause. Take a moment to complete Worksheet 3–1 at the end of this chapter.

SYMPTOM RELIEF

Estrogen provides relief of hot flashes, moodiness, depression, vaginal and skin changes, urinary changes, insomnia, and thought process disturbances (brain fog, forgetfulness). It appears to reduce incidence of dementia and Alzheimer's disease

TABLE 3–1	**Hormone Replacement Therapy Options**

SYNTHETIC ESTROGENS

Cenestin	Conjugated estrogens
Menest	Esterified estrogens
Ortho-Est	Estropipate
Ogen	Estropipate
Estratest	Esterified estrogen plus methyltestosterone
FemHRT	Progestin-estrogen combination

COMBINATIONS

Ortho-Prefest	Estradiol plus norgestimate
Activella	Estradiol plus norethindrone acetate
Combi-Patch	Estradiol plus norethindrone acetate patch

SYNTHETIC PROGESTINS

Cycrin	Medroxyprogesterone acetate
Provera	Medroxyprogesterone acetate
Aygestin	Norethindrone acetate

ANIMAL DERIVED HORMONES

Premarin	Conjugated equine estrogens (from pregnant mare's urine)
Prempro	Conjugated equine estrogens plus medroxyprogesterone acetate (progestin)
Premphase	Conjugated equine estrogens plus medroxyprogesterone acetate (progestin)

HUMAN IDENTICAL HORMONES

Triestrogen	Compounded estrone, estradiol and estriol
Biestrogen	Compounded estradiol and estriol
Estrace	Estradiol
Alora	Estradiol patch
Climara	Estradiol patch
Estraderm	Estradiol patch
Vivelle	Estradiol patch
Estring	Estradiol vaginal silicone ring
Prometrium	Micronized progesterone
Progesterone	Micronized compounded progesterone
Testosterone	Compounded testosterone

Note that **progestin** is not the same as **progesterone**. Here are the differences:

• Progesterone is the body's native hormone
• Progestin is a powerful synthetic that mimics the action of progesterone
• Human identical hormone progesterone is chemically identical to native progesterone (that your body makes), produced from soy or wild yams
• Progestin contributes to congestion effects and depression, and counteracts some of estrogen's good effects on cholesterol and blood vessels
• Progesterone often relieves congestion, enhances positive moods, builds bone, and supports many body functions (thyroid, libido, blood sugar, cell oxygenation, adrenals, fat metabolism)

(see Chapter 4). It provides anti-aging effects such as smoother, plumper skin. Progesterone balances the effects of estrogen, brings cell cycles to completion, and offers protection to breast tissue. It may help increase libido and energy, reduce congestive symptoms (breast swelling, PMS), and promote a sense of well-being.

There are three regimens (dose schedules) for taking HRT:

1. Monthly cyclic regimen—estrogen is taken from day 1 to day 25, and progesterone is added from day 14 or 15 to day 25. This follows the usual hormone fluctuations during the menstrual cycle. Most women have their menses after stopping HRT on day 25, and wait until the menstrual bleeding stops before starting the next round of HRT. This regimen is used for women who are still having menses, even if somewhat irregular.

2. Continuous single ERT or combined HRT regimen—estrogen may be taken alone every day when women have had a hysterectomy. They may choose to also take progesterone for additional benefits. Women who still have a uterus need to use combined HRT, taking both estrogen and progesterone every day. Progesterone (or a form of synthetic progestin) is necessary to offset the effect of estrogen on the uterine lining. Estrogen by itself can cause abnormal cell growth that might lead to uterine cancer. This regimen is usually followed when women are no longer having menses.

3. Long cyclic regimen—used for women with a uterus who are sensitive to side effects of progesterone or progestins. Estrogen is taken every day, then every 2–4 months progesterone is added for two weeks. This is adequate to protect the endometrium from overgrowth, and can reduce the length of time women need to go through uncomfortable side effects.

Table 3–2 presents therapy choices by three perimenopausal women.

> . . . Before you decide to take powerful hormones to protect yourself against the possibility of acquiring a medical condition you do not yet have, it is important to assess your own risk of ever getting the disease. Saying every postmenopausal woman should take hormones is like saying every pregnant woman should get a cesarean section *in case* she encounters problems during her delivery.
>
> —Lonnie Barbach, *The Pause: Positive Approaches to Perimenopause and Menopause*

TABLE 3–2	Therapy Choices: Three Perimenopausal Women	

NAME	HORMONE PROFILE	THERAPY
Patty	Normal levels of estrogen, progesterone, FSH, LH	Evening primrose oil (EPO), Vitamin B_6, Vitex, Vitamin E improved her PMS Celexa 20mg daily (antidepressant medication)
Marianne	Normal estradiol, low progesterone	Progesterone dermal cream 30mg/gm, 1 gm twice daily improved her moodiness and hot flashes
Lisa	Normal estradiol, low progesterone, FSH and LH elevated	Prometrium 200 mg daily made her sleepy and dizzy; reducing dose to 100 mg at bedtime helped her to sleep with no dizziness

OSTEOPOROSIS

Osteoporosis is a complex condition. Only about 25–30 percent of women develop postmenopausal osteoporosis. The natural decrease of estrogen levels at menopause is not the cause of osteoporosis, although it can cause acceleration of bone loss. After age 35, the bone-building osteoblasts begin to slow down, while the osteoclasts that eat away old bone continue at the same pace. The result is that osteoblasts are unable to replace old bone fast enough to keep up with the osteoclasts. Eventually this leads to thinning bones, but usually not until very old age. Some people break bone down too fast, losing as much as 1 percent of bone density each year after middle age. For every 10 percent of bone density loss, the risk of fractures doubles.

Estrogen slows the rate of bone loss, but does not increase the rate of building bone. Studies suggest that progesterone will actually build more bone (Lee, Henley, & Hopkins, 1999), but others have not found this result (Leonetti, Longo, & Anasti, 1999). The effect of estrogen on bone takes a long time (more than 7 years). Taking estrogen more than 5 years increases the risk of serious side effects. When estrogen is stopped, a period of rapid bone loss occurs. There is little protection gained from taking estrogen after age 75. The lifetime risk of death related to osteoporosis is 1 in 6 women. Complications of fractures, such as pneumonia and blood clots from being immobile, are the usual causes of death.

Failure to absorb and metabolize calcium properly is a factor in osteoporosis. Building bone is nearly impossible without adequate calcium, plus the balance of other minerals and nutrients necessary for bone health. Diet (drinking too much soda and other forms of phosphates; excessive protein), taking steroids (prednisone, cortisone), and untreated or overtreated thyroid disease all cause accelerated breakdown of bone.

Table 3–3 presents therapy choices by three menopausal women.

HEART DISEASE

Observational studies through the mid-1990s found that estrogen therapy after menopause was associated with a 30 percent reduced risk of coronary artery disease (Barrett-Connor & Stuenkel, 1999) and other cardiovascular risks (Nabulsi et al., 1993). Some experts believe a "healthy user" effect is responsible (the "healthy user" effect means that the women participating in the studies had healthier lifestyles and diet). Once women stop taking estrogen, their risk returns to average for age within 10 years. The PEPI study (Postmenopausal Estrogen/

TABLE 3–3	**Therapy Choices: Three Menopausal Women**	
NAME	**HORMONE PROFILE**	**THERAPY***
Janice	Estradiol low normal, progesterone low, testosterone & DHEA low-normal	Estrace (estradiol) vaginal cream 0.1mg/gm and progesterone skin cream 40 mg/gm
Arlene	Estradiol low-normal, progesterone very low, testosterone & DHEA low-normal	Biestrogen 2.5 mg (estradiol 0.5 mg, estriol 2.0 mg) and progesterone 100 mg pills, plus testosterone skin gel, 2.5 mg daily dose, improved her symptoms. Fosamax 10 mg pill daily for building up bone
Rosalyn	Estradiol, progesterone and testosterone low, DHEA normal Estradiol, progesterone retested, still low	Estriol 4 mg pill and progesterone 100 mg pill did not relieve symptoms. Estradiol 0.5 mg was added to estriol 3.0 mg, with progesterone 150 mg but she still had symptoms. Changed to sublingual tablets and added pregnenolone 10 mg pills, now getting good results.

*Doses used in these examples were individualized for these women. Dose ranges vary; the doses shown here would not apply to every situation.

Progestin Interventions Trial) in 1995 reported that estrogen lowered cholesterol and blood pressure, but the study lasted only three years, a time period too short to fully examine the longer term benefits on heart health (Writing Group for the PEPI Trial, 1995).

Data from the HERS (Heart and Estrogen/Progestin Replacement Study), a large randomized clinical trial of 2,763 women with heart disease, failed to support the earlier studies. Women with established heart disease in the HERS actually had more heart attacks in the first year on HRT, although they had a modest benefit in reduced risk of heart attacks and other heart problems in subsequent years (Col, Legato, & Schiff, 1998).

Estrogen decreases LDL (low density lipoproteins—the "bad" type that builds plaque in arteries) and increases HDL (high density lipoproteins—the "good" type that removes cholesterol from the body), and so creates a healthy lipid profile. Adding synthetic progestins to estrogen decreases the beneficial effects of estrogen by lowering HDL. This is one factor that increases risk of heart disease. Estrogen has a direct effect on blood vessels by preventing the formation of plaques (which clog the arteries) and decreasing the danger of clot formation (which blocks arteries). It also prevents vasoconstriction, which causes vessels to become narrow and impede blood flow. These effects improve circulation and reduce risk of heart attack and stroke. Synthetic progestins, however, appear to increase vasoconstriction, thus offsetting the beneficial effects of estrogen therapy (Westermann, 1997).

The ideal level of LDL for women is 100 mg/dl or less, especially if they already have heart disease. To reach that goal, the "statin" drugs, such as lovastatin (Mevacor) or atorvastatin (Lipitor), are much more effective than estrogen. These drugs lower cholesterol 20–30 percent compared with only 10–15 percent for estrogen (Consumers Union, 2000). Lifestyle changes, such as avoiding cigarettes, exercising, and eating low-fat foods, are still the most effective methods for preventing heart disease for women after menopause. In fact, 20 years of data from the Nurses' Health Study on 84,129 women with no heart disease at the start of the study showed that heart disease risk *can be reduced by 80 percent* through these dietary and lifestyle practices: no smoking, moderate physical activity, normal weight, higher fiber, omega-3 fatty acids and folate in diet, and moderate alcohol use (Stampfer et al., 2000).

There's no question that heart palpitations at menopause are related to changing hormones. But they are also related to an increasing need for living from the wisdom of the heart at mid-life . . . you need to live your life as passionately and joyfully as possible.

—Christiane Northrup, "Heart Palpitations at Menopause: Your Heart's Wake-up Call!" *Dr. Christiane Northrup's Health Wisdom for Women*, 1999.

HEAVY BLEEDING AND FIBROIDS

Hormones often are used to control heavy, irregular bleeding during peri-menopause. The major reason for heavy bleeding is the action of high estrogen levels on the uterine lining (endometrium), without the balancing effects of pro-gesterone. As women get closer to the end of menstruation, the ovaries produce fewer eggs which leads to deficient progesterone levels. This is called the "unop-posed estrogen" effect, and the treatment is to use progesterone supplements. Usually progesterone or synthetic progestin pills are taken the last 10–12 days before the next menstrual period is due. Many women find this treatment very effective in slowing and regulating their bleeding. Low-dose birth control pills are another hormonal approach.

Fibroid tumors of the uterus are another cause of heavy, irregular bleeding in perimenopause. These are benign tumors of the uterine muscle, and can also cause pain or pressure in the pelvic area, and painful intercourse. Fibroids are common—30–50 percent of women in the United States have them (Northrup, 2001). There may be several of varying sizes or just one fibroid, felt as bumps of the uterus, or an enlarged uterus. Resulting from overgrowth of sections of the uterine muscle, fibroids rarely become cancerous. The great majority of fibroids do not cause any major problems or increase risk for endometrial cancer. Women can live for years with fibroids, managing symptoms with herbal, nutritional, or medical therapies. Fibroids will shrink after menopause when estrogen levels drop.

During perimenopause fibroids can grow dramatically in women who have estrogen dominance. The uterine muscle is very sensitive to estrogen levels, and the fibers increase when stimulated by unbalanced estrogen effects. Usually bleed-ing is heavier when fibroids increase in size. Health practitioners become con-cerned about possible uterine cancer if there is rapid growth of the uterus. Some fibroids get as large as soccer balls, causing the woman's abdomen to bulge out like a five to six month pregnancy. When heavy bleeding cannot be controlled with hormones, the fibroid is growing rapidly, or it is so big that it creates a great deal of pelvic pain and pressure, women often consider having a hysterectomy. Other options to shrink troublesome fibroids include: myomectomy to surgically remove just the fibroid and leave the uterus; the drugs Lupron or Synarel (GnRH agonists), which put the body into artificial menopause, lowering estrogen but causing hot flashes and bone loss; and uterine artery embolization with injection of polyvinyl alcohol particles into the uterine artery, causing fibroids to shrink by reducing their blood supply. This relatively new procedure has a good success rate, but long term problems are not known and some serious complications have occurred (Bradley & Newman, 2000).

Hysterectomy?

Because hysterectomies are so commonly performed in the United States (in the early 1990s, one out of four women became menopausal through surgery), you may well have had one, or you may be considering a hysterectomy.

Questions most asked

The big questions are: 1) Will I be thrown suddenly into menopause? and 2) Will I need to take hormones after this surgery? The answer is: It all depends on whether or not you keep your ovaries. If they are removed and you haven't yet gone through the change naturally, this catapults you into menopause. Hormones, then, are usually prescribed. The main difference in taking hormones after hysterectomy is that progesterone is not usually added to the estrogen, because without a uterus you do not have to be concerned about uterine cancer anymore (progesterone prevents overgrowth of the inner lining of the uterus, called the endometrium, which occurs if estrogen is taken alone; and it is this overgrowth that can increase the risk of uterine cancer). However, some women find that after surgery they feel more balanced with progesterone added to their estrogen supplements. It may also help maintain bone health. So it is important to be in touch with your body and your feelings, to help decide if adding progesterone would be helpful.

If, however, one or both of your ovaries are left, they will continue producing hormones, including androgens such as testosterone, that are helpful in maintaining muscle tone and overall vitality. Even after menopause, the ovaries continue making a small amount of estrogen and progesterone.

Why have a hysterectomy?

Fibroids are the main reason for hysterectomy, and they are common (30–50 percent of women in the United States have fibroids). Other reasons include a prolapsed uterus (sagging into the vagina), uterine or cervical cancer, severe pelvic pain or pressure, and frequent heavy bleeding to the point of anemia (see Sandra's story). Hysterectomy means removal of the uterus. When surgery is done to remove one or both ovaries, it is called oophorectomy. If hysterectomy is indicated, the two most common

(Continued on next page)

surgeries are: the uterus and both ovaries are removed; or the uterus is removed, leaving one or both ovaries in place. Surgery may be done abdominally or vaginally. Sometimes just the fibroid can be removed, called myomectomy. If fibroids are small, and on the inside of the uterus, laser surgery can remove them, using a long tube through the vagina.

Main points to keep in mind after hysterectomy:

- Your ovaries (if left in), body fat, and adrenal glands continue making hormones.
- Your sex life can stay satisfying, or even improve.
- Estrogen supplementation alone is acceptable (you may prefer to supplement with progesterone also).
- You will go through menopause symptoms, which may occur right away (when ovaries are removed) or after a length of time that varies for individual women (when ovaries remain).
- The quality of life improves when severely disruptive symptoms end.
- Your physical and energetic systems can maintain balance and harmony.

Sandra's Story: Hysterectomy as Liberation

Sandra had tried nearly every alternative therapy available over the 22 years she had struggled with her large uterine fibroids. As an aroma/ essential oils therapist skilled in the healing uses of flowers and plants, she firmly rejected the repeated recommendations from health practitioners that she have a hysterectomy. Each month, Sandra spent two weeks feeling miserable and two days totally unable to function. From ovulation until her period started, she had severe pelvic congestion, bloating, cramps, and moodiness. The first two days of her period, she flooded through a combination of both super tampons and maxipads. She would not go anywhere because she might bleed all over her clothes, and preferred not to because her cramps were so severe. She stayed in bed, feeling exhausted and depleted, until her bleeding slowed down.

Many forms of energy work, visualization, prayer, meditation, herbs, supplements, and special diets had little effect on Sandra's symptoms. At age 46, never having had children, she came to see me (Lennie Martin,

(Continued on next page)

RN, FNP) to discuss possible hormone therapy because she had heard I provided holistic women's care. Physical examination revealed that Sandra's uterus was very large, the size of a big cantaloupe, and it pressed downward in the pelvis, leaving little room for anything else. I asked if sex was painful, and she said it often was. We discussed hormone and herbal options for helping her symptoms. Then, in passing, I said "You might consider a hysterectomy," not really thinking she would, because of her background. But she later recalled, "The cells of my body leapt with joy at the idea of removing the uterus, which had for so long caused them such recurrent ordeals."

After more discussion and counseling, Sandra did choose a hysterectomy. She prepared carefully, communicating with her body and seeking blessings and support from friends. She intuited that energetically her uterus had become a repository of old, painful, sorrowful emotions and experiences. It had completed its service by holding pain and old patterns while the rest of the body-mind could heal and grow. Now the uterus, which she had valued, cherished, and supported for years, was ready to leave her body-mind system.

Although Sandra's surgery was more extensive than expected, because of adhesions and scar tissue, she recovered smoothly. Even though her ovaries had been left, she nevertheless began having hot flashes, fatigue, and sleep problems within a week after surgery. She began a regimen of estrogen and progesterone cream, which soon relieved her symptoms. To complete her process, Sandra asked the doctor for her uterus, which she blessed and buried ceremonially. Now free of life-disrupting symptoms, her energy has stabilized and she feels liberated. She has moved into the next phase of her life—the wisdom years of expanded vision and creativity.

URINARY DISCOMFORTS

Women having urinary symptoms often benefit from hormone therapy. At midlife many women experience decreased tone of the muscles that support the pelvic floor, the ones that surround the vagina and urethra (tube through which urine passes). Lower hormone levels leading to thinner urinary tissues and stretching of pelvic muscles during childbirth are both factors. Symptoms include loss of urine when you cough or sneeze, needing to go again right after emptying your bladder, sensations of urgency to get to the bathroom, burning and discomfort when urinating, and frequent urinary tract infections. By age 60, 13–24 percent of women have urinary incontinence (leaking urine) (Thom, 2001).

Stress incontinence is the most common type in menopausal women. Urine leaks when women increase abdominal pressure by laughing, coughing, sneezing, standing up too fast, or exercising. The tiny sphincter muscle that closes off the urethra may be weakened, or the bladder may have sagged down because of poor pelvic muscle tone, causing a sharper angle of the urethral tube, which prevents the sphincter from working properly. Urge incontinence occurs when abnormal bladder contractions force urine into the urethra, causing the sensation of urgency (needing to urinate right away). This is caused by a hyperactive bladder, and it can be related to thinning tissues in the bladder and urethra. Some women have a mixture of both types of incontinence (Wein, 2001). Cigarette smoking, obesity, major pelvic surgery, and neurological disorders may also be factors in urinary incontinence.

Estrogen vaginal cream provides effective relief for stress incontinence in about 50 percent of women who have estrogen depletion (Northrup, 2001). It may also help reduce urge incontinence. The lower urethra is estrogen sensitive, and lies very close to the vagina. Applying estrogen cream to the top wall of the lower vagina allows the hormone to diffuse through the tissues, improving nerve function and blood supply. This often leads to better muscle size, tone, and strength. Estriol vaginal cream is frequently recommended, as it is highly effective and very little is absorbed into the blood stream and taken to other areas of the body. Estradiol vaginal cream may also be used with good effects. Taking HRT pills can help with urinary symptoms, but this is not as effective as vaginal cream (see Helen's and Hanna's stories).

The main self-care method to improve leaking urine is practicing pelvic floor muscle exercises. There are three ways to do these:

1. Kegel exercises, named for the doctor who invented them, may be done almost any time or place: Squeeze the vaginal muscles tightly and hold for a count of 10, relax for a count of 5, and repeat 15–25 times daily. To get the feel of proper vaginal squeezing, stop the flow of urine when voiding. These are the same muscles you want to squeeze when doing Kegel exercises. Up to 75 percent of women can control stress incontinence by doing regular Kegel exercises (Nygaard et al., 1996).

2. Vaginal weights are cones of various weights (15 to 100 gm) that are inserted into the vagina and held in place for increasing time periods. Start with 5 minutes and work up to 15 minutes twice daily. Gradually increase the cone weights. After 4–6 weeks of consistent use, about 70 percent of women have improvement or resolution of incontinence (Singla, 2000).

3. Biofeedback techniques are used to strengthen vaginal muscles and train them for better control. You need to see a trained therapist for this technique, and it requires using vaginal probes. A relatively new method directs magnetic energy to the pelvic and vaginal muscles, causing them to contract and relax in a proper rhythm. Both of these have high success rates.

Medications such as Detrol (tolterodine) may be taken to help stop spasms of the urethral sphincter muscle which cause irritable bladder and urge incontinence. Its side effects are headache, dry mouth, constipation, indigestion, and dry eyes. Injections of collagen or body fat around the urethra increase tissue volume and help withstand the pressure of coughing or laughing. A number of surgical techniques can be used to reposition the bladder neck and elevate a sagging bladder, so that the urethra can function normally.

Helen and Hanna: Helped by Vaginal Hormone Creams

Helen had a hysterectomy at age 46 for heavy bleeding and endometriosis (tissue from the uterine lining that has passed upwards through the tubes, and implanted itself on the ovaries, outside of the uterus and inner abdomen). Each menstrual period had become more painful, with increasing pelvic pressure. One ovary was also removed during her surgery, because it was covered with endometrial implants and scar tissue. The other ovary had only a few small implants, and was left to provide Helen with hormones. Now, at age 49, Helen is starting to experience hot flashes and mood swings, but her most troublesome symptom is feeling the urge to urinate all the time. She has slight burning and leaks urine at times, but a urine test did not show infection. Helen does not want to take oral estrogen because it might make her endometriosis worse. Her health practitioner treated her with estriol vaginal cream, 0.5 mg/gm. She puts 1 gm into the lower vagina 3 times per week, rubbing it onto the upper wall closest to the urethra. This relieves her urinary symptoms, and also helps lessen her hot flashes.

Hanna is now 53 and married her second husband Alan three years ago. They share a loving and mutually supportive relationship. Hanna's concern is vaginal dryness and discomfort with sex. She has less sex drive than she would like. Fifteen years ago Hanna had a lumpectomy for an early stage, small breast cancer. She has been cancer-free since then. She is worried about taking estrogen because of increased breast cancer risk (she does not know if her cancer was estrogen receptor positive or not). Using vaginal lubricants and herbs did not improve her symptoms much. After talking things over with her health practitioner, Hanna decided to use prescription grade progesterone vaginal cream, 10 mg/gm applied 3–4 times per week. Within 5 weeks she noticed more vaginal moisture, her discomfort with sex disappeared, and her libido improved.

LIBIDO

Many women have less interest in sex as they negotiate the physical and emotional shifts of menopause. One study found that 86 percent of women reported sexual problems during the years just before and after menopause, most commonly loss of desire, vaginal dryness, painful intercourse, and decreased responsiveness to sexual stimulation (Sarrel & Whitehead, 1985). While falling hormones, especially progesterone and testosterone, can set the stage for less libido, this is far from the whole story. Sexuality is complex and integrated with emotions and attitudes. It is influenced by social conditioning, family values, personal experiences, biological functions, and a vast array of psychological factors.

Hormone levels are affected by a woman's state of mind, emotions, and physical vitality. Often the problems with libido and physical responses that occur during the menopause phase are powerfully influenced by the quality of relationships. Women who were having sexual problems with one partner may find these disappear when they enter a relationship with a new sex partner. Resolving conflicts in the current relationship may also lead to much improved sex. Developing a real, caring partnership with the man or woman you love gives a terrific boost to vital energy, and this supports gratifying sexual expression. Also, it is not necessary to have a partner to experience your own sexuality.

For a small number of women, libido does not change during menopause. But for most, it seems to simply disappear for a while. Partly this is caused by a need to refocus life force energy on the challenges of managing the menopause transition. Sexual energy is used to fuel women's inner transformation, almost like a phase of "celibacy" on the path of spiritual development. After things become more settled in postmenopause, most women find their sexual interest and responsiveness increase once again.

Hormones can be helpful in supporting sexual function during menopause. Estrogen and/or progesterone deficiency can decrease libido through the vaginal changes that make sex less pleasurable. Saliva estradiol levels lower than 1 pg/ml or blood levels below 50 pg/ml usually have dampening effects on libido (Sarrell & Whitehead, 1985). Using estradiol and/or progesterone dermally or orally often leads to improvement. Estriol vaginal cream is especially good for plumping up thin membranes and increasing natural moisture. Testosterone is called the "hormone of desire," but its influence on libido falls behind that of relationship issues, estrogen, and progesterone decline (Northrup, 2001). Most women do not have significant drops in testosterone levels at menopause. However, they do have a gradual decline starting in the late 20s, so it is possible for some women to be at low levels when they reach menopause. In 65 percent of women whose testosterone levels are low at menopause, testosterone replacement does lead to increased libido and sexual responsiveness (Sarrell et al., 1998). Natural testosterone used as a gel or cream has minimal side effects when doses are appropriate.

Using a lubricant can be very helpful with vaginal dryness and discomfort. Those with a water-soluble base are recommended, as an oil base tends to get sticky and weakens the latex in diaphragms and condoms. Some commonly used lubricants are K-Y jelly, SYLK (made from kiwi fruit), Replens, Women's Group Formulas Vaginal Lubricant (contains herbs and marigold), and others with herbs or Vitamin E.

HORMONES AND CANCER

Uterine Cancer   If a woman needs estrogen support and still has her uterus, she also needs to use progesterone or progestin supplements to protect the lining of her uterus. Estrogen, used alone, may cause a buildup of tissue in the uterine lining (endometrium) which can predispose the woman to uterine cancer in later years. The most common symptom of uterine cancer is irregular bleeding and spotting. If women who are still menstruating have recurrent bleeding/spotting between periods, or if postmenopausal women have more than two to three episodes of bleeding/spotting, they should see a practitioner for evaluation. Usually an endometrial biopsy will be done to take samples of tissue, which are examined for abnormal or cancerous cells.

The addition of either progesterone (Prometrium) or a progestin (Provera, Cycrin) will balance the estrogen levels and prevent this unhealthy buildup of endometrial tissue.

Breast Cancer   For many years, both women and practitioners have been concerned about possible relationships between hormone therapy and breast cancer. Over one-third of women in the United States ages 45–65 (around 16 million women) use hormones. However, over 70 percent of postmenopausal women stop using hormones within six months (Nawaz & Katz, 1999), and 75 percent stop within 3 years, mostly because of the side effects that cause unpleasant symptoms and the fear of cancer (Ettinger, Li, & Klein, 1996). A survey of postmenopausal women found 38 percent were currently using hormone therapy. Those most likely to be using hormones were better educated, lived in the South and West, and were health conscious enough to be taking such things as calcium supplements (Keating et al., 1999).

Studies going back as far as the 1960s have conflicting and confusing findings about breast cancer–hormone connections. Scientists do not completely understand why in some studies estrogen and progestins seem to increase breast cancer risk, while in others there is no association. In a comprehensive re-analysis of over 90 percent of the world's epidemiological studies on breast cancer and HRT, researchers found there was a small increased risk when women were currently using hormones for longer times. Past use of hormones did not increase risk (Collaborative Group on Hormonal Factors in Breast Cancer, 1997).

A large data base has been assembled by the National Cancer Institute, through its Breast Cancer Detection Demonstration Project. A follow-up study of participants published in January, 2000 reported a substantial increase in breast cancer among women using hormones, especially estrogen-progestin combinations. The hormones used by most women in the study were Premarin and combined Premarin-Provera. Drawing from over 46,000 postmenopausal women, data from 1979 through 1995 were analyzed using telephone interviews and mailed questionnaires. A total of 2,082 cases of breast cancer occurred among these women. After adjusting for age at menopause, regular mammograms, body mass index, education and age, the study found that the risk for breast cancer was 20 percent higher for recent users of estrogen alone, and 40 percent higher for recent users of estrogen-progestin (Schairer et al., 2000).

Put another way, this study used a prediction model that showed women had a 1 percent per year increased risk of breast cancer using estrogen alone, and an 8 percent per year increased risk using estrogen and progestin. This held true only for recent hormone use, defined as current or past use within the prior four years, and for thinner women (who accounted for two-thirds of the cancers). Heavier women did not have the same increased risk when taking hormones. After stopping hormones, the good news was that breast cancer risk promptly fell.

The Nurses' Health Study showed very similar results. Women taking estrogen alone had an increased breast cancer risk of 3.3 percent, and those taking combined hormones had a 9 percent increased risk (Aeron LifeCycles Clinical Laboratory, 2000). In both the National Cancer Institute and the Nurses' Health Study, progestin was used (the synthetic version of progesterone), and Premarin was the predominant form of estrogen. Doses were standardized, meaning all women received the same dose of hormones. New understanding of hormones points to every woman having a unique hormone profile, with highly individualized responses to HRT. Some women metabolize hormones more quickly than others. Standardized HRT doses are often higher than women actually need. Women are not statistics, but rather living biochemical individuals. Many unique factors influence how they respond to hormones, making results of studies not necessarily applicable to a large number of menopausal women. This emphasizes the importance of individualized approaches to HRT based on each woman's own hormone profile.

Premarin (conjugated equine estrogens) and progestins are different from the body's own hormones; although they work in similar ways, it is not exactly the same physiologically. The 1995 Postmenopausal Estrogen/Progestin Intervention (PEPI) Trial showed that bioidentical progesterone works more effectively than synthetic progestins in maintaining healthy cholesterol profiles (Writing Group for the PEPI Trial, 1995). This might indicate that bioidentical hormones interact more compatibly with the body's physiology and could have fewer metabolic consequences that might lead to cellular damage.

Cellular research has indeed begun to point in this direction. Several biochemical studies on the metabolites (breakdown chemicals from the body's metabolism of hormones) of Premarin suggest that certain metabolites may be carcinogenic (cancer causing). Some of Premarin's metabolites appear to cause damage to strands of DNA (Zhang et al., 1999). By taking cultured human breast tumor cells and exposing them to metabolites of Premarin, researchers found a 30-fold increase in cell toxicity compared to estrone (one of the bioidentical estrogens) (Chen et al., 1998). This showed that some metabolites of Premarin have the ability to damage breast tissue, at least in cellular culture conditions.

Statistics from research studies are hard to understand, unless translated into more common terms. Here's another way to understand the National Cancer Institute study, which reported increased risk of breast cancer of 1 percent per year with estrogen alone and 8 percent per year with estrogen-progestin, compared to women's overall breast cancer risks: Among women not taking any hormones, 77 out of 1,000 will get breast cancer by age 75. In women taking HRT, 79 out of 1,000 will get breast cancer after 5 years, and 89 out of 1,000 will get breast cancer after 15 years (Northrup, April, 2000). The increase in risk is small. The vast majority of women who take HRT of all kinds do not get breast cancer. Some women who never take hormones do. Each woman needs to decide what this risk means to her. To some, even a small increase in risk is too much. To others, the benefits from using hormones are well worth the small risk.

Table 3–4 presents options for natural hormone therapy with human identical hormones (HIH).

Reasons Not to Take Premarin

- Premarin is a complex mix of conjugated equine (horse) estrogens, and also contains progestin-like substances and androgens (DuraMed, 1999)
- Some of these hormones break down into dangerous metabolites in the human body, which can damage cells and DNA
- Studies have found significant relationship between use of Premarin and breast cancer
- Animal rights groups have identified issues of how the pregnant mares are treated in the process of collecting urine
- Issues of animal cruelty arise from the sale of foals to foreign meat markets
- There is a soy-derived substitute which contains most of the conjugated estrogens (without the progestins and androgens) called Cenestin
- There are many other soy- and yam-derived human identical estrogens that provide relief of symptoms without creating dangerous metabolites

TABLE 3–4	**Natural Hormone Therapy with Human Identical Hormones (HIH)**

Hormone replenishment therapy using human identical hormones, made by compounding pharmacy or drug company from soy or wild-yam base.

Estrone (E1): Predominant form of estrogen synthesized in fat cells after menopause.

Estradiol (E2): Primary premenopausal form, made by ovaries, stronger estrogen

Estriol (E3): Produced by placenta during pregnancy, and made by the liver after menopause by converting estrone; less stimulating to breasts and endometrium; better for bones and for vaginal and urinary symptoms

PRESCRIPTION ESTROGENS

Triestrogen (E1–10%:E2–10%:E3–80%) 1.25–5.0 mg oral dose	Compounded
Biestrogen (E2–20%:E3–80%) 1.25–5.0 mg oral dose	Compounded
Estriol 2–4 mg oral dose	Compounded
Estradiol 1–2 mg oral dose Oral and patches	Drug company

Creams and sublingual forms of all types of estrogens can be compounded in individual doses that are lower than oral forms.

PRESCRIPTION PROGESTERONE

Micronized progesterone 100–200 mg oral	Compounded
Prometrium 100–200 mg oral	Drug company
Progesterone cream, up to 100 mg/oz	Compounded
Progesterone sublingual 25–50 mg	Compounded

OVER THE COUNTER

ProGest cream (16 mg/gm)	Over the counter
Progonol cream (30 mg/gm)	Over the counter
Progestone-900 (16 mg/gm)	Over the counter
Resolve (25 mg/gm)	Over the counter

Note: There are many brands of progesterone and wild yam creams. If you cannot tell how much progesterone is in the cream by reading the label, it probably does not have a reliable dose level. Prescription creams provide the exact dose per gram your health provider orders. Some commercial brands have guaranteed potency of the dose per gram on their label.

How Long to Take HRT

How long women continue taking HRT is an individual decision. Your purpose for using hormones is the key factor. If you started hormones to get relief from symptoms such as hot flashes, insomnia, and memory loss, you may want to taper off in two to five years. Most women have these symptoms over a five to ten year period, but the most intense phase often ends within a couple of years. It is best to taper off rather than suddenly stop HRT. The rapid fall in hormone levels from an abrupt cutoff usually causes a resurgence of symptoms. Your health practitioner can order reduced doses, and you can use hormones every other day, then every third day, for a few weeks to let your body gradually get used to lower hormone levels. If you have increased symptoms that make you uncomfortable, adding herbal support at this time can be quite helpful.

Women who take HRT to achieve a health benefit have other factors to consider. If you take HRT to help maintain bone density, you may do just as well without it if you are willing to do weight training and the nutritional and lifestyle practices that support bone health. If you have osteoporosis, and HRT is part of the treatment plan, you need to assess the results of your entire regimen periodically. If bone density is not improving, you may need to consider adding bone building medications, such as Fosamax. If density has improved and you are no longer at risk for fractures, you could do a trial off HRT for two years, then test bone density again.

Taking HRT to protect your heart is controversial, as previously discussed. If this is your main reason for using hormones, you may want to rethink that decision. There are many more effective ways to support heart health. If Alzheimer's is your concern, you may want to continue estrogen supplements until there is more definitive research.

Here are some principles for using HRT:

- Know your body's hormone levels by testing (saliva is most accurate).
- Replace only those hormones that are low.
- Use human identical hormones (HIH) that are biologically identical to your body's own.
- Take HRT for the shortest time needed to meet your goals.
- Know your risks for osteoporosis, heart disease, dementia, and cancers.
- Use other methods to provide bone, heart, and brain support, such as diet, nutrition, exercise stress management, and lifestyle.
- Phase off HRT gradually if you choose to stop.
- Follow your intuition and listen to your inner voice.

THE DECISION IS YOURS

As you take charge of the changes happening in your body, you will become more comfortable with its shifting landscape through the menopausal transition. Your hormone status, symptoms, and hormone replacement needs probably will change. Listen to your body as it communicates through sensations, and get a sense of what your inner wisdom advises. If you use HRT, periodic hormone testing will help you understand your body's responses, and provide data for making decisions. Work with your health provider in fine-tuning your regimen by adjusting doses, changing hormone combinations, or using a different delivery system (pills, creams, patches, or sublingual). Worksheet 3-2 on page 110 can be helpful in keeping track of the different therapies that you use.

When you feel ready, you may choose to discontinue HRT. Whether or not you have medical "indications" for using HRT, it is still your right to make this choice. Take a holistic approach, be informed, and tap into your wisdom. Then you can be at peace with your choice.

MANAGING MENOPAUSE NATURALLY

This material represents information collected from written resources, from our own experience, and from other women's experiences shared personally and in classes. It emphasizes complementary therapies and includes brief mentions of conventional therapies—all of which are being used by women to help manage symptoms of perimenopause, menopause, and postmenopause. It is a sampling only and is not exhaustive (note the absence of such things as homeopathy or herbs from other traditions; you are encouraged to see a practitioner trained in these remedies or to get a good book about them).

This discussion is not intended as medical advice, only as educational food for thought for you and your health practitioner. As always, if you are or might be pregnant or are nursing, be especially careful, checking first with your health practitioner. You should be able to find much of the foodstuffs, herbs, and supplements mentioned below at a good health food store.

> I urge all women to take particular care of themselves for a few years before they expect to go through menopause. I'd say from age 45 on. That means proper diet, supplementary vitamins, sufficient exercise, and I'd add, avoidance of chemical pollutants. This kind of care is very important because, I believe, if you have a fuse to blow, a weak link in your body, you'll blow that fuse in menopause.
>
> —Elaine Goldman Gill, "Blowing the Fuse," in *Women of the 14th Moon*

Nutrition

Many nutritionists agree that as a general rule of thumb an overall healthy diet consists of :

60 percent complex carbohydrates (vegetables, whole grains, beans, etc.)

20 percent protein (Dr. Andrew Weil [2000] advises between 10 and 20 percent is enough)

20–30 percent fats (the good ones, that is; keep the "bad" saturated fats really low—below 10 percent.)

These recommendations have been challenged, especially by Barry Sears (of the famous *Zone* diet), who suggests a 40:30:30 ratio. Indeed, some women feel better when they eat more protein and less carbohydrate. So much seems to depend on the requirements of your individual physiology.

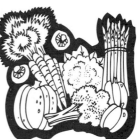

While controversy abounds in the field of nutrition, it is noteworthy that four of the nation's top health organizations have together endorsed an eating plan that helps stave off diseases that kill most people: heart disease, stroke, cancer, and diabetes. Called the Unified Dietary Guidelines (American Heart Association, 1999),* this plan suggests:

1. Eating a variety of foods
2. Choosing most of what you eat from plant sources
3. Eating five or more servings of fruits and vegetables each day
4. Eating six or more servings of bread, pasta, and cereal grain each day. (These are part of the family called complex carbohydrates, which are starches rather than sugars of simple carbohydrates. While six servings sounds like a huge amount, a serving can actually be small—a slice of bread, for instance. We, the authors, recommend that you choose the least processed carbohydrates; for instance, pasta is made of grain that has been milled into flour and has less food value than servings of "whole grain" forms of millet, rice, or barley, which have not been milled to lose their nutritious bran.)
5. Eating high-fat foods sparingly, especially those from animal sources (meat or whole dairy—these are saturated fats)
6. Keeping your intake of simple sugars (juices, sweets of all kinds, alcohol) to a moderate or even a low level.

*Unified Dietary Guidelines, developed by the American Heart Association's Nutrition Committee with the cooperation of the American Cancer Society, American Academy of Pediatrics, and National Institutes of Health; published in the July 27, 1999 issue of *Circulation: Journal of the American Heart Association* (Deckelbaum et al., 1999).

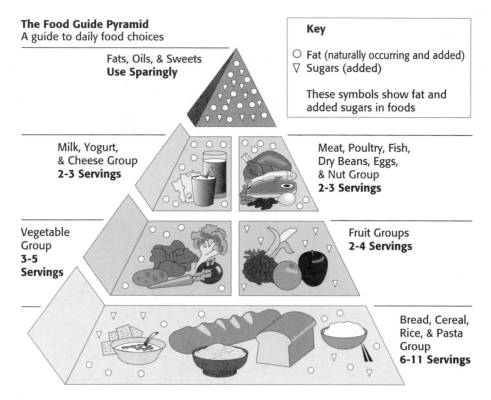

The Food Guide Pyramid
A guide to daily food choices

Key
○ Fat (naturally occurring and added)
▽ Sugars (added)

These symbols show fat and added sugars in foods

Fats, Oils, & Sweets
Use Sparingly

Milk, Yogurt, & Cheese Group
2-3 Servings

Meat, Poultry, Fish, Dry Beans, Eggs, & Nut Group
2-3 Servings

Vegetable Group
3-5 Servings

Fruit Groups
2-4 Servings

Bread, Cereal, Rice, & Pasta Group
6-11 Servings

Figure 3–1 The Food Guide Pyramid. Diet based on a foundation of grains and wheat products, with fruits, beans, legumes, and vegetables at every meal. Cheese, milk and yogurt, fish, eggs, lean meat and poultry several times a week. Oils, fats, and sweets used sparingly, a few times a week. *Courtesy of U.S. Department of Agriculture.*

Also see the Food Guide Pyramid, Figure 3–1.

Murray and Pizzorno (1998) add to the above: drink 32 to 48 ounces of water daily, reduce exposure to pesticides and herbicides, keep salt intake low and potassium high, eliminate intake of food additives and coloring agents, and identify any food allergies* one might have.

Andrew Weil (2000) says that the optimum diet also should provide the pleasure you expect from eating, as well as promote social interaction.

With the exception of your particular food intolerances or the special dietary requirements involved in certain diseases, the usual recommendations about diet around the time of menopause are to eat the following:

---

*For a good description of food allergies and intolerances, how to identify them, and what to do about it, see Balch and Balch (1997) *Prescription for Nutritional Healing* (2nd Ed.).

MORE OF

- Vegetarian foods for protection against development of chronic degenerative diseases (Murray & Pizzorno, 1998)
- Vegetables high in antioxidants (which inactivate damage-causing free radicals), especially dark leafy greens, a source of calcium
- Whole fruits; as juices can provide too much sugar too fast in the body, try watering juices down
- Organic foods ("organic" means grown without chemical fertilizers or pesticides)
- Foods high in phytoestrogens (*phyto* means plant); this includes flaxseed (oil and seeds), nuts, whole grains, and legumes, such as lentils, chickpeas, and, of course, soy, which research has shown to provide many benefits, including enhanced bone density to protect against osteoporosis (Arjmandi, et al., 1996; Barnes, 1998) and decreasing hot flashes
- Seaweeds, which provide natural iodine for thyroid, and are high in calcium and magnesium for stronger bones
- Sesame seeds, an excellent source of calcium if unhulled
- Whole, unprocessed grains, sprouted if possible which makes them less acid-producing (helps in bone health, among other things)
- "Good" fats, such as olive oil (monounsaturated) and omega-3 essential fatty acids; the latter are found in cold-water fatty fish, such as ocean salmon, tuna, and mackerel; in flaxseeds and flaxseed oil; and in the oils of evening primrose and black currant, which are also high in another beneficial fatty acid called gammalinoleic acid (GLA)
- Pure water, which helps the kidneys do their job of eliminating toxins and prevents dehydration, which is a component of aging (Batmanghelidj, 1997)

LESS OF

- Acid-producing foods (processed foods, sweets, meats, dairy; these are bad for the bones, among other things)
- Carbonated drinks with high phosphorus, such as colas (bad for bones)
- "Bad" fats, such as saturated animal fats and oils (coconut and palm), and vegetable oils that are hardened, such as margarine (trans-fatty acids have been implicated in cancer and heart disease)
- Caffeine and refined carbohydrates (deplete vitamins and minerals; acidic; cause insulin spikes, which can result in weight gain)

- Sugar (acidic; affects insulin; blocks transport of vitamin C; depletes vitamin B; prevents many minerals from being absorbed; bad for bones)
- Salt (while you need a small amount of iodized salt to help prevent goiter, excess salt robs bones of calcium)
- Dairy products (acid-producing; contain hormones; form mucus; the best dairy products are live, unsweetened yogurt, soft cheeses (such as ricotta, which has more calcium in ½ cup than 1 glass of milk, and goat products, which are easier to digest)
- Foods you have an intolerance/allergy to; this can best be determined by the elimination and rotation diets (Balch & Balch, 2000)

See the boxed material in this chapter on vegetarian diet, soy products, and flaxseeds.

Herbs That Play a Major Role in Menopause

The reason several herbs are often mentioned under a given symptom is twofold. Often they may be used together, working synergistically to increase symptom relief. Also, as herbalists know, not every herb is right for every woman, so a choice is given. Herbology is both a science and an art, so experimentation and intuition have to be included in herbal regimens. That being said, the following herbs are some of the ones most often mentioned in Western herbal books as being important to midlife women in managing some of the most troublesome of the menopausal symptoms. It certainly is not an exhaustive list and it leaves out many Chinese herbs, Ayurvedic herbs, and so on. You might first try the herbs that are listed here to see if they work for you.

GUIDELINES IN TAKING HERBS

Become knowledgeable about the herb you wish to try (even if you are working with an herbalist, it is important to be educated about the remedy you may be taking). Follow directions on the package. Patiently wait for results. Be aware of the reaction of your mind and body to the herb.

At health food stores or herb farms you may buy herbs in several forms:

- Capsules (ground herb put into a capsule; standardized extracts)
- Liquid extracts and tinctures (usually made with alcohol, although some may be made with glycerin)
- Loose plant materials for making teas, infusions, and decoctions

Make sure the herbs are organic and not grown with chemical fertilizers or pesticides.

Would You Benefit from Taking Herbs for Menopause?

Herbs have been used for thousands of years to ease perimenopause and menopause symptoms, and provide support for the female system during this transition. You might consider taking herbs for your menopause if some of these situations apply:

- You are having mild to moderate symptoms and want some relief.
- You feel your system would be more balanced taking female support herbs.
- You believe herbs are a safer, gentler, and more natural way to relieve symptoms than HRT.
- You do not want to take HRT because of your risks for breast cancer, or other health concerns.
- You are using HRT, but feel you would get better support or symptom relief by adding herbs.
- You cannot take HRT because of contraindications (such as blood clots or breast cancer), or you had significant side effects.

The dosages that follow have been gleaned from several sources and are meant only as guidelines. Check directions on the herbal package or check with your herbalist. If not otherwise specified, all dosages mentioned here are given on a daily basis and usually spread out over the day; thus, if a dosage says 40 drops of tincture, that would mean 20 in the morning and 20 in the evening, or even 13 drops three times a day. Alcohol-based tinctures are not taken straight, but rather diluted in ½–1 cup of water.

Herbs commonly used for menopausal symptoms are listed below.

VITEX (*VITEX AGNUS CASTUS*)

Called Chaste Tree or Chasteberry, vitex has anti-inflammatory and progesterone-like effects (Fetrow & Avila, 1999). It affects pituitary hormone regulation (FSH, LH) and restores estrogen-progesterone balance (Wright & Morgenthaler, 1997). Used for many years in Europe, vitex has been effective for PMS, estrogen dominance conditions, breast pain, fluid retention, headache, depression, and menopause symptoms. A German clinical trial found 77 percent of women taking vitex showed improvement of PMS symptoms (Lauritzen et al., 1997). Vitex can improve heavy menstrual bleeding and short cycles, regulating the menstrual flow (Hoffman, 2000).

As a female system balancer, spread out over the day in 2 or 3 doses. Recommendations are 40 drops of tincture (Weed, 1992; Firshein, 1998); 20 mg (Bender, 1998); 30–40 mg (*PDR*, 1999); and 30–40 mg (German Commission E, Blumenthal et al., 1998). Vitex has not caused significant side effects at recommended doses.

BLACK COHOSH (*CIMICIFUGAE RACEMOSAE*)

This is a very popular herb, especially in Europe, where it has been used for over 40 years for control of hot flashes, insomnia, depression, anxiety, and forgetfulness. According to German Commission E, its actions are estrogen-like, binding to estrogen receptors, and suppressing luteinizing hormone. Remifemin is a well-known brand, used in most studies on black cohosh. Clinical studies with menopausal women have found 80 percent improvement of symptoms after a month of taking 40 drops of Remifemin twice daily (Daiber, 1983) and improvement in mood after the same dosage for 3 months. In a comparison study with estrogen and placebo, black cohosh improved menopause symptoms as much as estrogen and had better effect on thickening the vaginal cells (Stoll, 1987).

Commission E recommends 40 mg daily. For depression, Bender (1998) recommends two 40 mg tablets. No health hazards or serious side effects have been reported using recommended doses.

Contraindications: Use cautiously if taking antihypertensive medications (Fetrow & Avila, 1999).

ST. JOHN'S WORT (*HYPERICUM PERFORATUM*)

Called nature's antidepressant, St. John's wort seems to act like Prozac without the side effects (Firshein, 1998). Several clinical trials have shown this herb to be effective for mild to moderate depression (Volz, 1997; Wheatley, 1997). The herb has several active compounds, which have a variety of effects on brain chemistry and receptor activity, including actions on monoamine oxidase, serotonin, GABA, and interleukin-6 (Glisson, Crawford, & Street, 1999). A large randomized clinical trial is underway through the National Institutes of Health comparing St. John's wort with a selective serotonin reuptake inhibitor (SSRI) antidepressant medication, and placebo.

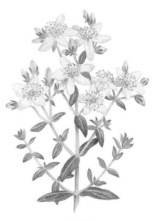

St. John's wort

Most experts agree that tinctures/capsules should be standardized at 0.3 percent hyperacin, although some researchers say the key active ingredient may be something else. This is one reason why many herbalists choose to use the whole plant in making their preparations, so that all "active" ingredients are included. The recommended dosage is 300 mg three times a day for at least 4–6 weeks to gauge effect. As a tea, use 1–2 teaspoons per cup, 3 cups a day (Bender, 1998).

Contraindications: Do not take with MAO (monoamine oxidase) inhibitors. These medicines include Marplan, Nardil, and Parnate. If you are taking an SSRI antidepressant, consult your health practitioner before using St. John's wort. If you are particularly sensitive to the sun and are taking this herb for a long time, you might develop photosensitivity and have to cover up with a shirt and hat, and wear sunscreen. There have been no reports of serious side effects among long-term users.

KAVA-KAVA (*PIPER METHYSTICUM*)

Kava is used for anxiety, stress, restlessness, nervousness, and insomnia. Kava-lactones, the active compounds, are taken rapidly into the brain with soothing effects on the alarm center in the amygdala. Its effects include sedation, relaxing muscles and mind, elevating mood, and promoting sleep (Singh & Blumenthal, 1997; Bloomfield, 1998). In clinical studies, kava was effective in reducing anxiety, tension, and excitation (Lehman, Kinzler, & Friedemann, 1996). A multicenter clinical trial found improvement in anxiety, fear, tension, and insomnia with both short- and long-term kava use (Volz & Kieser, 1997).

The recommended dosage for capsules and tincture is 100 mg of dry extract standardized to 70 mg kava lactones three times daily for four weeks (Lehmann, Kinzler, & Friedemann, 1996). Firshein (1998) doubles that to 210 mg of kava extract capsule 3 times a day. Bender (1998), who recommends 180–210 mg before bed, claims that women in her practice often take kava-kava instead of Valium or Xanax.

Contraindications: Do not take if you have Parkinson's, have endogenous (defined as physiologically-based) depression, are pregnant or nursing, and do not take for longer than 3 months without a doctor's supervision (*PDR,* 1999).

GINKGO BILOBA (*GINKGO BILOBA*)

Ginko is widely used to enhance mental functions. There is some controversy about the effectiveness of this herb for menopause-related forgetfulness, because it has not been studied for this purpose (Murray & Pizzorno, 1998). The main active compounds are flavone glycosides and terpene lactones. These appear to work by increasing blood flow to the brain, enhancing energy production within the brain, increasing the uptake of glucose by brain cells and improving the transmission of nerve signals. They also reduce blood thickness and clotting factors, promote free-radical scavenging, and strengthen tiny blood vessels (Glisson et al., 1999). German Commission E (1998) says that ginkgo is approved for treatment of memory impairment, problems of concentration, and depression from organic brain disease.

Dosage recommendation (Murray & Pizzorno, 1998) is 40 mg of extract standardized to 24 percent ginkgo flavone glycoside content. The *PDR* (1999) recommends 120 mg a day of the dried extract for at least 12 weeks. This should be divided into 2 or 3 doses daily as the effects do not last very long.

Contraindications: Should not be taken with anticoagulants (Coumadin, Ticlid, Plavix); use carefully with aspirin and NSAIDs such as ibuprofen.

VALERIAN (*VALERIANA OFFICINALIS*)

German Commission E says that this herb is used for restlessness and sleeping disorders based on nervous conditions. It acts mainly as a sedative. Firshein (1998) reports one double-blind study that found 89 percent of subjects treated with valerian reported improved sleep (reducing night-time awakenings). He reports this herb is particularly potent when combined with other calming herbs such as kava, St. John's wort, or passionflower. Bender (1998) suggests that the *dried* root preparation has a stimulating effect that counters extreme fatigue.

In tincture form, the recommend dose is ½ to 1 teaspoon (1–3 ml), once to several times a day (Commission E). The fresh root tincture, standardized to contain 0.8 percent valeric acid, 150–300 mg; ½–1 teaspoon of tincture, is dosed one to several times a day (*PDR,* 1999). Weed (1992) recommends 20–30 drops just before bed and repeat, if needed, in 30 minutes.

SIBERIAN GINSENG (*ELEUTHEROCOCCUS SENTICOSUS*)

This herb can be an invigorating tonic in times of fatigue/debility, stress, or declining capacity for work and concentration. It acts to support the adrenals. Take 2 to 3 grams of powdered/cut root decocted in water as a tea throughout the day (*PDR,* 1999; Bender, 1998); also available in tablets, capsules, and glycerin extracts.

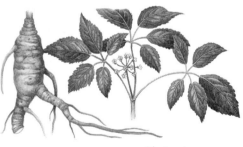

Siberian ginseng

Contraindications: Northrup (September, 2000) reports she does not prescribe this herb for patients with hot flashes.

DONG QUAI (*ANGELICA SINENSIS*)

This herb has a long-standing reputation for relieving hot flashes, vaginal dryness, menopausal achiness, and insomnia, and is used for regulating menses and reducing palpitations. Tincture: up to 120 drops (to 6 teaspoons, says Crawford, 1996) using the fresh root tincture (Weed, 1992). As a decocted tea taken throughout the day: 1 to 6 cups a day, using 1 teaspoon (2 grams) of root slice crumbled into 1 cup boiling water and allowed to steep for 20 minutes (Crawford, 1996).

Contraindications: Do not use if bleeding heavily, have fibroids, take blood-thinning drugs, are bloated, have diarrhea; or, if after taking it, you experience breast tenderness or soreness (Weed, 1992).

MOTHERWORT (*LEONORUS CARDIACA*)

Motherwort is used for hormonal imbalances, especially hot flashes, and nervous tension causing such symptoms as heart palpitations and rapid pulse. It is helpful for PMS with delayed menses. It combines well with dong quai. Dosage is 10 drops to ¾ teaspoon of tincture in water 3 times per day (Crawford, 1996).

HOW TO PREPARE HERBS

The most common methods for preparing herbs include teas, decoctions, infusions and tinctures.

Tea   This is the most gentle way of brewing an herb; used mostly with blossoms and leaves, either fresh or dried, pour water just at the boil over herb and steep for minutes only.

Infusion   Pour boiling water over dried herb and brew for 10 or 15 minutes; stronger than tea; used with leaves and stems.

Decoction   Barks, roots, dried twigs steeped for 20–40 minutes in water that has been brought to a boil then removed from heat.

Tincture   It is easiest to buy these already made. The label will let you know the ingredients and if the active ingredient has been standardized. If, however, you want to make them the way a backyard herbalist does, follow Susun Weed's directions in *Menopausal Years* (1992): Pick the herb, then chop it coarsely; do not wash. Fill any size jar with the plant material, then pour 100 proof vodka (or grain alcohol) over it, filling the jar to the top. Cap tightly. Label with date and name of plant. Your tincture will be ready to use in six weeks but is stable for as long as you wish.

OTHER COMPLEMENTARY/ALTERNATIVE THERAPIES

There are many other approaches to relieving symptoms and maintaining health. The following are some favorites. Find qualified practitioners in your area.

Hatha Yoga

This method integrates physical movement with breathing and conscious direction of energy. Yoga postures generally maintain flexibility, balance moods, massage internal organs, and can help with bone health and endocrine gland regulation. Stretching, bending, and holding postures increases circulation, which brings more nourishment and oxygen to tissues, and enhances removal of waste products. Yoga keeps muscles and connective tissue supple, improves function of joints, and supports bone strength. Postures which put weight-bearing demands on hips, spine, arms, and wrists are especially helpful for maintaining bone density. Yoga practice enhances balance and coordination, and modulates stress hormones by balancing the nervous system and promoting relaxation. Deep slow breathing increases oxygenation of tissues and has a calming effect on the mind and nervous system. Specific postures for different menopausal symptoms are pictured and described in Appendix A.

Acupuncture

This ancient Chinese healing art has received considerable acceptance by many health practitioners. Research has been able to trace acupuncture points, and clinical studies have shown excellent results for many conditions. Stimulation of acupressure points on the skin by fine needles or other forms of pressure causes energy (chi) to flow along pathways called meridians. This normalizes or redirects the flow of vital energy to various body parts, aiding healing and healthy function. Acupuncture has been used successfully to treat many menopause symptoms, including hot flashes, night sweats, insomnia, anxiety, moodiness, and headaches. It is particularly effective for regulating heavy menstrual bleeding and cramps. In some instances, it has been able to shrink fibroids. Increasing the flow of chi supports the adrenals, which may be very helpful during the menopausal journey. Cortisol balance, which enhances immune function and helps control addictions to cigarettes and alcohol, may be improved through acupuncture.

Ayurveda

Ayurveda, the "Science of Life," is an ancient natural healing system from India. It is a complex blending of diet, herbs, bodywork, yoga, and lifestyle practices with a spiritual perspective on health and illness. Life energy (prana) can be enhanced through these techniques and made more available for healing. This life force is expressed by three biological "doshas" of the body. The three doshas represent primary biological types in temperament, body characteristics, digestion, and metabolism. When unbalanced, the doshas cause symptoms and, ultimately, disease. The Ayurveda practitioner assesses the client's dosha, then suggests ways to help keep the doshas balanced. For menopause, special herbs are used for strengthening or rejuvenating the female organs, and others for regulating hormones and calming emotions.

Naturopathy

This approach to natural medicine follows principles of body-mind interconnection, holism, and treating underlying causes. The primary focus is on diet, lifestyle, and preventive measures to promote good health. Naturopathic physicians are trained in clinical nutrition, botanical medicine, homeopathy, traditional Chinese medicine, acupuncture, hydrotherapy, physical modalities, and counseling. In some states, they can prescribe naturally derived and plant-based drugs such as hormones. For menopause a diet with increased phytoestrogens and soy foods, and nutritional supplements are recommended. Botanical medicines include herbs that support hormone balance and improve menopause symptoms (dong quai, licorice, vitex, black cohosh, and ginkgo).

Body and Energy Work

Midlife women are turning to these alternative therapies for relaxation, toning tissues, and promoting energy flows. In addition to the physical benefits, body and energy work provide nurturance and emotional support. Many women feel in better body-mind balance with regular sessions. There are many techniques for therapeutic massage, including light and deep tissue work, lymphatic drainage, and energy balancing. Some forms of energy work include Polarity, Reiki, Shiatsu, Touch for Health, Therapeutic Touch, Jin Shin Jyutsu, T'ai Chi, Bowen, and many others. Most therapists include several massage or energy techniques, often combined with essential oils and music. For women going through the stresses of perimenopause, these sessions can be a real treat.

HEALTH MATRIX

This is a compilation of some of the many options available to you to consider for symptom relief or enhancing health.

If you are taking medications, have a disease, or suspect a food intolerance, you should check with your health care practitioner first. We have included some obvious contraindications, but not all that might exist. What follows simply alerts you to a range of possibilities to consider.

Herbs, like any medicines, should be taken with care. Follow label instructions. You might consider buying one good herb book as a reference (see References and Suggested Reading). When not specifically referenced it means that the same herbal remedy was found in at least two references and often three or four, making this very reliable information.

Matrix at a Glance

How to use this matrix   We have included the heading **Medical**, even though most of the matrix is devoted to natural or alternative therapies. Under this heading we include, when appropriate, a category of hormones—the prescribed synthetic kind that are used by much of the medical establishment today under the rubric ERT or HRT. The human identical hormones (HIH)—which include both the estrogens and progesterone—on the other hand, are given their own heading **Hormones**, because they fit in better with our philosophy. For specific names of HIH, some of which are given only by prescription and some of which can be bought over the counter, see the section on hormones and Table 3–1.

BONE HEALTH

Diet   Sesame seeds, seaweed, soy products; dark leafy greens; eat *sprouted* grain products when you can, which are less acid producing; avoid excess protein (red meat especially) because it is acid forming and leaches calcium from the bones; cut down on sodas (especially colas), coffee/alcohol (which inhibit calcium absorption), excess salt

Supplements/nutrients   Calcium (as citrate, maleate, or asporatate because these are the forms that are best used by the body), magnesium, boron, and vitamin D; beta-carotene, antioxidants. Ipriflavone, a synthetic isoflavone, has been found to reduce bone loss and increase bone mass in small studies. A recent large clinical trial, however, did not find any improvement in bone density by using ipriflavone (Alexanderson et al., 2001)

Herbs   Horsetail, oat straw, nettles, alfalfa, dandelion

Hormones   HIH (estrogen and progesterone)

Exercise   Weight-bearing (or resistence training) exercises strengthen bone

Tests   Bone scans (DEXA); urine test (Dpd—deoxypyridinoline excreted in urine) measures a marker of bone reabsorption and indicates how rapidly bone is being broken down

Medical   For preventing osteoporosis: selective estrogen receptor modulators (anti-estrogens) such as raloxifene (Evista); for treating once osteoporosis develops: estrogens, calcitonin (Miacalcin), and bisphosphonates (Fosamex).

Protein and Bones

Great controversy rages over how much protein a person should have and from what sources it should come. What your goal is—strong bones or weight loss—will influence you in making this choice. Some researchers say that Americans eat far too much protein and that the protein we need can be totally obtained from a vegetarian diet (Edell & Schreiberg, 1999). Others, such as the doctor behind *Dr. Atkins' New Diet Revolution* (1997) contend that eating lots of protein, mostly in the form of meat, is good for health and weight loss. However, at least one highly visible researcher, agreeing with Atkins that we need a high protein to carbohydrate ratio, also agrees with those who say that plant-based protein is best (Sears, 2000). Confusing it is.

While eating fewer pasta meals and more lean steak probably helps with weight control, on the issue of healthy bones the evidence is pretty clear that the source of protein is critical; that is, a vegetarian diet is associated with a lower risk of having osteoporosis (Ellis, Holesh, & Ellis, 1972; Marsh et al., 1983).

What about the amount of protein? What is adequate? Fifty grams is enough, according to Balch and Balch (2000); indeed, they contend that Americans eat too much protein. So do Murray and Pizzorno (1998), who claim daily protein intakes of 140 grams are common in the United States. Figure out how much you need, advise Edell and Schrieberg (1999), by body weight: one gram of protein per 2.2 pounds. Thus, if you weigh 154 pounds you would need 70 grams of protein daily.

Is there a problem with getting too much protein? Earlier research does show that excessive protein might lead to loss of bone minerals. High protein diet results in chronic acid load, which must be buffered by drawing calcium from the skeleton. Too much protein may cause hypercalciuria (excess calcium in urine) and a negative calcium balance which may reduce bone mineral density (Tesar et al., 1992). As to the source, red meat especially contains high levels of phosphorous, which is yet another factor that has negative effects on bones.

If bone health is your major interest, then weight-bearing exercise and a diet with moderate intake of plant-based protein is probably the best regimen to follow.

CARDIOVASCULAR HEALTH

Diet   Reduce/eliminate "bad" fats; eat "good" fats (Omega-3 essential fatty acid found in flaxseed oil and fatty ocean fish, and monosaturated fats, such as olive oil); soy products; mostly vegetarian diet with lots of fruits and vegetables, and garlic (for blood pressure)

Herbs   Motherwort and hawthorne berries strengthen heart muscle and blood vessels, and thus are good for palpitations and blood pressure; ginkgo biloba, black haw, green tea; ginseng (for blood pressure)

Supplements/nutrients   Vitamin E (experts agree you should not waste your money on the cheap kind; rather buy the brand that has all 4 tocopherols and 4 tocotrienols—this may help to prevent stroke); soy protein powder (lowers LDL, the so-called bad cholesterol); avoid excess iron when you finally stop bleeding; antioxidants; Coenzyme Q_{10}, the B vitamins (especially B_6 and B_{12}; folate)

Other   Feeling loved/loving, supported and connected keeps the heart healthy, as shown by Dr. Dean Ornish (1990), the well-known heart researcher; exercise: 30 minutes of vigorous exercise daily (even a brisk walk) can reduce incidence of stroke—the third leading cause of death in women—by 30 percent (Hu et al., 2000)

Tests   Cholesterol (total, low-density, high-density); triglycerides; blood pressure; possibly electrocardiogram or stress-echocardiogram if you have chest pain, pressure, or other heart symptoms

Medical   Cardiovascular problems come in numerous forms, with many different types of medications for each (such as coronary artery disease, high blood pressure, arrhythmias, high cholesterol or triglycerides, atherosclerotic plaques, angina, heart attack, and so on), you will need to talk this over with your health care provider.

Flaxseed

Along with soy, flaxseed ranks high in the dietary recommendations for women. In her newsletter, Dr. Christiane Northrup (July, 2000) presents a good summary of the benefits of this food by giving six reasons to include it in your diet.

- Potent anti-cancer agent for both breast and colon cancer
- Acts like soy in decreasing estradiol levels (the most potent of the body's natural estrogens, which has been implicated in breast cancer and blood clots)

(Continued on next page)

- Has antioxidant properties, which help prevent damage of tissues associated with aging and disease
- Is good for the heart, lowering bad cholesterol (LDH) and raising the good (HDL)
- Good source of fiber, helps prevent and treat constipation, and reduces the risk for cardiovascular disease
- Has a very low glycemic index and promotes feeling of fullness, both of which are good for weight control

DIGESTION

This includes flatulence and bloating; check with your health care specialist.

Diet   Check for food intolerances/allergies; try seaweeds

Herbs   Bitters, such as dandelion greens (or take tincture of dandelion root right before eating); Swedish Bitters

Other   Avoid antacids which soak up hydrochloric acid (which decreases as we age); consider going on a liver detoxification program (see Balch and Balch [2000], for a thorough detox program)

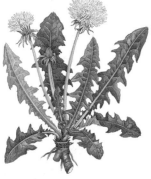

Dandelion

Tests   Upper GI X-rays, colonoscopy, bowel flora, or parasites

Medical   There are many types of gastrointestinal problems, with numerous medications such as H2 blockers for gastritis (Tagamet, Zantac), proton pump inhibitors for reflux (Prilosec, Propulsid), antispasmodics for cramps, antiflatulants for gas, antiparasitics, and so on.

FATIGUE/LOW ENERGY

Diet   Give your adrenal glands a rest by eliminating caffeine and sugar; generally eat a better diet; in other words, cut out junk foods and highly processed foods with their empty calories that fill you up but do not give you energy; experiment with increasing your protein intake slightly

Herbs   Ginkgo biloba, Siberian ginseng (do not take if you have hypoglycemia, high blood pressure, heart disorder, or thyroid diagnosis), green tea; nourish adrenals with astragalus and stinging nettles

Supplements/nutrients   Full complement of vitamins, including the Bs and the antioxidants C and E; and minerals (including magnesium)

Other   Try sleeping more; minimize stress; shift attitude from resistance to acceptance; exercise

Tests   Thyroid panel and TSH (thyroid stimulating hormone), thyroid antibodies, immunoglobulins, HIV testing, hepatitis testing; test for DHEA levels (go through health care provider because of potential adverse effects of overdosing)

Medical   If your thyroid tests low, thyroid hormone may be prescribed (Synthroid, levothyroxine); there are medical protocols for treating HIV and hepatitis.

FIBROCYSTIC BREASTS

Includes breast soreness

Diet   Avoid caffeine (coffee, black tea, chocolate, cola drinks)

Hormones   HIH (especially progesterone, according to Dr. John Lee, 1999)

Tests   Clinical breast exam by healthcare provider, mammograms to distinguish between fibroglandular tissue and tumors, and breast ultrasound when indicated.

FLOODING

(heavy menstrual flow)

Diet   Bioflavonoids, as found in the inner skin or white inner coating of citrus peel

Herbs   Vitex, wild yam, lady's mantle, shepherd's purse (a good source of bioflavonoids; other good sources are horsetail and elder). Avoid: blood thinning herbs, such as red clover, alfalfa, dong quai, and willow bark (has same active constituent as in aspirin, which is also to be avoided)

Supplements/nutrients   Oils of evening primrose and black currant

Hormones   HIH (progesterone)

Tests   Endometrial biopsy for repeated heavy or irregular bleeding; pelvic ultrasound to detect uterine enlargement, fibroids, or tumors

Medical   Birth control pills; some practitioners prescribe Provera (medroxyprogesterone) or natural HIH progesterone.

GENERAL ACHES AND PAINS

Diet   Seaweeds; eliminate sugar

Herbs   Red clover (Promensil is a brand name which has had many clinical trials)

Hormones   HIH (progesterone)

Supplements/nutrients   Evening primrose oil; flaxseed oil, glucosamine

Exercise   Swimming; yoga

Tests   If joints are red and swollen, arthritis or Lyme antibody testing may be indicated

Medical   NSAIDs (non-steroidal anti-inflammatories) are used for joint and muscle pain, but can cause gastritis (stomach inflammation) or ulcers; excess use stresses the kidneys and the liver (includes ibuprofen class of drugs).

GENERAL PMS SYMPTOMS

Hormones   HIH (estrogen and progesterone)

Herbs   Vitex, licorice root, black cohosh

Supplements/nutrients   Evening primrose oil; minerals chromium, selenium, zinc

Other   Keep a symptom diary through your cycle

Tests   Saliva hormone levels, or blood (serum)

Medical   Birth control pills, diuretics, estrogen-progestin regimens.

HOT FLASHES/FLUSHES/POWER SURGES

Diet   Soy products (tempeh, soy butter, soy milk, tofu); eliminate or reduce caffeine (coffee, tea, chocolate, cola drinks), very hot (temperature) foods/beverages, and spicy foods

Supplements/nutrients   Good multivitamin plus extra, if necessary, of the following: 400–800 I.U. vitamin E (avoid if diabetic or taking digitalis); 400–800 mg of magnesium, 200 mg four times a day of citrus bioflavonoids and vitamin C; antioxidants

Hormones   HIH (estrogen with progesterone)

Herbs   Vitex, black cohosh (Remifemin is one form), dong quai, motherwort

Other   Yoga and deep breathing; deal with anger/anxiety through therapy; keep your body cool (cotton clothes, layered clothes; room temperature; layers of bedding, not just one big quilt; cool things to eat and drink)

Tests   Serum (blood) or saliva hormone levels

Medical   Synthetic estrogen-progestin regimens; human identical estrogen-progesterone regimens.

Soy Products

Over 7,000 citations (circa 1997–1998) are available concerning different pharmacologic aspects of soy, according to *The Review of Natural Products* (1998). Of special interest to the menopausal woman is the estrogenic influence soy exerts on the body. Bioflavonoids are a large family of plant compounds that have estrogenic activity. Legumes such as soy contain isoflavones (one class of bioflavonoids). The main isoflavones in soy are genistein and diadzein. Women who have diets high in soy have less bone turnover, better bone density, and healthy lipid (cholesterol) profiles (Barnes, 1998). Soy products can relieve estrogen deficiency symptoms, including hot flashes and vaginal thinning. Postmenopausal women who consumed enough soy foods to get 200 mg of isoflavones per day had thickening of vaginal mucosa cells, which reduced dryness and irritation. This dose of isoflavones is comparable to 0.45 mg of conjugated estrogens (average dose of conjugated estrogens is 0.5 to 2.5 mg daily) (Murray & Pizzorno, 1998).

Interest in soy foods has increased in the past decade, because of their many health benefits, and the good quality low-fat protein provided. Soy has been called a super-health food, and the FDA has even allowed claims about promoting heart health. Many studies found soy foods can reduce risk for heart disease and cancer (breast, colon, uterus, prostate), and improve menopause symptoms (Aldercreutz & Mazur, 1997; Burke, 1996; Messina & Barnes, 1991). Women in Asia and Japan who eat traditional soy-rich diets have the lowest risk of hormone-dependent cancers (Knight & Eden, 1996). Some questions have been raised about soy products leading to dementia, endocrine problems, and decreased absorption, but the data appear unreliable (*UCB Wellness Letter,* August, 2000). The research on soy is overwhelmingly positive, including reducing risk of osteoporosis and breast cancer, and improving cholesterol profile (Lindsay & Claywell, 1998).

(Continued on next page)

Soy, like other plant foods, is a complex mixture of substances. Products made from whole soybeans are higher in isoflavones than those produced from soy protein concentrates. Using whole soy foods is the safest approach. Cooking soy will inactivate the trypsin inhibitors that might block absorption and utilization of amino acids and minerals. On balance, soy foods offer many health and nutritional benefits, therefore:

- If soy agrees with you, continue taking it
- The closer the food product is to the whole soy bean, the better
- Remember that cooked soy foods are safer
- Isolated soy constituents (soy protein powder, soy bars, capsules with certain isolated isoflavones) may have fewer health benefits

LIBIDO (SEXUAL DESIRE)

Hormones   Human identical progesterone (Lee & Hopkins, 1999) or estrogen; DHEA or testosterone

Herbs   Siberian ginseng, vitex

Tests   Estrogen, progesterone, testosterone, and DHEA levels (saliva best)

Medical   Viagra is sometimes used for women with severe problems; this is not an FDA-approved use.

MEMORY LOSS/CONCENTRATION DIFFICULTIES

Herbs   Siberian ginseng, ginkgo biloba, gotu kola

Hormones   HIH (estrogen with progesterone)

Supplements/nutrients   Lecithin (standardized to contain 30–55 percent of phosphatidyl choline—1500 mg/day), antioxidants, omega-3 essential fatty acid; vitamin E is said to increase brain circulation, which may be helpful; the mineral manganese

Tests   Check thyroid; mental status assessment tools, tests for dementia (if symptoms are severe).

MOODS/ANXIETY/DEPRESSION

Diet   Fermented foods such as miso can sometimes help, as can clams and oysters; foods high in calcium/magnesium, such as dark leafy greens; minimize processed foods; avoid sugar, caffeine, alcohol, and highly saturated fatty foods; eat small, frequent, high complex-carbohydrate meals balanced with a small amount of protein, according to Dr. Judith Wurtman of MIT (1986); this helps assure adequate serotonin levels in the brain, which contribute to a calmer feeling

Supplements/nutrients   B vitamins (including GABA); the minerals calcium and magnesium; local bee pollen (if not allergic to); SAM-e (S-adenosyl-L-methionine) (Clouatre, 1999)

Herbs   St. John's wort (don't take with pharmaceutical antidepressants or with MAO inhibitors); kava-kava, vitex, nutritive herbs, such as alfalfa and stinging nettle, which help strengthen the nervous system

Hormones   HIH progesterone (the synthetic form, called progestin, often prescribed under the brand name Provera, has been linked with the blues in some women according to Dr. John Lee, 1999)

Exercise   Most forms of exercise help release endorphins into your body and, thus, act as a mood enhancer.

Other   Yoga and meditation; dealing with anger/anxiety/grief through counseling or support groups; get thyroid checked

Tests   Thyroid tests, psychiatric evaluation if severe

Medical   Antidepressant or anti-anxiety drugs; commonly used are SSRIs (selective serotonin uptake inhibitors), such as Prozac, Paxil, Zoloft, and Celexa; tricyclics, such as Elavil, Triavil, Pamelor, Deseryl; benzodiazepines, such as Xanax, Valium, Restoril (only for short-term use, as these have habituating qualities); counseling or psychotherapy.

NIGHT SWEATS

Hormones   HIH (estrogen, per Bender, 1998)

Herbs   Dong quai, motherwort, garden sage, black cohosh

Other   Cotton nightgown, sheets; layered blankets instead of one huge quilt

Tests, Medical   See hot flashes

SKIN AND HAIR

Diet   6–8 glasses of pure water daily and a healthy diet

Hormones   HIH (estrogen and progesterone; helps with "crawly" skin, thinning, and drying)

Supplements/nutrients   Flaxseed oil and evening primrose oil; vitamin E; anti-oxidants

Herbs   For ingesting: stinging nettles (Weed, 1992), wild yam root (Crawford, 1996); moisturizing herbs to apply as skin preparations: comfrey, chamomile, sandalwood, and calendula (Crawford, 1996)

Other   Exercise; stop smoking; Northrup (September, 2000) advises limiting sun exposure to a 15-minute sunbath in the early morning or late afternoon from mid-March to mid-October in northern latitudes, and using skin products that contain alpha- or beta-hydroxy acids.

SLEEP

Diet   Do not drink before bedtime, especially caffeinated drinks (black tea, hot chocolate, coffee, colas—within 6 hours of bedtime), or alcohol; do eat complex carbohydrates at dinner for increased serotonin in the brain, which promotes relaxation (do not go to bed hungry, rather eat a light snack); milk warmed up (to activate the calming amino acid tryptophan)

Herbs   Valerian, kava-kava, chamomile, oat straw, lemon balm, hops, skullcap, passion flower; lavender oil in a warm, not hot, bath

Supplements/nutrients   Calming calcium/magnesium tablets around dinner time and before bed (good for bones, too)

Hormones   HIH (estrogen and progesterone)

Other   If you cannot get to sleep after 15 minutes, go to another room and read for a while. No television in your bedroom

Medical   Sleeping medications such as Ambien, Dalmane, Halcion, or benzodi-azepines (Restoril, Ativan, Xanax, Valium) may be used, but this is not considered good practice because of their habituating qualities. Any drug used to aid sleep should be used for very short times (only a few days). Prolonged use disturbs sleep patterns even more, and can lead to dependence.

URINARY TRACT PROBLEMS

Includes incontinence and infections

Diet   Drink lots of pure water at first sign of urgency or burning to head off infection (Weed, 1992); cranberry juice (brands without glucose and corn syrup); seaweeds; bioflavonoids (inner skin of citrus or buckwheat greens in tablet form)

Herbs   Specifically for incontinence: black cohosh helps stop spasms in the urinary tract; a tea of dried teasel root (Weed, 1992); wild yam root cream/progesterone cream applied to strengthen bladder tissue; other helpful herbs include yarrow or bearberry leaf (disinfectants); echinacea (antibiotic action)

Other   Biofeedback, Kegel exercises

Tests   Urinalysis for blood, leukocytes (pus cells), and bacteria; urine culture for bacteria; tests of urodynamics to identify problems with sphincters, bladder sagging, changing urethral angle

Medical   Antibiotics for urinary tract infections; urethral and bladder antispasmodic drugs (Ditropan or Detrol); surgery (bladder suspension, pelvic muscle repair to reduce sag); estrogen applied as creams or vaginal ring (Estring, releases estradiol over 3 months).

UTERINE FIBROIDS

Diet   Anti-estrogenic lignans found in whole grains, such as flaxseed, rye, buckwheat, millet, soy, oats, barley, corn, rice, and wheat (in descending order—Weed, 1992). Avoid or eat less animal protein with high fat content (red meat, for instance) and dairy products

Herbs   Vitex (also has an anti-inflammatory effect on the endrometrium), cotton root bark (stops flooding caused by fibroids—a dropperful of tincture every 5–10 min. until hemorrhage stops, according to Weed, 1992), red clover (Trifolium pratense—use freshly dried flower heads per Crawford, 1996). Avoid dong quai

Other   Acupuncture; increase pelvic circulation/tone with exercise and Kegels

Tests   Pelvic ultrasound, pelvic exam by health care provider to detect uterine enlargement

Medical   Depends on symptoms; if prolonged heavy bleeding, prolapsed uterus, severe pelvic pain and pressure, then hysterectomy or myomectomy using laser procedure to remove fibroids may be indicated. Fibroids shrink after menopause, so waiting will usually resolve symptoms if not unduly severe.

VAGINAL DRYNESS AND ITCHING/THINNING

Painful sex included

Diet   Soy products; omega-3 essential fatty acid; foods rich in phytosterols (beans, legumes, sprouted seeds, nuts, dates, carrots, yams, real licorice candy); seaweeds; bioflavonoids; water (see urinary). Cut down on or eliminate alcohol and caffeine (diuretics and antihistamines, too, says Ojeda, 2000)

Hormones   HIH estrogen ingested or applied vaginally, as in estriol or estradiol creams

Herbs   Vitex, dong quai, oatstraw, stinging nettles, elder, St. John's wort oil

Supplements/nutrients   Vitamins C and E (500 I.U. a day internally and the oil applied to vaginal tissue; beware possible irritation or allergic response); evening primrose oil; flaxseed oil

Exercise   Kegel exercises

Other   Do not douche or use bath bubbles; use water-soluble lubricants in the vagina

Medical   Estrogen-progestin regimens, local use of creams or Estring (vaginal ring that releases estradiol over 3 months) are especially good for vaginal and bladder symptoms.

TAKING CHARGE OF THERAPIES

At a glance, here are our general recommendations for staying healthy during your perimenopause and menopause transitions. Through these self-care measures you can take charge of your experiences and symptoms.

Diet

Emphasize vegetables (leafy greens included), whole grains, fruit, soy products. Restrict animal protein, alcohol, caffeine, sodas, fats (especially the "bad" ones, such as margarine, animal fats/butter, vegetable oils), sugar, simple carbohydrates.

Exercise

Stretching (yoga), 4–5 times per week.
Aerobic and weight bearing, 20 minutes, 4–5 times per week.

Supplements

These are drawn from recommendations by Drs. Christiane Northrup (1999), Andrew Weil (2000), Jonathan Wright and Alan Gaby (1997), and Michael Murray and Joseph Pizzorno (1998). The amounts of each nutrient recommended by different experts varies.

Calcium citrate, maleate, or ascorbate 600–1500 mg

Magnesium 400–800 mg

Zinc 15–30 mg

Boron 2–12 mg

Antioxidants:

   Vitamin E 400–800 IU

   Vitamin C 1000–2000 mg

   Beta-carotene 5000–15,000 IU

   Folic acid 400 mcg

   Vitamin B_6 3–35 mg

Others:

   Omega-3 fatty acids, 3 gm

   Grapeseed extract (dose depends on preparation)

The amount of calcium needed varies, with some controversy as to how much. Women with good dietary calcium, who are taking estrogen, are physically active, have more bone mass, and few factors that leach calcium from bones or reduce absorption, need lower amounts of supplements.

Hormones

Human identical hormones (HIH) are recommended, because they have identical molecular structure to women's own native hormones. HIH are made from plants (soy, yams). Both estrogens and progesterone are available by prescription (see Table 3–1); progesterone creams may be purchased at health food stores or by mail order.

PROGESTERONE CREAM

(USP) 20–30mg/gram (2–3 percent)

Use 1–2 grams per dose. 1 gram equals ¼ tsp.

Apply to areas where skin is thin (wrists, neck, back of hands, abdomen, breasts, inner thighs) once or twice daily. If still having menstrual cycles, use the last 2 weeks (days 15–25 of cycle). If not having periods, you may use the cream every day, although some believe you get better long term effects by taking four to five days off a month.

Prescription creams guarantee dose; over-the-counter creams have less reliable doses. When using over-the-counter creams, look for brands that contain 400–500 mg of USP progesterone per ounce. If the jar does not give a dosage, then it probably contains very little progesterone and effects on symptoms will be less.

ESTROGEN CREAMS

Prescription creams usually have 80 percent estriol and 20 percent estradiol (biestrogen) or may have either hormone alone. Vaginal estrogen creams have lower doses.

Use 1–2 grams per dose for skin creams. 1 gram equals ¼ tsp.

Apply as above for progesterone cream, once or twice daily. If still having menstrual cycles, use from days 1–25 of cycle. If not having periods, use 3 to 3½ weeks per month.

Phytoestrogen creams contain herbs and isoflavones, and are available at your health food store.

WILD YAM CREAM

The active ingredient is diosgenin, and strengths vary; some yam creams contain progesterone and some do not. Most authorities state that diosgenin is not active in the body, and does not convert to any active hormones. Many yam creams contain small amounts of progesterone.

Usual dose is 1/4 to 1/2 tsp. once or twice daily.

STRESS MANAGEMENT

Regular, daily meditation or centering practice (minimum 10–15 minutes).

Relaxation techniques, such as imagery, breath exercises, progressive muscle tensing and relaxing, taking walks, and being in nature.

Maintaining positive attitudes and self-talk.

Having a support system and feeling connected with others.

HABITS

No cigarettes. Minimal alcohol.

REFERENCES

Aeron LifeCycles Clinical Laboratory. (2000). The HRT controversy. *Hormonal Update, 1,* 1–2.

Aldercreutz, H., & Mazur, S. (1997). Phyto-estrogens and Western diseases. *Annals of Internal Medicine, 29,* 95–120.

Alexanderson, P., Toussaint, A., Christiansen, C., Devogelaer, J.P., et al. (2001). Ipriflavone in the treatment of postmenopausal osteporosis: A randomized controlled trial. *JAMA, 285,* 1482–1488.

Arjmandi, B.H., Alekel, L., Hollis, B.W., et al. (1996). Dietary soybean protein prevents bone loss in ovariectomized rat model of osteoporosis. *Journal of Nutrition, 126,* 161–167.

Atkins, R. (1997). *Dr. Atkins' new diet revolution.* New York: Avon Books.

Balch, J.F., & Balch, P.A. (2000). *Prescription for nutritional healing* (3rd Ed.). Garden City Park, NY: Avery Publishing Group.

Barback, L. (1995). *The pause: Positive approaches to perimenopause and menopause.* New York: Plume.

Barnes, S. (1998). Evolution of the health benefits of soy isoflavones. *Proceedings of the Society for Experimental Biology and Medicine, 217,* 386–392.

Barrett-Connor, E., & Stuenkel, C. (1999). Hormones and heart disease in women: Heart and Estrogen/Progestin Replacement Study in perspective. *Journal of Clinical Endocrinology and Metabolism, 84,* 1848–1853.

Batmanghelidj, F. (1997). *Your body's many cries for water: You are not sick, you are thirsty!* (2nd Ed.). Falls Church, VA: Global Health Solutions, Inc.

Bender, S.D. (1998). *The power of perimenopause: A woman's guide to physical and emotional health during the transitional decade.* New York: Three Rivers Press.

Bloomfield, H.H. (1998). *Healing anxiety with herbs.* New York: HarperCollins.

Blumenthal, M., Busse, W.R., Goldberg, A., Klein, S., Riggins, C., & Rister, R. (1998). *The complete German Commission E. monograph therapeutic guide to herbal medicines.* Austin, TX: The American Botanical Council.

Bosarge, P.M. (2000). Helping patients assess HRT options. *Transitions: Menopause News for NPs and PAs, 1,* 1–5.

Bradley, L., & Newman, J. (2000). Uterine artery embolization for treatment of fibroids: From scalpel to catheter. *The Female Patient, 25,* 71–78.

Burke, G.L. (1996). The potential use of a dietary soy supplement as a post-menopausal hormone replacement therapy. *Second International Symposium on the Role of Soy in Preventing and Treating Chronic Disease, Program and Abstract Book,* 40–41. Brussels, Belgium.

Chen, Y., Shen, L., Zhang, F., Lau, S.S., van Breemen, R.B., Nikolic, D., & Bolton, J.L. (1998). The equine estrogen metabolite 4-hydroxyequilenin causes DNA single-strand breaks and oxidation of DNA bases in vitro. *Chemical Research Toxicology, 11,* 1105–1111.

Clouatre, D. (1999). *Sam-e (S-adenosyl-L-methionine): What you need to know.* Garden City Park, NY: Avery Publishing Group.

Col, N., Legato, M., & Schiff, I. (1998). HRT: New data, continuing controversies. *Patient Care Nurse Practitioner, 1,* 18–34.

Collaborative Group on Hormonal Factors in Breast Cancer. (1997). Breast cancer and hormone replacement therapy. *Lancet, 350,* 1047–1059.

Consumers Union. (2000). Estrogen: Shifting recommendations. *Consumer Reports on Health, 12,* 8–9.

Crawford, A.M. (1996). *The herbal menopause book: Herbs, nutrition & other natural therapies.* Freedom, CA: The Crossing Press.

Daiber, W. (1983). Menopause symptoms: Success without hormones. *Arztl Praxis, 35,* 1946.

Deckelbaum, R.J., Fisher, E.A., Winston, M., Kumanyika, S., Lauer, R.M., Pi-Sunyer, F.X., St. Jeor, S., Schaefer, E.J., & Weinstein, I.B. (1999, July 27). Unified dietary guidelines. *Circulation: Journal of the American Heart Association, 100,* 4.

DuraMed. (1999). *Cenestin: A safe and effective alternative to Premarin.* Cincinnati, OH: Duramed Pharmaceuticals.

Edell, D., & Schreiberg, D. (1999). *Eat, drink and be merry: America's doctor tells you why the health experts are wrong.* New York: HarperCollins.

Ellis, F., Holesh, S., & Ellis, J. (1972). Incidence of osteoporosis in vegetarians and omnivores. *American Journal of Clinical Nutrition, 25,* 55–58.

Ettinger, B., Li, D.K., & Klein, R. (1996). Continuation of postmenopausal hormone replacement therapy: Comparison of cyclic versus continuous combined schedules. *Menopause, 3,* 185–189.

Fetrow, C., & Avila, J. (1999). *Professional's handbook of complementary & alternative medicines.* Springhouse, PA: Springhouse Corporation.

Firshein, R. (1998). *The nutraceutical revolution: 20 cutting-edge nutrients to help you design your own perfect whole-life program.* New York: Riverhead Books.

Gill, E. (1991). Blowing the fuse. In D. Taylor & A. C. Sumrall (Eds.). *Women of the 14th moon.* Freedom, CA: The Crossing Press.

Glisson, J., Crawford, R., & Street, S. (1999). The clinical applications of ginkgo biloba, St. John's wort, saw palmetto, and soy. *The Nurse Practitioner, 24,* 28–47.

Goldman, E.G. (1991). Blowing the fuse. In D. Taylor & A. C. Sumrall (Eds.). *Women of the 14th moon.* Freedom, CA: The Crossing Press.

Hoffman, D. (2000). Chaste Berry. Herbal Materia Medica. Accessed 3/00: *http://www.healthy.net/hwlibrarybooks/hoffman/materiamedica/chaste.htm.*

Hu, F.B., Stampfer, M.J., Colditz, G.A., Ascherio, A., Rexrode, K.M., Willet, W.C., & Manson, J.E. (2000). Physical activity and risk of stroke in women. *Journal of the American Medical Association, 283,* 22, 2961–7

Keating, N.L., Cleary, P.D., Rossi, A.S., Zaslavsky, A.M., Ayanian, J.Z. (1999). Use of hormone replacement therapy by postmenopausal women in the United States. *Annals of Internal Medicine, 130,* 545–553.

Knight, D.C., & Eden, J.A. (1996). A review of the clinical effect of phytoestrogens. *Obstetrics and Gynecology, 87,* 897–904.

Lauritzen, C., Reuter, H.D., Repges, R., et al. (1997). Treatment of premenstrual tension syndrome with Vitex Agnus Castus. Controlled, double-blind study versus pyridoxine. *Phytomedicine, 4,* 183–189.

Lee, J., Henley, J., & Hopkins, V. (1999). *What your doctor may not tell you about menopause: Balance your hormones and your life from thirty to fifty.* New York: Warner Books.

Lehmann, E., Kinzler, E., & Friedemann, J. (1996). Efficacy of a special Kava extract (*Piper methysticum*) in patients with states of anxiety, tension, and excitedness of non-mental origin—A double-blind placebo-controlled study of four weeks treatment. *Phytomedicine, III* (2), 113–119.

Leonetti, H.B., Longo, S., & Anasti, J.N. (1999). Transdermal progesterone cream for vasomotor symptoms and postmenopausal bone loss. *Obstetrics and Gynecology, 94,* 225–228.

Lindsay, S.H., & Claywell, L.G. (1998). Considering soy: Its estrogenic effects may protect women. *AWHONN Lifelines, 2,* 41–44.

Marsh, A.G., Sanchez, T.V., Chaffee, F.L., Mayor, G.H., & Mickelsen, D. (1983). Bone mineral mass in adult lacto-ovo-vegetarians and omnivorous males. *American Journal of Clinical Nutrition, 37,* 453–56.

Massoudi, M.S., Meilahn, E.N., & Orchard, T.J. (1995). Prevalence of thyroid antibodies among healthy middle-aged women. Findings from the thyroid study in healthy women. *Annals of Epidemiology, 5,* 229–233.

Messina, M., & Barnes, S. (1991). The roles of soy products in reducing risk of cancer. *Journal of the National Cancer Institute, 83,* 541–546.

Murray, M., & Pizzorno, J. (1998). *Encyclopedia of natural medicine* (Rev. 2nd Ed.). Rocklin, CA: Prima Publishing.

Nabulsi, A.A., Folsom, A.R., White, A., et al. (1993). Association of hormone-replacement therapy with various cardiovascular risk factors in postmenopausal women. The Atherosclerosis Risk in Communities Study Investigators. *New England Journal of Medicine, 328,* 1069–1075.

Nawaz, H., & Katz, D.L. (1999). American College of Preventive Medicine Practice Policy Statement: Perimenopausal and Postmenopausal hormone replacement. *American Journal of Preventive Medicine, 17,* 250–254.

Northrup, C. (1998). *Women's bodies, women's wisdom: Creating physical and emotional health and healing.* New York: Bantam Books.

Northrup, C. (1999). *Dr. Christiane Northrup's Health Wisdom for Women, 6,* 1.

Northrup, C. (April, 2000). HRT and breast cancer: Getting terms straight. *Dr. Christiane Northrup's Health Wisdom for Women, 7,* 1–2.

Northrup, C. (July, 2000). Flaxseeds: Super source of lignans and omega-3 fatty acids. *Dr. Christiane Northrup's Health Wisdom for Women.* Potomac, MD: Phillips Publishing.

Northrup, C. (September, 2000). How to protect and improve your skin with antioxidants, part 1. *Dr. Christiane Northrup's Health Wisdom for Women.* Potomac, MD: Phillips Publishing.

Northrup, C. (2001). *The wisdom of menopause: Creating physical and emotional health and healing during the change.* New York: Bantam Books.

Nygaard, I.E., Kreder, K.J., Lepic, M.M., et al. (1996). Efficacy of pelvic floor muscle exercises in women with stress, urge, and mixed urinary incontinence. *American Journal of Obstetrics and Gynecology, 174,* 120–125.

Ojeda, L. (2000). *Menopause without medicine.* (Rev. 4th Ed.). Alameda, CA: Hunter House Publishers.

Ornish, D. (1990). *Dr. Dean Ornish's program for reversing heart disease.* New York: Random House.

PDR for herbal medicines (1st edition). (1999). Montvale, NJ: Medical Economics Co.

The review of natural products (September, 1998). St. Louis, MO: Facts and Comparisons Publishing Group.

Sarrell, P., & Whitehead, M.I. (1985). Sex and menopause: Defining the issues. *Maturitas, 7,* 217–24.

Sarrell, P., Dobay, B., & Wiita, B. (1998). Estrogen and estrogen-androgen replacement in postmenopausal women dissatisfied with estrogen-only therapy. *Journal of Reproductive Medicine, 43,* 847–856.

Schairer, C., Lubin, J., Troisi, R., et al. (2000). Menopausal estrogen and estrogen-progestin replacement therapy and breast cancer risk. *Journal of the American Medical Association, 283,* 485–491.

Sears, B. (2000). *The soy zone.* New York: Regan Books.

Singh, Y.N., Blumenthal, M. (1997). Kava: An overview. *Herbalgram* (Special Review Herbalgram No. 39), *39,* 33–55.

Singla, A. (2000). An update on the management of SUI. *Contemporary Ob/Gyn, 45,* 68–85.

Stampfer, M.J., Hu, F.B., Manson, J.E., et al. (2000). Primary prevention of coronary heart disease in women through diet and lifestyle. *New England Journal of Medicine, 343,* 16–22.

Stoll, W. (1987). Phytotherapy influences atrophic vaginal epithelium. *Therapeutikon, 1,* 23.

Tesar, R., Notelovitz, M., Shim, E., et al. (1992). Axial and peripheral bone density and nutrient intakes of postmenopausal vegetarian and omnivorous women. *American Journal of Clinical Nutrition, 56,* 699–704.

Thom, D.H. (2001). Overactive bladder: Epidemiology and impact on quality of life. *Patient Care for the Nurse Practitioner* (Suppl.), 6–14.

UCB Wellness Letter. (August, 2000). Are those tofu rumors true? *16,* 1.

Volz, H.P. (1997). Controlled clinical trials of hypericum extracts in depressed patients—an overview. *Pharmacopsychiatry, 30*(Suppl.), 72–76.

Volz, H.P., & Kieser, M. (1997). Kava-kava extract WS 1490 versus placebo in anxiety disorders: A randomized placebo-controlled 25-week outpatient trial. *Pharmacopsychiatry, 30,* 1–5.

Weed, Susan. (1992). *Menopausal years: The wise woman way.* Woodstock, New York: Ash Tree Publications.

Weil, A. (2000). *Eating well for optimum health: The essential guide to food, diet, and nutrition.* New York: Alfred A. Knopf.

Wein, A.J. (2001). Putting overactive bladder into clinical perspective. *Patient Care for the Nurse Practitioner* (Suppl.), Spring 2001, 1–5.

Westermann, C. (1997). Pharmacology and selection of postmenopausal estrogen replacement therapy. *Female Patient, 22,* 15–25.

Wetzel, W. (1998). Human identical hormones: Real people, real problems, real solutions. *Nurse Practitioner Forum, 9,* 227–235.

Wheatley, D. (1997). LI 160, an extract of St. John's Wort, versus amitriptyline in mildly to moderately depressed outpatients—a controlled 6-week clinical trial. *Pharmacopsychiatry, 30*(Suppl.), 77–80.

Wright, J.V., & Gaby, A.R. (1997). *Dr. Jonathan V. Wright's Nutrition & healing with Alan R. Gaby, M.D.* Phoenix, AZ: Nutrition & Healing Corp.

Wright, J.V., & Morgenthaler, J. (1997). *Natural hormone replacement for women over 45.* Petaluma, CA: Smart Publications.

Writing Group for the PEPI Trial. (1995). Effects of estrogen or estrogen/progestin regimens on heart disease risk factors in post-menopausal women. *Journal of the American Medical Association, 273,* 199–208.

Wurtman, J., with Danbrot, M. (1986). *Managing your mind and mood through food.* New York: Rawson Associates.

Zhang, F., Chen, Y., Pisha, E., Shen, L., Xiong, Y., van Breemen, R.B., & Bolton, J.L. (1999). The major metabolite of equilin, 4-hydroxyequilin, autoxidizes to an o-quinone which isomerizes to the potent cytotoxin 4-hydroxyequilenin-o-quinone. *Chemical Research Toxicology, 12,* 204–213.

SUGGESTED READING

Brostoff, J., & Gamlin, L. (2000). *Food allergies and food intolerance: The complete guide to their identification and treatment.* Rochester, VT: Healing Arts Press.

Checking Your Hormone "Bank Account"

Take a moment to take a quick inventory of your hormone "back account" during your life:

	Teens	20s	30s	40s	Current
Withdrawals					
poor diet & nutrition	☐	☐	☐	☐	☐
not enough B vitamins	☐	☐	☐	☐	☐
excess alcohol	☐	☐	☐	☐	☐
cigarette smoking	☐	☐	☐	☐	☐
excess caffeine	☐	☐	☐	☐	☐
sodas with phosphates	☐	☐	☐	☐	☐
lack of proper rest	☐	☐	☐	☐	☐
stressful lifestyle	☐	☐	☐	☐	☐
Deposits					
healthy, nutritious diet	☐	☐	☐	☐	☐
supplements, B vitamins	☐	☐	☐	☐	☐
enough rest	☐	☐	☐	☐	☐
regular exercise	☐	☐	☐	☐	☐
short daily sunlight exposure	☐	☐	☐	☐	☐
take it easy during menstruation	☐	☐	☐	☐	☐
regular spiritual practice	☐	☐	☐	☐	☐

Do you have more checkmarks in "withdrawals" or "deposits?" If your body was well-nourished during puberty and teen years, especially with B and C vitamins, minerals, and essential fatty acids, then you had the foundation for healthy bones, adrenal glands and ovaries—and a smoother menopausal transition. If you had more "withdrawals" in early years, you can regain balance by making healthful changes in the 30s and 40s. If you continue a health-depleting lifestyle, you'll age more rapidly, especially after menopause.

Adapted with permission of Phillips Publishing, Inc. *Dr. Christiane Northrup's Health Wisdom for Women.* (January 1998). To subscribe to *Health Wisdom for Women,* or for more information, call 1-800-211-8561.

Worksheet 3–2

Therapy History: The Physical Experience

This history may serve as your medical profile to take with you to health care practitioners. Record when you start (and end) taking a drug or herb, for example; or when you start and complete a series of visits to the acupuncturist or masseuse. Then, most important, record the results. Over time you'll get a clearer picture of what is working for you and what isn't.

Symptom Treated	Kind of Therapy	Date Started	Date Stopped	Results

The Mental-Emotional Experience

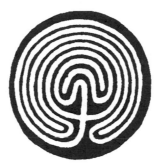

Labyrinth.
Reproduced with permission.
Copyright © Kate Cartwright.

Menopause changes the way women's minds work. The hormone patterns during this time affect brain functions by altering connections between brain cells (neurons) and the chemicals that flood through the brain. One result of this process is major shifts in women's outlook on life. The dance of the hormones during perimenopause and menopause has many effects on women's mental and emotional experiences. This may lead to feeling out of balance, with moods often becoming less predictable. Some women feel a stranger to themselves. Through the three phases of women's menopause transition, the various physical, mental, and emotional experiences are preparing for the emergence of a new self. These experiences serve as springboards to acquaint women with their new potential, and provide opportunities through which unprocessed emotions and unresolved situations may be worked out. Biologically, during menopause the brain is programmed to focus inward, re-examine issues, and find novel solutions (Northrup, 2001). After menopause the emotional terrain smoothes out, and women enter the phase of postmenopausal zest, creativity, and new horizons.

> Our deepest fear is not that we are inadequate. Our deepest fear is that we are powerful beyond measure.
>
> —Nelson Mandela

A powerful connection exists between the mind and the body, often leading to a wake-up call during perimenopause. Women who have intensely uncomfortable PMS during perimenopause, or severe mood symptoms, probably are being urged by their inner wisdom to deal with and resolve old emotional baggage. Contrary to popular belief, the fluctuating hormones during this time are not solely responsible for distressing emotional and psychological symptoms, such as anger and depression. Research has not shown substantial differences in hormone levels between women who suffer from PMS and those who do not. The important difference found, however, is that the brains of women with severe PMS are more susceptible to the effects of fluctuating hormone levels. A woman's preexisting brain chemistry, combined with her life experiences and present situation, interact with changing hormone levels to cause amplified PMS symptoms (Schmidt et al., 1998; Novaes & Almeida, 1999).

The symptoms of perimenopause have complex origins, well beyond simply fluctuating levels of estrogen and progesterone. Women who have undergone hysterectomies with removal of both ovaries, and who have been on full hormone replacement therapy for 10 to 20 years, nevertheless may still experience symptoms such as hot flashes and mood swings in their late 40s (Northrup, 2001). These women's brain chemistry and neural pathways still change, triggered by biological programming that signals the mind and body that a new developmental stage has been reached.

The mandate for psychological change is very strong as women approach menopause. It appears that women's brains and bodies are activated to set in motion a process that allows them to heal and integrate the past. Hormonal effects on brain structures permit retrieval of memories long buried, along with more energy and motivation to deal with these issues and bring them to resolution. In a sense, women at menopause pick up the self-development that was initially shaped during adolescence, and now feel propelled to bring it to completion. The adult years certainly hone aspects of women's identity, but at menopause a new intensity calls forth the next stages of expression.

Midlife is the critical time when completing unfinished emotional business, learning to relate more fully to our physical vessel, the body, and anticipating further development set the stage for the Wise Woman to emerge. The storms of menopause may be seen, in retrospect, as the testing ground for the new capacities being birthed. . . . In menopause, the birthing is of a new woman who will mother herself and the greater community.

—Maura Kelsea, "Beyond the Stethoscope: A Nurse Practitioner Looks at Menopause and Midlife," in *Women of the 14th Moon*

In Western culture there is a tendency to seek a quick fix, something that will make the pain, whether physical or emotional, go away so that we can get on with our lives. There is benefit in relieving symptoms, but that is only the beginning. It buys time to do the real work. Menopause signals a time for introspection, gaining deeper understanding of who you truly are, and what your life means. By manifesting physical or emotional symptoms, it may be that your higher self is trying to get your attention.

Before one can begin introspection, however, it helps to have knowledge about how the different phases of the midlife woman's mental and emotional development affect our minds and our hearts. It often surprises women to learn that their states of mind and feelings are not unique; rather, these are shared by many women going through perimenopause and menopause. Some women in the authors' classes have almost wept with relief upon hearing that the disturbing symptoms they are experiencing are felt by others in the class. Nods of recognition, laughs of relief, and a sense of sisterhood emerge with this honest sharing.

PHASES OF THE MIDLIFE WOMAN'S MENTAL-EMOTIONAL DEVELOPMENT

Women are aware of cycles as their bodies change during the monthly menstrual "moon cycle." Women also have longer rhythm cycles that encompass several years, perhaps 7 to 12 years, and sometimes longer. These are phases of physical, mental, and emotional development, moving from childhood to adolescence, young adulthood, adulthood, midlife, and older age. Exactly when these phases start, and how long they last, varies for different women. For women at midlife, there are three phases in the menopausal transition:

Perimenopause—Entering Midlife

Menopause—Metamorphosis

Postmenopause—Fullness/Wisdom.

Perimenopause—Entering Midlife

Women enter the significant midlife change cycle around age 35 to 40, the perimenopause, which may last 10–15 years. This is a time of bodily and emotional changes, of major transitions in self-concept as we move from being young adults to mature women.

The main mid-life developmental mandates are:

- Emotional healing of our wounds and traumas from earlier life
- Mastering the lessons of these life challenges: "spinning straw into gold"
- Living authentically in growth-promoting relationships

- Reviewing priorities in our work and inner balance
- Sharing our psychological and spiritual growth with others

Women need to bring to closure the experiences of the first part of their lives. Integrating the lessons from this time is necessary to emergence of the authentic self. Many women revisit or discover early traumas during this phase. They may have vivid dreams, or begin to remember details about difficult situations, such as parents divorcing, the death of a friend or family member, or conflicts with parents or siblings. It is common for memories of childhood abuse to surface now. Many of these memories were deeply repressed into the subconscious and stored as images, because the child does not have enough psychological strength to deal with them directly. In the late 30s and 40s, the mind censors weaken their hold, and deeply buried memories begin to push upward toward consciousness. The accumulated stresses of midlife wear down defenses, and women re-experience many of these earlier emotions. Having access to memories and associated emotions is the start to healing them. Verbalizing these traumas in appropriately supportive circumstances helps transfer the deep images (icons) from the lower brain structure where they are stored (amygdala) into the cerebral cortex where we may deal with them rationally. When women are heard, find meaning, and gain different perspectives, this enables them to grow from these traumatic experiences.

Women naturally begin to examine relationships and look at their past behaviors and motivations. The inner mandate for honoring the authentic self focuses a laser-like beam on ways women have sold themselves short, compromised too much, or put up with disrespect. The feminine values of relationships and interdependence are still important, but within the context of greater self-authenticity. Women are less willing to remain in relationships that do not support their growth. Whether primarily homemakers or career women, in this phase women prefer to take their chances with economic insecurity rather than stay in hurtful or loveless situations. Husbands, partners or friends who do not contribute to these life values have to go.

> . . . [T]he danger zone through which most women will pass in their late forties . . . (leads to) a profound change in self-concept. . . . They often break the seal on repressed angers. They overcome the habits of trying to be perfect and of needing to make everyone love them. They may shed the terror of living without a man that trapped them in a dead or destructive marriage. Many . . . find the sustained courage to extricate themselves from lives of desperate repetition.
>
> —Gail Sheehy, *The Silent Passage: Menopause*

Is Divorce Inevitable?

Divorce during the menopause transition is a common occurrence. Virtually every marriage/partnership, even good ones, needs to undergo change in response to the rewiring of women's brains and the deep inner processes occurring at this time. Taking an honest look at all aspects of your relationship is essential to staying healthy, physically, emotionally, and spiritually (Northrup, 2001). Over 20 years of research on relationships at the University of Washington showed how some key health areas affected the success or failure of intimate relationships:

1. Healthy relationships are based on kindness. If positive interactions outnumber negative ones by a critical ratio of 5 to 1, the relationship has a high probability of continuing. If there are more "nasty" than "nice" moments, it is headed for breakup.
2. Husbands who do housework are happier, healthier, have better sex lives, and are more likely to stay married.
3. Women married to belittling, contemptuous men are much more likely to become ill with a wide variety of problems.
4. Disrespectful wives who express disgust or contempt are more likely to separate or divorce within a few years.

John Gottman, University of Washington, in J. Borysenko, *A Woman's Book of Life,* 1996

All types of inauthentic relationships become harder to tolerate. Women become more emotionally astute and clarify their values. They are less inclined to continue friendships, jobs, clubs, groups that are one-way, that take more than they give, or that do not support these values. Questions about life purpose, the meaning of success, or the measure of a life well-lived arise. Priorities are reassessed, and women seek balance between their inner and outer lives.

Menopause—Metamorphosis

The changes that occur during the late 40s and early 50s herald the metamorphosis of menopause, which is often referred to as the "Change of Life." When our bodies are behaving differently, and we are beginning to look and feel different, it is impossible to be unaware that we are moving into another phase. While some women have a smooth passage, this time of transition can be deeply disturbing emotionally. Through this upheaval, we are being primed for coming more fully into our creativity and making an expanded social contribution. We

> I feel a certain new detachment. I watch with surprise and sometimes dismay as my old motivations begin to seem inadequate. I am becoming less patient with what does not seem deeply important to me.
>
> —Connie Batten, "A Journey Homeward," in *Women of the 14th Moon*

can think of menopause as an initiation into the most powerful, exciting, and fulfilling part of women's lives.

The developmental issues during the menopausal phase include:

- Managing physical and emotional changes to maintain balance
- Accepting and embracing our emerging new identities
- Emptying out what no longer serves our growth or essence
- Finding the strong voice of authenticity blended with compassion
- Enhancing our receptivity to intuitive ways of knowing

The many emotional and physical changes of the menopausal metamorphosis can motivate women to enter new relationships with their bodies, minds, energy systems, and often with partners. Some women have changes in sexual preference. When the body-mind becomes less predictable or reliable, we reconsider the importance of health. This can serve as a wake-up call to live healthier lifestyles. We become intensely aware that just as we cannot abuse our biological systems without facing the consequences, neither can we ignore our feelings. It becomes essential to learn stress management and boundary-setting. Women often recommit to health practices, or begin an intense process of learning how to live in greater balance.

At this time menopause symptoms may be redefined. Hot flashes become the inner fires of transformation, a rising and rebalancing of life-force energy that burns off stress or unnecessary encumbrances. Increased or redistributed body fat becomes a valuable source of estrogen once the ovaries decrease production. The relative

> In contrast to . . . fearful expectations about menopause . . . my actual experience has been a positive one in some very surprising ways. My accustomed sense of who I am has begun to slip, and while I feel a threat to my sense of security, I also feel a kind of excitement about my new awareness.
>
> —Connie Batten, "A Journey Homeward," in *Women of the 14th Moon*

> More and more frequently nowadays, my hot flashes have begun to feel like urgent communiqués from the interior of a vast, dark continent—fast breaking news items from my heart of darkness.
>
> —Barbara Raskin, "These Fevered Days," in *Women of the 14th Moon*

increase in testosterone (as estrogen and progesterone fall) helps women develop inner masculine qualities of strength, courage, assertiveness, and authority. Mental fog heralds rewiring of the nervous system, as elevated levels of FSH and LH, acting as neuropeptides or molecules of emotion, help open new pathways for intuition.

Self-definitions change. We begin to look and feel different. The process of growing older cannot be denied. This can throw us into fear and depression or propel us forward to more expanded concepts of ourselves. Women often develop a fierce resolve to reclaim their lives and power. They have reached a saturation point. There is a need to empty out all that is unnecessary and discordant and to find our true essence. This emptying and cleansing process creates space for our new selves to emerge. It has been called "holding the pause" as the new is born.

There is a triad of values that characterizes the wisdom of middle-age women: love, peace of mind, and service to others. Women become more concerned with the well-being of people, animals, plants, and the entire planet. Of course, this happens along a continuum, with some women just starting the exploration of these values while others are steeped in them. This is no time for nonsense, lack of tolerance, and the selfish disregard of others. Women often show a fiery directness, a new boldness that speaks up and asserts their truths in personal, family, and social arenas. This signals movement into the "Guardian" role for higher social purposes, often protecting the weak, challenging injustices, and working for ecological balance.

While this is a time of expanding awareness, the opposite can happen. If women fall into negativity, this fierceness may turn inward and be expressed as fear of aging, self-criticism, deepening depression, or the need to control situations and others.

> We Americans, with our terrific emphasis on youth, action, and material success, certainly tend to belittle the afternoon of life and even to pretend it never comes. We push the clock back and try to prolong the morning, over-reaching and over-straining ourselves in the unnatural effort. . . . In our breathless attempts we often miss the flowering that waits for afternoon.
>
> —Anne Morrow Lindbergh, *A Gift from the Sea*

Postmenopause—Fullness/Wisdom

Within the decade after menses stop, women have the opportunity to enter into the wisdom and vision years of postmenopause. During this phase, women are capable of expressing the fullness of their feminine potential, the consciousness of being in relation with all, and the interdependence of all. To reach this stage of fullness women need to attain emotional maturity, heal old wounds, find inner balance and harmony, reach deep self-knowledge, and integrate body-mind-spirit.

The developmental focus of this phase includes:

- The blending of authenticity with compassion.
- Expanding and refining intuitive and creative processes.
- Establishing unshakable inner peace and harmony.
- Using wisdom, clarity, and strength in service of others.
- Expanding and expressing spirituality.

Women in the wisdom years become the truth-tellers for society, and the preservers of the planet for future generations. Their concern is for the well-being of others and the environment, for encouraging the best to emerge. Because truthfulness begins within, deep self-honesty is required. When you define and honor your values, you are defining your truth. If you have the courage to speak and act on this truth, a sense of serenity comes from this authenticity. As we live more consistently connected to our inner self, we establish inner peace and harmony.

Many older women may speak the truth bluntly, much like young girls. If empathy and compassion have been nurtured, this truth will be full of wisdom. If not, these blunt words may be bitter, carping or destructive. The expression of authentic self can bring out the highest in others. By opening to another and connecting to her or his potential, we encourage creativity and happiness. There is great satisfaction through this giving, and an experience of the interrelatedness of all. From deep within, the inner voices of clarity, wisdom, and compassion guide us in the daily acts of kindness and encouragement that express universal love in action.

Research shows that people who send healing energy, prayers, or kind thoughts to others have enhanced immune function themselves. Greater longevity and fewer illnesses are associated with healthy immune function (Quinn & McClelland in Borysenko, 1996). The basic energy principle "What you put out, you get back" works here. A ripple effect takes place; those who receive kindness are better able to pass it on to others. In this way we can help create an emotionally healthy earth.

After a woman passes menopause she really comes into her time. I feel that. I've never felt so well or had so many images before me.

—Meridel Le Sueur, "Indian Summer," in *Women of the 14th Moon*

> Everyone comes into this world with a work to do, and there are special forces to guide in accomplishing that work. To truly do this work with the purest expression, you must be with the spirit, mentally and physically.
>
> —Unnamed Native American woman, in Wall, *Wisdom's Daughters*

Elder women have traditionally been the visionaries of society. Their mental and psychological processes naturally encode intuition, drawing from deeper levels of consciousness and tapping into spirituality. Research indicates that the female brain continues to evolve throughout the life cycle in ways that support interdependent, oracular thinking (Diamond in Borysenko, 1996). Wise women hold the vision of an interrelated world, respect for nature and all life, honoring diversity, encouraging each person's highest potential, and being connected to our spirit self. Prophecies from many cultures, including the Hopi and the ancient Mayans, indicate that around the millennium there is a "shift of the ages" (Braden, 1997) with heightened planetary consciousness. The planet is entering the "time of the wise woman."

MENTAL AND EMOTIONAL CHANGES

Many women find the changes in their inner world of feelings, thoughts, and responses more challenging than physical symptoms during the menopause transition. Sometimes women may experience such disconcerting symptoms that they wonder "Am I developing Alzheimer's?" or "Maybe I'm going crazy." Alterations in brain functions combine with hormonal changes to re-pattern how women's brains and minds work at menopause. This results in heightened memory activation, greater sensitivity to emotional states, less inhibition of feelings,

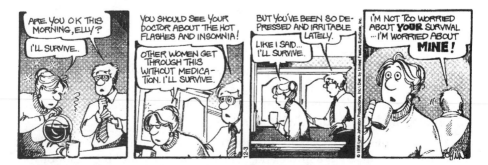

Figure 4–1 For Better or Worse. Copyright © Lynn Johnston Productions Inc./Dist. by United Feature Syndicate, Inc.

For the Partner of My Life: Accompany Me Through Menopause

While I'm coping with my symptoms and am having lots of emotional ups and downs, here are some ways you can help us both:

- Take time to learn about menopause. I'm not making this thing up—there are physical causes for these symptoms.
- Imagine having to walk in my moccasins for a week. I don't think you would like it.
- Practice patience with me, please.
- I hope you will not clam up and withdraw from me.
- Express your frustrations to a therapist, friend, or pastor to relieve stress and gain clarity. Then we can talk about it.
- Please don't tease me.
- Know that this is not forever. One day I will be back to "normal."
- I appreciate your efforts. What can I do for you in return?

more clarity of perceptions, and lower tolerance of discrepancies between inner values and outer conditions.

The Brain, Hormones, and Emotions

The midbrain, called the limbic system, is the primary site of human emotions. It interweaves emotional impulses with thoughts from the higher brain, or cerebral cortex. Although memories are held in many parts of the body and mind, two limbic structures, the amygdala and hippocampus, are especially important for encoding and retrieving memories. They work in conjunction with the hypothalamus. See Figure 5–2, page 189, for a diagram of the brain.

- The **amygdala** is a very old brain structure, with a watchdog function and rich neural networks to other areas of the brain. It expresses subtle emotional nuances such as love, affection, friendliness, and distrust. It is always watching for signals of opportunity or danger, so it can activate the hypothalamus, which then sets off action in the autonomic nervous system (controls the flight or fight response).
- The **hippocampus** acts in a complementary way with the amygdala to focus the mind's attention and regulate emotions, linking emotions to images, memory, and learning. It regulates autonomic nervous system action to avoid extreme responses and maintain emotional equilibrium.

- The **hypothalamus** is the master control for the autonomic nervous system, and helps create basic emotions such as rage and terror, as well as positive states ranging from pleasure to bliss. It links with higher structures in the cerebral cortex, and through various neural pathways can affect any organ or part of the body. States of mind, such as that created by meditation, act on the hypothalamus and affect its influence on certain hormones, such as thyroid stimulating hormone, growth hormone, testosterone, and vasopressin (which regulates blood pressure).

The amygdala and hippocampus are especially rich in receptors for estrogen, progesterone, and GnRH (gonadotropin releasing hormone), which fluctuate the most during perimenopause. GnRH, produced by the hypothalamus, signals the pituitary gland to release FSH and LH (see Chapter 2, pp. 25–27). The heightened activity of these hormones, which affects the brain's memory centers, leads to enhanced short-term and long-term memory during these years (Northrup, 2001). Losses, traumas, and disappointments that we thought were long forgotten may be remembered, renewing pain from the past. These processes can also give women new insights into their past experiences, and a suddenly clear understanding of their meanings. New connections are made between our own behaviors, the choices we made, and our current issues.

The hypothalamus not only influences regulation of hormones, but it is also influenced by hormones and many other neurotransmitters. It has receptors for the hormones progesterone, estrogen, DHEA, and testosterone, and for the neurotransmitters norepinephrine, dopamine, and serotonin that regulate mood and well-being. These hormones and neurotransmitters are affected by states of mind, thoughts, beliefs, diet, stress, and environment.

Another area of the brain that changes at perimenopause is the temporal lobe of the cerebral cortex. It is closely connected with the limbic system. The temporal lobe is the seat of language and conceptual thinking, and is also associated with enhanced intuition. Differences in relative levels of estrogen and progesterone affect the temporal lobe and limbic systems, leading to emotional volatility and the common experiences of irritability and anxiety. High levels of FSH and LH have neurotransmitter-type action, flooding these brain structures and driving the changes taking place in women's brains at midlife. It is of interest that FSH and LH levels remain high for many years after menses have stopped. The body probably does not expend the energy to produce these pituitary hormones for such a long time, unless they are serving another purpose than stimulating the ovaries to produce eggs (Northrup, 2001; Schultz, 1998).

The constant, high levels of FSH, LH, and GnRH beginning in perimenopause and continuing after menopause enhance the brain's intuitive capacities. These neuropeptide hormones also communicate to organs and cells throughout the body, providing a constant flow of intuitive communication and knowledge. This is thought to be the biological basis of mature women's wisdom. The ancient traditions which honored the "wise elder woman" or "wisdom of the crone" reflect the understanding that once women were able to "hold the pause" of their monthly cycles, they became imbued with insight and ways of knowing beyond what is ordinarily available. Now we understand this wisdom is not only drawn from age and experience, but also from the biological condition of the body after menopause.

These brain changes, and their effects on mental functions and the mind, give the menopausal woman a powerful opportunity for making major transformations. In the process, women gain the perspective to see their lives clearly, and the courage to face wounds of the past. The inner fire is there to take necessary steps that can break up destructive patterns, and support deep healing. Women can remold their lives to create fullness and satisfaction.

Mental Functioning

During perimenopause, women may begin to notice difficulty concentrating and staying focused on a task. Indeed, researcher and psychologist Claire Warga (1999) outlines seven categories of symptoms, including changes in thinking, speech, attention, short- and long-term memory, behavior, spatial skills, and sense of time that can bedevil women at this time. Forgetfulness occurs more often, sometimes to the point that you may need to make a list for nearly everything, or check two or three times to be sure the lights or stove burners are turned off. Many women say their mind is just not as sharp, and their brain seems to be functioning differently from before. Some call this "mental fog" or "fuzzy brain" and it is a very common symptom caused by hormones acting on the thinking sections of the brain. Fortunately, our brains and minds do recollect themselves as the hormones stabilize, and after a few years of fuzziness, women usually find that concentration and memory improve. Insight, the ability to see connections, clarity of vision, and enhanced intuition begin to emerge as women integrate the experience of menopause.

Moods and Depression

Moodiness and emotional reactivity increase during the transition through menopause. We may find ourselves crying or frustrated by small things that never set us off before. One women reported, "I cry about dog food commercials." Moods may swing from feeling bright and happy to sad and depressed in rapid order, often without any clear reason. Many women report feeling depressed. Going through menopause may bring on a first episode of clinical depression, even in women with no previous depression problems. Those with a history of depression are at even greater risk for developing it again during the menopause transition. All the hormonal, physiological, psychological, and emotional stresses during this time can destabilize one's body-mind system. If there is a weak link, menopause is sure to find it. The positive side to this is the opportunity women have to revisit old issues and wounds, using their accumulated life wisdom to bring these to higher levels of resolution.

Insomnia and Fatigue

Insomnia is a major problem for many women during menopause. It may be set off by night sweats and hot flashes that waken them five to ten times nightly. Needing to get up to use the bathroom is another cause of interrupted sleep. Often insomnia is caused by the mind staying too active, and not relaxing and letting go of problems and issues. Anxiety may flare up during the night, with rapid heartbeat, dizziness, and shakiness. Anxiety is the flip side of depression, and they often go together in alternating cycles. Frequently there is less energy and stamina and an overall feeling of being more tired than usual. For some women, this becomes profound fatigue that interferes with the ability to work and carry out activities.

Body Image Issues

Issues often arise around body image. Women may worry about being too fat, gray, wrinkled, sagging, or flabby. Around menopause many report gaining weight around the abdomen, hips, and thighs even though their diet and exercise have not changed. Metabolism appears to slow down around middle age, and routines that helped to lose weight and tone muscles in the past may not be as effective. Deeper issues around self-worth may be triggered, especially in Western society where older women are devalued and disempowered.

Many women entering midlife maintain trim figures and good muscle tone. In part this is caused by heredity, but the baby boomer generation tends to have lifestyles that support continued health and well-shaped body structures. It may be that this group of women is changing the way that Americans age. The woman who is attractive, shapely, productive, and functioning well into her 60s or 70s and beyond may be the norm for this group.

Change and Uncertainty

A type of "soul yearning" emerges at this time, a longing for something else or more in women's lives. We feel the need to be somehow different, and sense that menopause is propelling us toward change. You may feel that you just do not fit in your life any more. You may be disoriented, or feel discomforted about yourself. Women often ask themselves questions such as: "Where am I going? What is my life all about? Isn't there anything more?" These questions can precipitate spiritual crises or propel women on the path of spiritual unfolding (see Chapter 5).

STRESS

The far-reaching effects of stress may come home to roost during menopause. The body's stress response includes over 1,400 physical and chemical reactions, and over 30 different hormones and neurotransmitters (Childre & Martin, 1999). These messages, carried through the bloodstream and nervous system, affect almost every system in our bodies. When we are stressed, adrenaline quickly raises heart rate and blood pressure, tenses our muscles, and speeds up breathing, preparing us to confront the danger or run for our lives. The hormones noradrenaline and cortisol are also activated to prolong our state of heightened awareness and vigilance against danger. Even hours after the stress occurs, these hormones may remain high.

Cortisol, secreted by the adrenal glands, is known as the "stress hormone" because of its extensive role in the stress response. Balanced levels of cortisol are essential for the body to function normally, but levels that rise and stay high can damage many body systems. When we are under chronic stress and our bodies produce high levels of cortisol over long periods of time, the brain's internal thermostat resets and tells the adrenal glands to maintain this higher level of cortisol as though it were the normal amount. Chronically elevated levels of cortisol have been found to impair immune function, reduce proper glucose use, increase bone loss and promote osteoporosis, reduce muscle mass, inhibit skin regeneration, increase fat, especially around waist and hips, impair memory and learning, destroy brain cells, cause anxiety and sleep problems, and damage stomach, kidneys, and heart tissues (Childre & Martin, 1999).

Little daily stresses, accumulating day by day, week by week, and year by year take a greater toll than big disasters. We adjust to everyday stress, often coming to see it as the norm. But, our bodies are flooded by neurotransmitters and hormones that can destablilize our coping abilities. The body does not distinguish among the causes or reasons for stress. The exact same physiologic response is triggered by physical stressors such as cold and excess physical exertion, illnesses with fevers and pain, and emotional stressors such as anger, grief, fear, and despair. Even if we have a "good" reason for being stressed, the body still gets the message "danger, fear, alarm" and goes through its cascading stress response.

Just the Facts on Stress

According to the American Institute of Stress, up to 90 percent of all visits to primary care physicians result from stress-related disorders (Childre & Martin, 1999). In an article "Stress Busters" in *Psychology Today* (March/April, 2000), psychiatrist Robert Epstein writes that 40 percent of employee turnover is stress-related. In a Mayo Clinic study of people with heart disease, psychological stress was the strongest predictor of future heart attacks, cardiac arrest, and cardiac death (Allison et al., 1995). The medical community and public generally agree

> Usually, when there is some pathologic hindrance to the flow of blood in the heart vessels in humans it is associated with some psycho-social stress, such as bereavement, job insecurity, or marital strife. And in the vast majority of cases, heart palpitations at midlife are also associated with some types of psycho-social stress that may have been bearable before, but which are no longer tolerable.
>
> —Christiane Northrup, *Health Wisdom for Women*, May, 1999

that stress is a major contributor to heart disease, high blood pressure, ulcers, and nervous disorders (Shealy & Myss, 1993).

The litany of symptoms we humans experience as a result of stress in our lives is impressive: fatigue, headaches, irritability, changes in appetite, memory loss, low self-esteem, tooth grinding, cold hands, shallow breathing, nervous twitches, lowered sexual drive, changes in sleep patterns, illness caused by impaired immunity, back problems, anxiety, and depression (Balch & Balch, 2000). Bourne (1995) adds to this list adrenal exhaustion, sensitivity to light, worsening allergies or asthma, and low stress tolerance. Nutritional disorders both arise from and perpetuate stress. Examples are deficiencies of B vitamins, which are important for nervous system function, and buildup of free radicals that damage cell membranes.

Stress and Emotions

Emotional tension and strong emotional reactions are disruptive to our bodies. Research by the HeartMath Institute has found that negative emotions produce incoherent heart rhythms with imbalances in the heart's electromagnetic field. Resentment, anger, frustration, worry, disappointment, in fact, all negative emotional states, take a toll on the heart, brain, and body (Childre & Martin, 1999). The majority of illnesses result from an overload of emotional, psychological, and spiritual crises: emotions exert a controlling influence on the physical body. People who become ill identify with one or more of these eight stress patterns, according to Shealy and Myss (1993):

1. Unresolved or deeply consuming emotional, psychological, or spiritual stress

2. Disempowering belief patterns (low self-esteem, feeling unworthy)

3. Inability to give and/or receive love

4. Lack of humor, making everything a big deal

5. Not having choice about responses to and flow of events in life (conversely, trying to control events and people in one's life)

6. Abuse or neglect of physical body health, nutrition, exercise
7. Absence or loss of meaning in life
8. Denial of problems, issues, and situations that need attention

Adrenal Fatigue

Unrelenting, chronic stress over years usually leads to decreased adrenal gland function, called adrenal fatigue or "burn-out." The adrenals produce a significant proportion of the body's stress hormones and neurotransmitters. According to pioneer adrenal-stress researcher Hans Selye, the adrenals go through 3 phases: normal responses to stress, heightened secretion after prolonged stress, and decreased capacity to respond after long-term chronic stress (Hafen et al., 1992). When adrenal fatigue sets in, other endocrine glands such as the thyroid, pancreas, and ovaries/testes are affected. The adrenals are important in keeping up our energy level, assisting energy metabolism, and supporting sexual desire. By the time of menopause, many women have already reached the stage of adrenal fatigue. This further aggravates estrogen and progesterone imbalances, leading to many menopausal symptoms.

In healthy women, cortisol levels are highest on awakening in the morning, then slowly decrease over the day, reaching their lowest level around midnight. This pattern provides energy to get going and accomplish the day's activities, then allows for winding down in the evening, and easing into restful sleep for rejuvenation. For stressed-out women, however, this cortisol pattern may become inverted, with higher levels in the evening and night making restful sleep nearly impossible. In the mornings these women wake exhausted, with no energy to face the day. The nervous system of chronically stressed women causes decreased production of progesterone, which is one of the body's calming agents. This also leads to imbalances among estrogen, progesterone, and testosterone.

Chronic stress and adrenal fatigue may be exacerbated by inadequate nutrition, impaired digestion, and lower assimilation of nutrients. These less than optimal nutritional and digestive patterns often occur in people with high stress. Over time, these patterns can lead to immune system suppression, which increases

Keeping your adrenal glands healthy is important all through life because they assume a starring role at menopause: the primary producers of estrogen. Many symptoms we attribute to menopause—fatigue, lethargy, dizziness, headaches, forgetfulness, food cravings, allergies, and blood sugar disorders—may actually be more related to reduced adrenal function.

—Linda Ojeda, *Menopause Without Medicine*

susceptibility to infections, inflammatory conditions, autoimmune disorders, and cancers.

HOLISTIC APPROACH TO MOOD DISORDERS

Mood disorders are usually caused by both physiologic and psychologic factors. Holistic treatment addresses both of these aspects. Taking an antidepressant without attending to diet, exercise, and counseling may be like putting a Band-Aid on a bruise: the root cause is not addressed. The medication is often essential to provide stability and support so that a person can then work on the things that need to be changed in her life. Those who provide care to patients with mood disorders, from holistic practitioners to psychiatrists, seem to agree on this mind-body approach (Brody, 2000). Harvard-educated psychiatrist Jim Gordon, M.D., who directs the Center for Mind-Body Medicine in Washington, D.C., reports that even chronically depressed patients can be transformed by the physiologic effects of exercise, dietary changes, herbal supplements, and regular sessions of acupuncture and psychotherapy to the point that they may discontinue chemical antidepressants. In a *People* interview, Gordon said, "We have a great and largely untapped capacity to improve our own health" (Aug. 14, 2000).

Applying the mind-body approach specifically to women's emotional and physical health, Sichel and Driscoll (1999) have designed a program that may be used at all stages of a woman's life, but most effectively during the rigors of perimenopause. It is called NURSE, which translates into Nourishment, Understanding (study/learning), Rest and Relaxation, Spirituality, and Exercise. Cousens (2000) adds the importance of touching and being touched in a nurturing way, breathing correctly, cultivating a sense of humor, having a creative outlet, and staying connected to close friends and family. Such holistic lifestyle choices sometimes can resolve emotional problems. If not, they certainly support medical therapy.

Holistic treatment of mood disorders most often begins with nutrition which affects biochemistry. Maintaining normal blood sugar is essential, according to physician Linda Ojeda (2000) and health researcher Ann Louise Gittleman (1998). When blood sugar levels are controlled, claims Gittleman, depression may resolve in some individuals.

In his compelling book *Depression-Free for Life* (2000), psychiatrist and holistic practitioner Gabriel Cousens outlines a five-step program: four steps deal with what we ingest, and the fifth step focuses on an uplifting lifestyle. The rate at which you oxidize your food (slow, fast, or balanced) is the foundation for his program. Another holistic doctor, Rudolph Ballentine (1999), adds a good detoxing regimen (see Resources) to his program, maintaining that you need to get rid of the old before taking in the new.

The mind-body connection is critical to health and healing, according to Candace Pert, Ph.D., a ground-breaking biochemistry researcher. Pert first discovered brain receptors for opiates while working for the National Institutes of Health, and is a pioneer in the field of psychoneuroimmunology (PNI). This highly respected scientist proclaims the incredible interconnectedness of the body and the mind in her book, *Molecules of Emotions: Why You Feel the Way You Feel* (1997). She devotes an appendix to lifestyle choices that can help promote feelings of well-being. In summary, these are:

- meditation.
- movement (yoga, walking, and so on).
- spending time in nature.
- diet (when and what to eat; avoid refined sugar).
- avoid drugs (legal and illegal).
- drink water.
- when upset, try getting to the bottom (or core) of your feelings.
- wind down gradually at night (with bath, book, loving thoughts).
- live in an unselfish way.

The connections between thoughts and stress, and between temperament and stress levels are described by Dr. Christiane Northrup (2001). People are born with temperament types that generally persist throughout life. At one end of the spectrum, there are people who seem happy and positive regardless of what happens, and at the other are people who are anxious, worried, and fearful no matter how well their lives are going. This accounts for a good deal of individual responses to life events, although one can move along the spectrum with effort and intention toward greater positivity. Basic temperament colors women's responses to stress, and it does no good to deride yourself if your tendency is to worry. Taking actions to counteract stress is important, however, because women showing exaggerated responses to stress are at greater risk for depression, anxiety, and other emotional illnesses in later life (Heim et al., 2000).

Working with your perceptions is one way to counteract the effects of stress. If your thoughts and attitudes around events, demands, and challenges in life have a negative spin, your body keeps getting the message to prepare for danger. This sets in motion the adrenal hormones epinephrine and cortisol, with long-term effects that can lead to illness. Learn how to perceive things differently, to shift your definitions of events. Instead of thinking about emotions as good or bad, see them as messengers that are giving you guidance about the situation. Persistent negative emotions need to be resolved, or they become toxic to the body and mind. When emotions flow freely and find suitable expression, they are cleansing. Both happiness and sadness are necessary for the full human experience. For health, we need balance in emotions and their messenger molecules that carry biochemical communications throughout the body.

> It (menopause) has opened the doors to Pandora's box, and brought
> me to the threshold of a higher consciousness and increased self-
> understanding. Like Pinocchio, I am in the process of becoming more
> real, more human than ever before.
>
> —Geeta Dardick, "Opening Pandora's Box," in *Women of the 14th Moon*

REMEDIES AND THERAPIES

What might be a general prescription for finding emotional and mental balance as you enter menopause? Start with getting to know yourself better. Pay closer attention to your thoughts, feelings, and intuition (the small guiding voice within); become aware of the inner critic; practice gentleness and forgiveness with yourself.

Moodiness seems to be part of the territory for many women at this time of their lives. For this, as well as mild depression, we have some suggestions on managing symptoms. However, depression can be complicated. It is best to consult with your health care provider and not attempt to deal with it alone.

Here is a point worth noting for women who are considering only alternative therapies. One of the authors (Pam Jung) remembers going through a depression during menopause that left her rather nonfunctional. After she talked with a physician who explained what was happening chemically in her brain, she opted to forego her usual insistence on alternatives and started taking a pharmaceutical antidepressant. Over the course of three months, she was restored to normal and was then able to stop the medication, all the while feeling extremely grateful to Western medicine for getting her through this period.

Mood Disorders (Depression and Anxiety)

Mood symptoms during the menopausal journey are more the norm than the exception. Episodes of feeling panicky, sad, fearful, or unsure of being able to cope are common while hormones are gyrating, your lifestyle is changing, and questions such as "What am I going to do with the rest of my life?" are bubbling to the surface. If you have unfinished business (guilt, low self-esteem, or unresolved grief), this may be the time when your psyche prompts, "Here I am, deal with me." This may not be an easy opportunity, perhaps, but one that is staring you in the face.

Of course, there is a world of difference between feeling a little blue or anxious and being clinically depressed. Recognizing the difference is important. Treating yourself for mild depression with everything from herbs to talks with a good friend may work. But depression can be far reaching. New research indicates that

The Physiology of Depression

Depression is Western countries' second most disabling condition after heart disease (Marano, 1999). It is twice as common in women as in men (Balch & Balch, 2000). About 30 percent of patients seeking medical care report having depression. Overall, 23 percent of people have experienced some depression during their lifetime, and 6 percent of those have major depression (Marano, 1999).

Depression results from brain neurotransmitter dysfunctions, personality and childhood developmental problems, and psychosocial stresses such as divorce, unemployment, and bereavement. Lower levels of neurotransmitters (serotonin, norepinephrine, and beta endorphins) are circulating in the brain and tissues of depressed people. Many factors can affect our levels of these "feel-good" neurotransmitters, including chronic stress, unresolved issues, and poor nutritional patterns. Counseling or psychotherapy, antidepressant medications, and nutritional approaches can be helpful in resolving depression.

Serotonin comes primarily from tryptophan, an amino acid contained in most protein foods. We need to eat enough protein to supply tryptophan in the bloodstream. To move tryptophan from the bloodstream into the brain, we need carbohydrates by themselves. This is why a simple carbohydrate such as sugar improves mood—temporarily. Sugars cause a spike of neurotransmitters, then a sudden drop that leaves us feeling tired and moody. Complex carbohydrates, on the other hand, are needed for sustained release of tryptophan and beta endorphins.

Beta endorphins have a huge effect on self-esteem. When levels are high in the brain, we feel confident, but when they drop we can feel the "bag lady" syndrome, fearing we may end up alone and destitute. Sugar invokes beta endorphins, but we incur mood swings if we eat simple sugars instead of complex carbohydrates. We need complex carbohydrates for a regular supply of glucose, and protein for amino acids (which include tryptophan, tyrosine, GABA, and phenylalanine.) Also, a regular supply of carbohydrates is needed to release neurotransmitters into the brain—but these should be from whole grains, beans, and vegetables instead of hot fudge sundaes and chocolate chip cookies.

Thus, to promote positive mood and combat depression, one should eat three meals, including a healthy breakfast, have protein (amino acids) at each meal, eat complex carbohydrates regularly, and cut down on simple sugars.

during a depressive episode, neural circuitry is impaired and the whole body appears to be afflicted, not only the brain. In other words, depression is more than just brain chemistry. Proper diagnosis and treatment can be essential in preventing future episodes (Marano, 1999). Anybody who is dealing with depression that is severe, or who is having suicidal thoughts should not self-medicate or self-treat or attempt to manage this condition on her own (see Table 4–1).

DYSTHYMIC DISORDER (MILD OR MINOR DEPRESSION)

Mild depression, called dysthymic disorder, can be a serious long-term problem. Symptoms include sad/low mood, sleep disturbances, fatigue, problems concentrating and making decisions, and less interest in life. People suffer for years with unhappiness and misery, often thinking that it is just their personality. Continued guilt, self-doubt, and low energy erode their interpersonal skills, reducing their chances of social and job success. Dysthymic disorder occurs two to three times more often in women than men. But, it is not diagnosed as easily as major depression. Often women repeatedly seek medical care for "physical" symptoms that are actually signals of depression. Once diagnosed, dysthymic disorder can be treated effectively with antidepressant medications, therapy, and lifestyle choices. Criteria for dysthymic disorder are shown in Table 4–1.

MAJOR DEPRESSION

Significant clinical depression affects over 19 million adults in the United States, striking women twice as often as men (Markowitz, 1999). There are many varieties of depression, classified by the American Psychiatric Association in the *Diagnostic and Statistical Manual of Mental Disorders* (1994). Major depression can bring a person's life to a grinding halt. There are "vegetative" symptoms such as too much/too little sleep, loss of energy or appetite, and loss of interest or pleasure in activities. Cognitive function decreases with poor concentration, pessimism, and negative

> Pain is the great teacher. I woke before dawn with this thought. Joy, happiness, are what we take and do not question. They are beyond questions, maybe. A matter of being. But pain forces us to think, and to make connections, to sort out what is what, to discover what has been happening to cause it. And, curiously enough, pain draws us to other human beings in a significant way, whereas joy or happiness to some extent, isolates.
>
> —May Sarton, in Pat Streep, *An Awakening Spirit: Meditations by Women for Women*

TABLE 4-1	Criteria for Depression and Dysthymic Disorder

- Depressed mood most of the day
- Loss of interest or pleasure in activities
- Insomnia or hypersomnia
- Low energy or fatigue
- Low self-esteem, feeling worthless, guilt
- Poor concentration, difficulty with making decisions
- Feelings of hopelessness
- Loss of appetite, weight loss or gain
- Recurrent thoughts of death or suicide

To be called major depression, at least one symptom must be "depressed mood" or "loss of interest/pleasure" nearly every day for two weeks or more, in combination with five other symptoms. To be called dysthymic disorder, there must be "depressed mood" for most days over two years, plus three other symptoms.

Adapted from American Psychiatric Association. (1994). *Diagnostic and Statistical Manual of Mental Disorders* (4th Ed.). Washington, D.C.: American Psychiatric Press.

outlook. Mood is sad, depressed, and hopeless. Criteria for the diagnosis of major depression are shown in Table 4–1. Major depression often improves or resolves within weeks to months with appropriate antidepressant medication and therapy. According to Mary Ellen Copeland in *The Depression Workbook* (1993), 80 percent of major depressive disorders are highly responsive to treatment.

PREMENSTRUAL DYSPHORIC DISORDER (PMDD)

About 5 percent of women suffer from PMDD during their menstrual years. Think of it as exaggerated PMS that seriously interferes with work, school, or usual social activities and relationships, to the point that you would avoid social contact and have markedly decreased productivity. Symptoms peak in the 30s and continue until menses stop at menopause. PMDD is caused by excessive hormone responses during 7–10 days before menstruation starts. Hormones alter serotonin, noradrenaline, and GABA systems in the brain, as well as directly affect pelvic and breast tissues (Shah & Gonsalves, 1999).

Criteria for PMDD include five or more of the following symptoms (American Psychiatric Association, 1994), occurring in the week or so before menstruation, which improve after bleeding starts, and are gone during the week after menstruation (must have at least one of the first four):

- depressed mood, hopelessness, self-deprecating thoughts
- anxiety, tension, feeling on edge
- emotional lability (sudden sadness, tears, sensitivity to rejection)
- anger or irritability, increased interpersonal conflicts
- less interest in usual activities
- difficulty concentrating
- lethargy, fatigue, marked lack of energy
- hypersomnia or insomnia
- feeling overwhelmed or out of control
- breast tenderness, headaches, joint/muscle pain, bloating, weight gain

For the diagnosis of PMDD, women need to work with their health practitioner to chart symptoms daily for at least two consecutive cycles. These other conditions must be excluded: major depression, thyroid dysfunction, gynecologic disorders, and premenstrual exacerbation of migraine headaches, seizures, asthma, allergies, or genital herpes. PMDD is treated with lifestyle changes, support groups, diet (reduce caffeine, salt, refined sugars, and eat small meals containing complex carbohydrates), micronutrients (vitamins B_6 and E, calcium, magnesium), and a variety of medications including diuretics, antidepressants, hormones, and anti-hormones (Shah & Gonsalves, 1999).

What to Do for Depression

Much has been written about what to do when you find yourself depressed. It can be confusing, to say the least. Should you go first to a psychotherapist, to your doctor, to a meditation retreat, or to the kitchen? It is hard to say, as so much depends on how bad you feel and what your natural proclivities are. Maybe, indeed, approaching depression on all fronts is advisable, as depression is a whole-body disorder. Certainly, the stress-busting strategies are part of this package because chronic stress can easily result in anxiety and depression.

Two books that give holistic coping strategy training to people who suffer from anxiety are *Women and Anxiety* by psychiatrist Helen DeRosis (1998), which gives a 20-step behavioral modification program, and *The Anxiety and Phobia Workbook* by Edmund Bourne, M.D. (1995). Dr. Bourne states, "Nearly all practitioners who specialize in working with anxiety disorders rely on the cognitive-behavioral approach because of its proven effectiveness." He lists 12 strategies, three of which—abdominal breathing, relaxation training, and regular aerobic exercise—are at the top of the lists of most experts who have researched this field.

Remember, if your depression/anxiety is interfering with your life, it is important to get professional evaluation. Many self-rating scales provide guidelines for figuring out just how serious your depression may be. We provide one as an example (see Worksheet 4–1: Depression Checklist, on page 170).

EFFECTS OF ATTITUDE

Understanding of self begins by increasing one's awareness of habitual thoughts, attitudes, beliefs, and behaviors, and then using your innate wisdom to determine what is changeable and what is more intractable. Developing your spirituality can help improve your attitude to the extent that it helps you find some peace of mind amidst the many fears that beset us all. Focusing on the larger picture of consciousness helps us to see things with more perspective. See Chapter 5 for more on this topic.

While the art of positive thinking can be elusive, especially at difficult times in our lives, research has shown that simply forming one's face into a smile can help lift moods. Indeed, a sage from India, the late Paramahansa Yogananda, includes this practice in his book *Man's Eternal Quest* (1982). While forcing a smile may be the last thing you feel like doing, and you may feel phony doing it, nothing works better than trying an experiment. Practice smiling while looking in a mirror. It might even get you laughing, thus releasing pleasure endorphins into your system.

Emphasis on the positive has even brought forth a new school of psychology, called positive psychology, which seeks to understand and build human strengths such as optimism, love, responsibility, altruism, and tolerance. The father of this movement, Martin E. P. Seligman (past president of the American Psychological Association and now a professor at the University of Pennsylvania) says, "what looks like a symptom of depression—negative thinking—is itself the disease" (Wellner & Adox, May/June, 2000). He is now devoting his life to finding ways to change patterns of negative thinking.

Many spiritual teachers and modern-day therapists agree that what you resist, persists. Sometimes calm acceptance is the only way. While not an easy thing to hear, and certainly not a popular stance in this age of "everything is fixable," Sichel and Driscoll (1999) suggest that emotional disorders can be long-term problems. "Think of it as living with an illness like diabetes, heart disease, or arthritis that flares up at intervals. Since the condition is ongoing, often there is no 'cure.' You learn to live alongside the disorder and find a way to accept it that doesn't victimize you." They then recommend psychotherapy to help in this process.

A form of psychotherapy, called cognitive therapy, aims to eliminate depressive thoughts and attitudes, while another form, called interpersonal therapy, focuses on conflicted relationships or other current interpersonal difficulties.

DIET

Your diet may need changing. Foods such as dairy and dark leafy greens are high in calcium and magnesium and, thus, are calming. Complex carbohydrates, such as in fruits and vegetables, are relaxing. You may want to minimize wheat products because wheat gluten has been linked to mood disorders in susceptible people. Focus on fruits and vegetables (some raw, organic if available); soy products (preferably non-genetically modified); brown rice, millet, legumes, salmon, and turkey (which are high in spirit-lifting tryptophan) (Balch & Balch, 2000).

Avoid the artificial sweetener aspartame (Equal, NutraSweet), and foods high in saturated fats (hamburgers, French fries), which lead to sluggishness, slow thinking, and fatigue. Also avoid sugars, alcohol, caffeine, and processed foods.

Chocolate is a mixed blessing. Touted for years as a mood booster, it does enhance serotonin activity in the brain. However, it contains fats, sugars, and xanthines that can make PMS and moodiness worse when its effects wear off.

Small, frequent meals high in complex carbohydrates, balanced with a small amount of protein, help assure adequate serotonin levels in the brain, which contribute to positive feelings (Wurtman, 1986). You may be sensitive to some foods, although true food allergies are not that frequent. Food intolerances may decrease digestive efficiency and contribute to feeling unwell, which may lower your emotional state. Find a health care practitioner who specializes in nutrition and food intolerances; also, see Suggested Reading at the end of this chapter.

VITAMINS AND MINERALS

A complete, high-quality vitamin and mineral supplement is practically essential, given today's eating habits, food supply, and method of preparation. The B vitamins, especially pantothenic acid, and vitamin C, are helpful for mood swings according to Gittleman (1998). She also recommends taking calcium and magnesium if you are feeling particularly irritable. Take 500–1000 mg of magnesium before going to bed for a more restful night. Depressed people are often zinc deficient, so taking a daily dose of 50 mg may be helpful (Balch & Balch, 2000). One efficient way is to take zinc gluconate lozenges that dissolve in your mouth (and which might also protect against cold viruses).

ESSENTIAL FATTY ACIDS (EFAs)

Several experts agree that essential fatty acids (Omega-3 and Omega-6 in proper proportion) are helpful in combating depression (Balch & Balch, 2000; Gittleman, 1998; Cousens, 2000). As the Western diet provides far more Omega-6 and far less Omega-3 than we need, taking 1–2 tablespoons of Omega-3-rich flaxseed oil daily, or eating cold water oily fish such as salmon, tuna, herring, and mackerel, can bring these into balance. Perimenopausal women often find great relief for mood

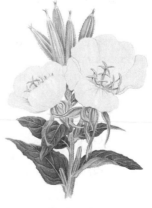

Evening primrose

changes, anxiety and irritability, and breast tenderness by taking evening primrose oil, a source of Omega-6 (Gittleman, 1998).

HERBS AND SUPPLEMENTS

Several herbs can be especially helpful for mood disorders during the menopause transition. The following mood modifiers need to be treated with respect. Even though they are "natural," they are also strong. The usual caveats apply; do not combine these with certain prescription drugs or with alcoholic beverages. Though this does not apply to most women at midlife, pregnant women or nursing mothers should avoid any herbs or supplements that have not been thoroughly researched or approved by their health care provider. Chronic symptoms that persist need to be evaluated by a health care provider.

St. John's wort, ginkgo biloba, and kava Richard Firshein, M.D., an expert in nutritional research and medicine, lists three herbs to ease mood disorders: St. John's wort, ginkgo biloba, and kava (dubbed the "feel-good herb of the South Pacific"); and two nutraceuticals: SAM-e and the amino acid tyrosine. In an interview in *Mother Earth News* (April/May, 2000), he discusses how he chooses what herb to recommend: "If someone comes to me and says they are depressed and are also feeling sluggish and have mental clouding or are not thinking clearly, that is when I start to think about ginkgo." He often recommends taking St. John's wort and kava together because, as he puts it, "Anxiety and depression often go together." Most often he prescribes kava when a person not only has a mood disorder but is also having insomnia. Kava is best when a person's anxiety is mild and of a short-term nature, such as when a particular event in his life causes stress. Gittleman (1998) recommends the herbs licorice root and vitex for mood swings.

Vitex (*Vitex agnus castus*)

Vitex has been used for centuries as a female balancing herb with primarily progesterone-like actions. Mood disorders may respond well, especially if low progesterone during menopause is an underlying factor. The benefits of vitex include the following:

- Promotes a healthy estrogen-to-progesterone balance.
- Helpful for PMS symptoms.
- Helpful for hormone and mood balancing; take 30–40 drops of tincture three to four times daily (Weed, 1992; *PDR for herbal medicines*, 1999).

St. John's Wort (*Hypericum perforatum*)

The scientific evidence for the effectiveness of this herb in treating mood disorders has been documented by a number of well-designed double-blind placebo-controlled trials and has received the stamp of approval from the German Commission E Report. Indeed, St. John's wort has been dubbed "Nature's Prozac" as its popularity in treating everything from the blues and PMS to moderate depression has increased with each published study. Davidson and Connor (2000) report that they are now conducting research to determine its effectiveness in major depression.

Some questions exist about which compound in this herb is the most effective in treating depression. While most St. John's wort extracts have traditionally been standardized to hypericin, new research (Laakmann et al.,1998) is pointing to hyperforin as the active compound in the therapeutic effect of the herb, especially at higher concentrations (5 percent hyperforin in 300 mg versus 0.5 percent). Reading labels on the preparations you buy is important, so that you know their ingredients and dosage recommendations. Taking an adequate dose of the herb for a long enough time (usually three months) is important also.

Summarized here are features, benefits, and dosages of St. John's wort:

- Mostly effective for mild to moderate depression, acting on serotonin in the brain
- Helps with SAD (seasonal affective disorder), anxiety, the "blues," and mild insomnia
- May be taken in many forms: as a tincture, tea, or in capsules
- Should not be taken with MAO inhibitors (a family of antidepressants); let your health care provider know you are taking this herb.
- May sensitize some to sunlight; use sunscreen and protective clothing.
- For depression most experts agree that tinctures/capsules of St. John's wort should be standardized (for either or both hypericin and hyperforin as noted above; take three times a day (for a total of between 900 mg and 1800 mg, depending on the standardization—read directions on the label) for at least four to six weeks to gauge effect. As a tea, take 1–2 teaspoons per cup, and drink three cups a day (Bender, 1998).

For comprehensive information about St. John's wort, read *Herbs for the Mind* by Drs. J. Davidson and K. Connor.

Kava (*Piper methysticum*)

Kava (also called kava-kava) is a good herb for easing anxiety, insomnia, and stress. There is considerable research on kava, and it has a long history of use by Polynesians for these purposes. Some researchers say the best results come from using a preparation standardized to 30–55 percent kavalactones; others say 70 percent. These chemical compounds have a soothing action on the amygdala, the brain's alarm center, thus modulating emotional processes. Kava enhances the action of other tranquilizers (it has been compared to Valium), as well as sleeping pills and antidepressants, so you may find it in combination with such herbs as St. John's wort. As there are some contraindications, it is important to read the manufacturer's recommendations.

- Do not use if you have Parkinson's disease, if you are pregnant or nursing, or if you have clinical depression (may increase danger of suicide) (*PDR for Herbal Medicines,* 1999).
- Do not take for longer than three months without a doctor's supervision.

For anxiety, stress, restlessness, nervousness, insomnia: capsules, tincture; extract of 70 percent kavalactones three times a day, 45–70 mg per dose, or 180–210 mg before bed. Bender (1998) reports that women in her practice often take kava instead of Valium or Xanax.

SAM-e   A substance our body synthesizes naturally, SAM-e (S-adenosyl-L-methionine), seems to relieve depression by boosting brain levels of serotonin and dopamine. "There's a correlation between low levels of SAM-e and depression," reports Richard Brown, M.D., associate professor of psychiatry at Columbia University in *Stop Depression Now* (1999). It is expensive and, according to Firshein (1998), "I have not, however, found that SAM-e is necessarily better or works in more patients than does St. John's wort. I can say that St. John's wort still holds its own and does quite well in comparison, and it's much cheaper."

Amino acid therapy   Amino acid therapy is mentioned by at least three experts (Firshein, Bourne, and Cousens) as important in alleviating mood disorders. Amino acids are the building blocks of proteins. Firshein (1998) recommends the amino acid tyrosine, which is depleted during stress, especially stress that is repetitive and ongoing, such as an exhausting work regimen. ". . . They get this sense of fatigue and depression, where they say, 'I just can't do anymore.' And they start to become anxious and depressed. Tyrosine can help alleviate that kind of problem." He recommends taking from 500 to 2,000 mg/day. In their discussion of tyrosine, Balch and Balch (2000) recommend 500 mg twice daily, during the day and at bedtime.

Edmund Bourne, M.D., director of the Anxiety Treatment Center in Santa Rosa, CA, reports that tyrosine is only one of four amino acids that he has used effectively in the treatment of depression and anxiety. The other three are:

- 5-hydroxy-tryptophan (different from the L-tryptophan that has been banned in the United States), which converts directly into serotonin. Fifty to 100 mg may be purchased over the counter, but higher doses require a prescription.

- Gamma amino butyric acid or GABA has a mildly tranquilizing effect, few side effects, and is non-addictive. He suggests 100–400 mg once or twice a day, taken with carbohydrates but not with protein (the first speeds up absorption, the latter competes).

- DL-phenylalanine (DLPA), as well as tyrosine, increases the neurotransmitter norepinephrine in the brain, which is depleted during times of stress.

Bourne reports that many of the depressed clients he has worked with have significantly benefited from taking one or the other of these amino acids (apparently not at the same time). He lists the guidelines to observe, such as taking them with carbohydrates and not protein, and starting with lower doses, then increasing the dose in four-day increments to a point where you feel relief. It takes a couple of weeks to determine if it is working, says Bourne. If one does not, then try another. Do not take these amino acids if you are pregnant, have PKU (phenylketonuria), are taking MAO-inhibitor antidepressants, or have high blood pressure.

While amino acid therapy seems to work, determining which amino acid to take for which condition can be confusing. Cousens's (2000) work is very user friendly, and also comprehensive. However, trying to figure out your personal profile may be too overwhelming, and you may want to enlist the aid of a practitioner.

LIGHT THERAPY

For those women who find that their moods seem to get worse during winter, getting more light may help. Balch and Balch (2000) suggest increasing the light in a particular room to 10,000 lux of full-spectrum light and spending at least ½ hour a day there. Full-spectrum lights are available on-line and in various catalogs (see Resources).

Painting walls or furnishings can also affect winter moodiness. According to Balch and Balch (2000), the colors green and sunshine yellow can help alleviate depression, and pink helps ease anxiety. The field of color therapy is rapidly expanding, and some hospitals are beginning to use blue ambient light or wall colors in surgery or emergency rooms for their calming effect.

COUNSELING AND SUPPORT

Seeking the assistance and support of others when coping with depression or anxiety can provide just the boost women need to get through this trying time. Many forms of professional therapy are available. Cognitive therapy is widely used, and helps you to identify destructive thoughts and defuse them. Insight therapy helps you identify what you are feeling, get some idea where it is coming from, and use various techniques to change your mental habits and reactions to more positive and effective patterns. Couples may want counseling to improve communication and enhance their relationship. Most therapists provide methods for emotional release and restructuring emotional responses to people and events.

Talk to trusted friends and advisors, especially if they are adept at mirroring techniques (reflecting back to you what they think they heard you say). Being heard by a caring person provides immense support when you are coping with emotional difficulties.

Deal with anger/anxiety/grief through support groups. Most communities have numerous types of support groups, many of which are free. Grief support groups have been gaining in popularity as people realize the importance of healthy grieving and completing the grief process in a way that brings positive resolution.

Down through the ages women have talked, shared, and congregated with other women, often around a task such as quilting, grinding grain, or preparing a meal. Indeed, it is this tendency for females to "tend and befriend" that seems to increase during times of stress, according to researcher Shelley Taylor, a psychology professor at the University of California, Los Angeles. This communing acts as a pressure release valve from social and psychological pressures. It can function as a tool of learning and training (as we hear how others have dealt with a challenge), a way to feel nurtured and reassured, a way to explore our perceptions and dream together, a place to give and to receive emotional support, to learn how to trust and how to handle conflict. Berry and Traeder (1995) explore the richness of friendship in *Girlfriends: Invisible Bonds, Enduring Ties.* (See Appendix B for Starting a Woman's Group).

Friends, you and me . . .
You brought another friend . . .
And then there were three . . .
We started our group . . .
Our circle of friends . . .
And like that circle . . .
There is no beginning or end.

—Anonymous. In Marilyn Nyborg,
Through Women's Eyes

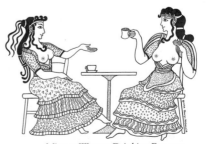

Minoan Women Drinking Expresso.
Reproduced with permission.
Copyright © 1994 Sharyn McDonald.

MEDITATION, RELAXATION, AND PRAYER

Spirituality is being recognized as an essential dimension of humans that influences our state of health and well-being. Larry Dossey, M.D., author of *Prayer Is Good Medicine: How to Reap the Healing Benefits of Prayer* (HarperCollins, 1997), provides many examples of how prayer affects both physical and emotional healing. Gregg Braden, author of *The Isaiah Effect* (2000), describes a "lost mode of prayer" and its effectiveness. The Essenes of biblical times blended mental intention with deep love to arrive at a heart-feeling state in which they experienced a person as healed. They held the vision that health and wholeness already existed within the person. According to Braden, this technique actually calls into expression a potential reality that is always present: that we *are actually already* healthy and whole. This is similar to Jesus Christ's instructions that we should "pray believing" and that our "faith has healed us."

Well-known scientist Candace Pert (1997) claims "meditation practiced early morning and early evening, routinely, even religiously, is I believe, the single quickest, easiest, shortest, and cheapest route to feeling good . . ." The benefits of meditation for physical and emotional relaxation, health and inner harmony have been extensively studied (Murphy & Donovan, 1997; Karpen, 1996; Austin, 1999). Chapter 5 covers spiritual practices and meditation in more detail.

Lifting the Black Cloud of Depression with Prayer

One man found his salvation from depression in a prayer meeting. After describing the history of his illness and his feelings of despair to the twelve people present at this meeting in 1997, author and counselor Douglas Bloch (2000) was then asked to shift away from his symptoms and imagine what wellness would look like to him. He then described in detail the thoughts, feelings, and behaviors he might experience if he were healed of his affliction, with the group affirming that his desire was already a reality and that they would hold this vision of his wellness in their consciousness until they met again in 30 days. To Bloch's amazement, the "black cloud of depression began to lift" within 72 hours after the prayer support began, and within 90 days he was "completely free of my symptoms." A miracle? Perhaps. Whatever the explanation, Bloch said his "struggles with depression are finally over."

Relaxation and breathing techniques are widely used to calm body and mind, to relieve muscle tension, and improve numerous ailments. These techniques use combinations of repeating a sound or phrase, focusing on the breath, quieting the thinking process, and tensing then relaxing body parts progressively. Heart rate, breathing, blood pressure, and muscle tension are reduced, and a calm mental state is invoked (Lesser, 1999; Kabat-Zinn, 1990; Benson & Stark, 1996; Sovik, 1997).

See Worksheet 4-2 on page 170 for a relaxation technique that you can practice on your own.

EXERCISE AND YOGA

Exercise to get those endorphins (the "feel-good" chemical messengers in the brain) flowing. Body tensions, which affect the mind, are released. Stuck energy gets moving. Start with a 25-minute walk three times a week, or a swim at the health club.

Hatha yoga, which is a combination of body postures and breathing techniques, is used in many programs to reduce stress, anxiety, and depression. Deepak Chopra, M.D., is a strong proponent, as is Jon Kabot-Zinn, Ph.D., of the University of Massachusetts, whose yoga Stress Reduction and Relaxing Program has been hugely successful over the past two decades. Amy Weintraub reports in *Psychology Today* (November/December, 2000) the compelling story of a woman with a history of paralyzing bipolar depression who, after she left a psychiatric hospital, decided to learn hatha yoga in a desperate attempt to stabilize herself. Her yoga practice, along with the antidepressant Paxil to which she had not responded before, put an end to her severe mood swings. A certified yoga instructor since 1994, she now teaches what she believes "has literally saved my life" to other depression sufferers.

SERVICE TO OTHERS

Give, as in service to others. This getting "out of yourself" not only helps the world in the larger sense, it helps us individually. According to Borysenko (1996), giving results in a stronger immune system and longer life, alleviates depression, and generates self-esteem.

NURTURE YOURSELF

Put things that make you happy onto your calendar, as you would any appointment or task. They may be something you do with others (a movie, lunch), or by

When you learn to live for others, they will live for you.

—Paramahansa Yogananda, *Man's Eternal Quest,* 1982

> What if a woman trusted her own tears enough to listen to them. . . .
> What if she trusted her anger, her irritation, her illness, even her
> depression, as signs that her own life was calling to her?
>
> —Judith Duerk, *Circle of Stones: Woman's Journey to Herself*

yourself (a hike, reading a good book, an evening of pampering). Some suggestions follow, but of course you will have many ideas of your own:

- Pamper yourself regularly (a soothing lavender oil bath in candlelight with
  classical music playing).
- Carve out some time to read—just for fun.
- Keeping a journal can be magical. Write in long hand or on your computer,
  at least a couple of times each week.
- Cry. Tears, research has discovered, soothe and relieve stress. The fear many
  women have is that once they start, they won't stop; trust yourself more
  than that.
- Drop "should" and "ought to" from your vocabulary.
- Read Judith Duerk's *Circle of Stones: Woman's Journey to Herself* (1989). It is
  a poetically sensitive, nurturing, and gentle treatment of depression that
  feels like a warm hug.

Handling Disempowering Thoughts

When you become aware of thoughts that do not enhance your life,
repeat the following steps over and over again.

- Take at least three deep, slow breaths, counting 10 on the inhale,
  hold for 10, and count 10 on the exhale. This is a powerful calming
  yogic breathing technique. The point is to relax and come into the
  present time (not past or future).
- Repeat something: a song, a chant, a mantra (such as "Om, peace,
  amen"). This also brings you into present time.
- Once relaxed and calm, become a nonreactive observer of your
  thoughts and feelings. Just notice them come and go, all the while
  trying to stay out of judging whether they are good or bad. You
  may be thinking you have failed and are feeling anxious about it.

(Continued on next page)

This thought could start a cascade of negativity, ending with a tight stomach and heart palpitations and a sense of utter worthlessness. The moment you become aware of this thought, become the neutral observer: "I am having this thought. It is only a thought. I am letting this thought go." All the while remember to breathe. The cascade slows or stops. This takes practice, so do not be hard on yourself if you do not "get it" for a while.

- Once you have applied this "first aid" and stabilized yourself, you can move into cognitive thinking (whereby you ask yourself a series of questions as to the validity of the thought you just had), or you can move into active creation of positive thoughts and feelings. An affirmation (I am safe, I am sound. All good things come to me; they bring me peace) can work wonders, as can a visualization (see yourself looking radiant as you contemplate breaking waves on the beach or walking through a lush colorful garden). Reassuring self-talk is yet another technique, as in "Millions of women have lived through this and are doing so now. They endured and so will I" (Warga, 1999).

CHECK OUT PHYSICAL PROBLEMS

Several physical problems may cause symptoms of depression and anxiety. If you have not had an examination or laboratory tests recently, it is a good idea to get these checked out. Sometimes a fairly straight-forward dysfunction of an organ or gland can underlie mood disorders. Some common problems are:

- Thyroid dysfunctions—too much thyroid hormone (hyperthyroidism) may cause anxiety and insomnia; too little hormone (hypothyroidism) may lead to lethargy, fatigue, low energy, weight gain, and depressed mood.
- Anemia—low hemoglobin or decreased numbers of red blood cells cause anemia, which leads to fatigue, loss of stamina, and slower healing.
- Diabetes—inability to properly metabolize and utilize carbohydrates because of pancreatic dysfunction may cause diabetes, leading to fatigue, lethargy, slow healing, and weight gain.
- Hypoglycemia—rapid drops of blood glucose following high carbohydrate meals or snacks lead to shakiness, irritability, poor concentration, anxiety, weakness, and dizziness.
- Hormone deficiency—dropping levels of estrogen or progesterone during menopause often affect mood and energy levels.

How to Test Your Own Thyroid

You may want to get a basal body thermometer. It is large and has more space between tenths of degrees for easier reading. For 30 days in a row, when you first wake up, do not move beyond putting a thermometer under your arm pit. Leave it there for 10 minutes (as you meditate or pray). Record results. If the average reading comes out to 97 degrees or below, you may have a thyroid deficiency and want to get more testing.

ADRENAL CARE

The adrenals are important in energy level and sexual desire. For most of us, the adrenals are already stressed by the time we get to menopause. Strengthening the adrenals naturally with diet and vitamins is a good starting point. Douglas Williams, M.D., responded in his newsletter to a medical journal report on DHEA, which claimed that women with adrenal insufficiency given 50 mg DHEA daily for four months had several of their adrenal hormones return to normal: "To me, using DHEA, an adrenal hormone, before trying to strengthen the adrenal glands, is putting the cart before the horse. . . . I recommend using them (hormones) as a last resort." (*Alternatives,* October, 2000)

To support the adrenals naturally:

- Nutritional researcher Gittleman (1998) recommends diet and supplements that include a good B complex, lots of vitamin C (500 mg every 3 hours), adrenal gland extract, green and yellow-orange vegetables, and sea vegetables as a condiment.

- Balch and Balch (2000) recommend vitamin B complex injections as well as a sublingual tablet, and 3,000–10,000 mg of vitamin C per day when the body/mind is under stress.

- Ojeda (2000) suggests at least 400 IU/day of vitamin E and 15–30 mg/day of zinc. She goes on to recommend avoiding or reducing sugar, fried foods, alcohol, tobacco, processed foods, and salt while emphasizing fresh, whole, raw fruits and vegetables, and whole grains. To add zinc to your diet, try eating oysters, beef, turkey, crab, sunflower seeds, almonds, and beans.

Reduce or eliminate caffeine to take care of your adrenals. According to Williams (October, 2000), studies have shown that adrenaline increased by 80 percent after three cups of coffee were consumed. That is equivalent to a stressful work situation or an emotionally-charged movie. Cola beverages are just as damaging to the adrenals. Find alternatives or drink caffeine-laced drinks in moderation.

A mind/body approach that elicits the relaxation response, through such techniques as meditation, visualization, and progressive relaxation, helps keep the stress hormones adrenaline and cortisol in check. This helps reduce chronic adrenal stimulation and the fatigue caused by over-secretion of adrenal hormones.

Hormones and Mood Disorders

Many women find relief from mood symptoms by taking hormones, either in pharmaceutical or phytochemical forms. However, are hormones helpful for women with clinical depression? Also, what are estrogen's effects on preserving mental functioning as women go through menopause and age?

HORMONES AND DEPRESSION

Estrogen enhances the action of the neurotransmitters norepinephrine and serotonin. These normal brain chemicals are known to create more positive feelings and mood. By keeping brain levels of these neurotransmitters higher, estrogen is acting to some extent as an antidepressant. As estrogen levels decline during menopause, women may experience symptoms of depression (Shah & Gonsalves, 1999). Lack of adequate estrogen causes lethargy and depression, while an excess of estrogen, which often occurs during perimenopause, can cause irritability, over-sensitivity, and insomnia (Lee, 1999).

Several studies have found that estrogen replacement therapy is associated with fewer depression symptoms (Palinkas & Barrett-Connor, 1992; Whooley, Grady, & Cauley, 2000). Women with Alzheimer's disease with higher levels of native estradiol had lower depression scores (Carlson, Sherwin, & Chertkow, 2000).

Progesterone is thought to enhance a sense of well-being and bring balance into women's hormonal systems. Pharmaceutical progestins (such as Provera), however, act differently than natural progesterone and often cause moodiness and depression (Lee, 1999).

ESTROGEN AND MENTAL FUNCTION

Estrogen seems to enhance some aspects of mental functioning. Women are eager to know if taking ERT will maintain memory and mental sharpness, and prevent Alzheimer's disease. Hormones such as estrogen act as powerful neurotransmitters, or messenger molecules, that communicate with the brain and endocrine glands as well as the reproductive organs. In the brain, estrogen increases the number of dentritic spines produced by neurons, and makes these branch-like projections from the nerve cells more flexible. Estrogen also increases serotonin (a "feel-good" neuropeptide) and acetylcholine (which aids communication between neurons). By keeping blood vessels flexible, estrogen helps prevent hardening of arteries, which may lead

Hormones Work Miracles for Ellen

Ellen is a vivacious, energetic woman in her late 40s. Her career in marketing has been going well. For about six months she has been in a new relationship with "a wonderful, kind and loving man," with hopes for a lasting and satisfying union. Always emotionally volatile to some degree, Ellen's mood swings have gotten much more severe since she entered perimenopause. For two or three years she had tried alternative remedies, such as herbs, relaxation, exercise, and meditation. These helped at first, but now they no longer keep her emotional outbursts under control, especially during the day or two before her period starts. She continues to have regular, monthly periods with heavier bleeding than before. Ellen sought help from me (Lennie Martin, RN, FNP) because she was afraid that her PMS symptoms were going to damage her relationship, saying: "I get so edgy and lash out at him about anything. I'm suspicious and jealous even though he doesn't give me any reason to think he isn't faithful. At its worst, I just want to curl up in bed and not face the world. I cry for no reason, and can't seem to stop." She also could not work as effectively, and often needed to take a day off. Since Ellen had tried alternative methods, we agreed that hormone therapy would be her best option now. She started on 1.0 mg estradiol with 200 mg progesterone added the last 10 days of her cycle—human identical hormones, to act more naturally in her body. Ellen noticed results right away. Her moods were more stable with much less irritability and reactiveness. She could continue working during the premenstrual phase. As she puts it: "The hormones worked miracles for me. I've got my life back, and my relationship is better than ever."

to a lack of oxygen and nutrient supply to brain cells. Estrogen also appears to limit deposition of a fatty substance (Beta-amyloid) that is key in developing destructive plaques leading to Alzheimer's disease (Col, Legato, & Schiff, 1998).

Despite these beneficial physiological effects, there are still questions about how much effect ERT actually has on improving mental function. Dr. Barbara Sherwin is a leading researcher on estrogen's brain and mental effects in postmenopausal women. She believes that estrogen does enhance some aspects of cognitive function in healthy women (Askew, 1998). Her research found that estrogen has a specific effect on verbal memory skills, and enhances capacity for new learning. Verbal memory includes recall of words, names, and sentences. Other mental functions such as spatial memory were not affected (Sherwin, 1998, 1999; Kampen & Sherwin,

Because of their tremendous range of effects—from beneficial to harmful—estrogens were dubbed the "angels of life and the angels of death," by Dr. Ercole Cavalieri, a scientist who has spent the last three decades studying their effects . . . we now know at least one gene-related mechanism of action that connects estradiol to cancer promotion.

—John Lee, *What Your Doctor May Not Tell You About Premenopause*

1994). Dr. Sherwin concluded that estrogen may prevent the decline in verbal memory that occurs with normal aging in women (Sherwin, 2000).

Other studies were not so conclusive. In one, higher estradiol levels improved verbal memory and recall, while lower estradiol levels were associated with better visual memory (Drake et al., 2000). Higher native estrogen levels provided no benefits for cognitive function in a study of 500 postmenopausal women not taking ERT (Yaffe et al., 1998). Data from the Nurses' Health Study (over 2,000 older women) did not find better cognitive function in hormone users, although they did have better verbal fluency (Grodstein et al., 2000).

ALZHEIMER'S DISEASE AND ESTROGEN

Changes in mental functions that occur during menopause, such as fuzzy thinking and forgetfulness, are not symptoms of Alzheimer's disease or dementia. By age 75, only about 12 percent of women have some form of dementia. Most women find their mental and cognitive abilities return to normal after the hormone fluctuations of perimenopause level out. There is some evidence that estrogen may decrease risk or delay onset of Alzheimer's (Sherwin, 1999). However, it cannot reverse memory loss, probably because too many brain cells have been damaged by the disease process (Science Daily, 2000).

Education level is a powerful predictor of cognitive function at any age. Estrogen therapy appears to have more impact on improving mental abilities in less-educated older women (Matthews et al., 1999). Brain training and continued use of mental abilities is a major factor in preserving cognitive function in later life. The normal decrease of brain cells with aging seems to be a pruning process, removing non-essential neural pathways while dendritic connections that help us make complex associations increase. These new connections help us synthesize our life experiences (Northrup, 1998).

Fatigue and Low Energy

Feeling tired may be caused by both physical stressors (such as disease) and mental/emotional stress. These are so intertwined as to be inseparable. The mind, however, plays a vital role in our management of energy resources. Remember what it feels like to come home from work exhausted, believing that the only thing possible is to eat and go to bed, only to discover an invitation to something fun on the answering machine. Exhaustion somehow flies away. Spirits are revived, fatigue is banished. This is a good indication that our mind and emotions are major factors in our tiredness. The key is the attitude with which we meet challenges in our lives. Perceiving events as too stressful can easily turn into a cascading effect: as we feel more emotionally drained, we do not take care of ourselves, and that contributes to our low energy, which makes us more tired. If it is difficult to minimize the stressful situations in life, we can at least learn how to relax and achieve a level of peace that comes in part through acceptance and in part through good coping strategies.

DIET AND SUPPLEMENTS

- Erratic blood sugar can cause a number of problems, including mood disorders and lowered vitality and stamina, which are often expressed as feeling fatigued. Moderate your intake of refined sugar and flour products, caffeine, and alcohol, because these disturb blood sugar and are energy robbers. Nutritional expert Gittleman (1998) recommends always eating a balance of protein and healthy fats to complex carbohydrates every time you eat, because protein and fats have a stabilizing influence on blood sugar, producing steady, long-term energy instead of a short burst followed by a quick letdown.

- You also may need more protein, especially if you are a vegetarian (there is some controversy about the types and amounts of protein, see Chapter 3).

- Specific vitamins (especially A, C, and the Bs) and minerals (magnesium, potassium, and chromium) are helpful in relieving fatigue. While chromium is best taken as a supplement, magnesium and potassium can both be obtained by eating dairy, fish, meat, avocados, apricots, bananas, and brown rice (Balch & Balch, 2000).

- Eat more live food, including fresh and organic vegetables and fruit.

- Food intolerances can cause lethargy. Test for intolerances by an elimination diet.

- Drink pure water, at least 8 glasses a day and more in hot weather; dehydration is common, according to some experts, and causes not only fatigue but aging (Batmanghelidj, 1995).

> When I am caught in a downward spiral of negative feelings, I instantly know that I am out of touch with my inner guidance and that I'm giving too much attention to what I don't want.
>
> —Christiane Northrup, *Women's Bodies, Women's Wisdom*

EXERCISE

Aerobic exercise gets the body oxygenated, thus adding to a sense of vitality. Smaller amounts done regularly are most beneficial; for example, walk 40 minutes three times a week.

HERBS

- Siberian ginseng (*Eleutherococcus senticosus*) is the herb most often recommended to alleviate fatigue and improve endurance, although those with hypoglycemia, high blood pressure, or a heart disorder should avoid this herb. Recommended dose: 70 mg of extract once in the morning and once in the evening. If taking powdered herb, the dose is ½ teaspoon twice a day. Buy a preparation that is standardized from 0.8 to 1 percent eleuthrocytes.
- Supporting the liver, which is a major detoxifier of the body, may be accomplished with dandelion.
- Ginkgo biloba has been shown in recent research (Ojeda, 2000) to increase the uptake of glucose by brain cells and improve the transmission of nerve signals.
- Chinese herbal formulas can be very helpful. See a health practitioner who specializes in these, as there are many herbs and understanding how to best use them is complicated. Michael Tierra's book *Planetary Herbology* can serve as a guide to Chinese herbs.

OTHER CONSIDERATIONS

- Take a series of deep breaths, slowly and deliberately, when you become aware that you are feeling stressed. Then do some easy stretching.
- Fear, resistance, sadness, grief, and unhappiness all can make you feel drained. You may need to resolve the pressures in your life around relationships, job, and lifestyle.
- An attitude adjustment may be needed to change a habit, such as from saying "no" to life (resistance) to saying "yes" (acceptance) instead. That does not mean to avoid taking action to try and change things. Rather, it refers to a state of mind that leads to serenity and peacefulness.
- Do your own preliminary home test of your thyroid functioning (see page 145), especially if your lethargy is accompanied by other symptoms, such as coldness, weight gain, depression, and inability to concentrate. If your thyroid is low, see your health provider or do a few months of thyroid support herbs and supplements.

- Check out acupuncture, which frees the body's chi (life force) to flow unimpeded, thus adding to your sense of vitality.
- You simply may not be getting enough sleep (see Chapter 3 for sleep aids).
- If fatigue is severe and persistent, see your health care provider for further testing.

Maca (*Lepidium meyenii* and *Lepidium peruvianum*)

This Peruvian herb dates back to the Incas 2,000 years ago. It helps balance the entire endocrine system, enhances vitality, and gives the libido a lift. Backing up claims from traditional cultures, studies today show that the benefits of maca include anti-fatigue and aphrodisiac effects, among others. According to Michael Gerber (November, 2000), doctors in South America have also used maca to treat PMS, osteoporosis, memory disorders, and such menopause symptoms as hot flashes, vaginal dryness, night sweats, depression, and male impotence.

Skin and Hair

The condition of the skin and hair are important to most women. Midlife women notice skin changes such as more dryness, fine wrinkles, and less fullness and resilience. Skin may tend to sag or appear slack. Hair becomes more coarse and dark on the face, and more thin and gray on the head. While you want to look your best, it is also important to make peace with skin and hair changes. Your inner beauty and joyfulness gives the face a glow that goes far beyond mere surface looks.

There are many approaches to preserving the health of skin at midlife, or healing skin damage that has occurred. Principles of skin care include daily cleansing using a pH balanced soap or cleanser, using a toner to close pores after cleansing, promoting skin turnover and new growth with an exfoliant and antioxidant, providing moisture to keep cells plumped up, and protecting skin from sun damage. The amount of moisturizing will depend upon whether your skin is dry or oily. Products that contain fruit acids (alpha hydroxy, beta hydroxy, glycolic acids) are good exfoliants, and you can gently scrub your face with a washcloth to remove dead cells and promote new cell growth. Antioxidants include creams with vitamin C, E, or A, and green tea extract. Retinoic acid derivatives are powerful antioxidants, but may cause redness and sun sensitivity. Topical estrogen or progesterone face and neck creams are also used by some women (most need a prescription). Here are some additional tips on skin and hair care from Dr. Ojeda (2000):

- Keep out of the direct sun; protect your skin with hats and sunscreen.
- Do not smoke. Nicotine and tars from cigarettes lead to significant skin damage, and are a leading cause of massive fine wrinkles and dry, sagging skin at midlife.
- Minimize chemical drinks (cola, diet drinks), coffee, tea, and alcohol.
- Drink plenty of water (at least two quarts of pure water a day).
- Do not lose weight too rapidly (two pounds a week at most), as this leads to sagging.
- Keep the air in your home moist; spray mists of water to help bring moisture back to your face (especially if you live in a dry climate, work in air-conditioning, or fly often).
- Exercise regularly.
- Diet: Eat high-quality protein and complex carbohydrates (the less processed the better); minimize your intake of excess oil, saturated fats, and hydrogenated spreads; reduce sugar and refined flours and grains in your diet.
- Supplement your diet with antioxidants (vitamins A, C, and E, and the mineral selenium) and oils such as flaxseed oil.
- Evening primrose oil, flaxseed oil, and olive oil are recommended by Gittleman (1998).

Sleep

Getting enough restful sleep is important for emotional balance and mental functioning. McCall (March/April, 2000) cites research from Stanford University and the *New England Journal of Medicine* emphasizing the sleep-robbing effects of the following:

- Medical conditions, such as depression, snoring/apnea, hormone changes, unrelieved pain
- Diet (caffeine, alcohol)
- Tobacco
- Medications, such as cold formulations and over-the-counter diet pills (which contain stimulants), and some prescription medications

The following are sleep-helping aids found in this research:

- Winding down, relaxing, and letting worry go in the evening by stopping work, food, exercise, and drinking a couple of hours before bedtime
- Making the bedroom a place for sleep only, not watching TV or doing projects

- Taking herbs (valerian root and kava tinctures, chamomile tea) and using fragrant, relaxing lavender oil in a bath or via a massage
- Doing calming yoga postures

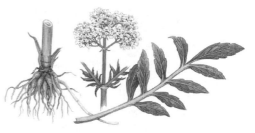

Valerian

Candace Pert (1997) suggests that neuropeptide informational molecules actually link our biological clocks to the motions of the planets. According to Pert "your quality of sleep—and wakefulness—is likely to improve the more closely your retiring and your rising are linked to darkness and daylight. If you get to sleep between 10 and 11 P.M., most of you will be able to wake up naturally and rested with the sunrise, if not before."

Gittleman (1998) reports that perimenopausal insomnia (as well as mood swings and anxiety) can be helped with vitamins and minerals: a good B complex; 1000 mg of vitamin C three times daily; 400–1200 IU of vitamin E daily; and 500 to 1000 mg of magnesium before bedtime. Once the hormones settle down and you are postmenopausal, cut back to 1000 mg of vitamin C and 400 IU of E daily.

Sex and Libido (Sex Drive)

It has been said that the most important sex organ is the mind. Libido and sexual response are affected more by emotions and mental states than by purely physical factors (see Chapter 3). Many women wonder what to do about their sexuality during menopause. It is not uncommon to feel as though one's libido has gone on vacation. We may wonder "is it all over? Is this part of my life done?" Actually, there are a number of ways that sexuality can be supported during this phase. Following are some suggestions for supporting healthy sexual functioning during and after menopause.

DIET

Keep your endocrine glands healthy and full of vitality by such methods as eating a nutritional diet (see Chapter 3), avoiding excesses of energy-sapping foods such as highly processed, fat-loaded junk foods, and minimizing stress.

VAGINAL DRYNESS

If this condition is present, as it often is as we achieve menopause, it can interfere with your sex life, causing painful intercourse and reducing sexual pleasure.

For the Partners in Our Lives: Sex

Women during menopause go through phases of decreased interest in sex (although for a few, the sex drive is higher). They may be less responsive both physically and emotionally, or, sexual desire can fluctuate—leading to confusion on the partner's part. The best approach is tolerance and understanding. These are challenging times for women, and a little support goes a long way in keeping the relationship on solid ground. Women may be more direct about likes and dislikes and less willing to engage in unsatisfying sex. Look at this as an opportunity to improve communication to give it a positive spin.

Around menopause, vaginal tissues are thinner and less moist. This can cause discomfort and further reduce interest in sex. You can use a good lubricant, such as Women's Group Formulas, Replens, or Sylk (see section on vaginal dryness). Water-based lubricants such as KY jelly or Astroglide are helpful. Take enough time in love-making to be well-aroused, and be gentler overall in sexual activity. Vaginal muscle tone and increased thickness and moisture of the vaginal mucosa (cells lining the vagina) may be aided by using estrogen vaginal cream, most often estriol or estradiol, or a combination of these. Vitamin E suppositories or oral capsules can also help. Increased intake of flaxseed oil and soy products provides nutritional support of vaginal tissues.

It may help to remember that in heterosexual relationships men and women often approach sex from different viewpoints. Men seem more interested in physical pleasure while women care more about a loving relationship. Understanding and honoring these different perspectives helps create the heart connection that keeps relationships healthy. Lesbian couples may also need to communicate with greater sensitivity, and to accommodate different sexual rhythms during the menopause transition.

There are several ways to ease the dryness. Keep the vagina lubricated, either by taking herbs such as vitex, motherwort, or dong quai, which nourish the vaginal tissues; or by applying vaginal lubricants. According to Notelovitz and Tonnessen (1993), the lubricant Replens is more effective than the water-based K-Y jelly because it gets to the root of the problem by lowering vaginal pH, increasing the quantity of vaginal secretions, and decreasing the fragility of the vaginal lining. However, some women report that Replens becomes sticky and flakes as it dries.

Remaining sexually active with a partner or through self-stimulation keeps tissues supple. Mind and muscle-relaxing practices such as a bath or a massage before sexual activity can be helpful.

HERBS FOR LIBIDO

- Siberian ginseng (see page 150)
- Vitex (see page 136; some women find sex drive is enhanced by vitex)
- Maca (see page 151)

KEGEL EXERCISES

Contracting then relaxing the vaginal muscles was suggested by Dr. Kegel as a way to maintain vaginal tone (see Chapter 3). Good vaginal tone increases ability to respond to sexual stimulation and enhances orgasm.

ACUPUNCTURE

Acupuncture can be helpful to all conditions of the sexual organs, according to Michael Gerber (January 2001), including sexual performance and lack of sex drive. If one has had surgery in the pelvic region, the surgical scars may dampen sexuality and sensitivity. Acupuncture can help correct these problems.

SENSUALITY

Sexuality comes under the umbrella of sensuality. Our sexuality is simply another expression of our sensual natures, albeit a powerful one. To a great extent, Western culture has reduced sensuality to a function of the sex organs, but there is so much more. Sensuality is responding to and getting pleasure from all the senses. Obviously, this may be broadly interpreted, such as the delicious feeling of warm fragrant water on the skin or the delight of eating a favorite meal by candlelight. Give and receive a massage; while a whole body massage is divine and may be downright sexy, a face massage or a foot massage is a wonderful feeling that is "safely sensual." Maybe you have a partner, maybe you do not. Be sensual either way. Practice. When you go for a walk, for instance, be aware of what you are smelling (pine needles, moisture in the air), seeing (notice how the sunlight backlights the leaves), hearing (the luscious sounds of Mozart on your Walkman, the waves receding from the beach), and touching (tree bark, stones, feeling the touch of silk on your body as you walk).

> The truth that I observe of all my women friends and many of my
> male friends, is that we become less sexual as we age. . . . For myself,
> I believe there is a vitality in continuing to be sexually active. However,
> by insisting that our sex drive need not change as we age, we probably
> deny reality. . . .
>
> —Jill Jeggery Ginghofer, "Sex, Sighs, and Media-Hype,"
> in *Women of the 14th Moon*

HORMONES FOR SEXUALITY AND LIBIDO

Decreased hormone levels around menopause commonly lead to reduced sexual desire and fantasies, slower sexual arousal, less intense or absent orgasm, and decreased frequency of intercourse. Estrogen and progesterone both are involved in sexual expression, although testosterone is considered the main "hormone of desire" in both women and men. During puberty, it stimulates development of sexual areas of the body, such as growth of pubic and underarm hair. Women have testosterone receptors in the nipples, vagina, clitoris, and brain (Rako, 1996). Testosterone also helps maintain muscle tone, bone strength, flexible ligaments, skin thickness and moisture, and healthy cholesterol. As an anabolic (building) hormone, it can generate energy for stamina and endurance, and gives a sense of overall vitality (Ahlgrimm & Kells, 1999).

Once testosterone levels have dropped by about 50 percent, menopausal women begin to get deficiency symptoms. Although loss of libido is the best known, other signs of testosterone deficiency are general lack of energy and vitality, loss of muscle tone, and dry thin skin. Around menopause, the ovaries stop producing testosterone. This is compounded by the adrenal glands producing less androstenedione and DHEA, which the body uses to make testosterone (see the description of the hormone cascade in Chapter 2). The sex steroid hormones work together like a symphony, as estrogen primes brain cells to respond to testosterone, progesterone converts to testosterone via androstenedione, and testosterone cascades into estrogen. If you have too much estrogen, testosterone can desensitize your tissues to its effects (Ahlgrimm & Kells, 1999).

If hormone levels fall enough, or get really unbalanced, the cascade cannot work to convert them back and forth to meet body needs. Then symptoms of deficiency occur. According to Dr. Lee (1999) progesterone is the best hormone to start with to improve libido. Many women do find that adding progesterone cream or pills does help with sexual functions, muscle tone, and skin changes. If vaginal dryness and thinning cause discomfort with intercourse, adding estrogen vaginal cream is often very effective.

For other women, testosterone supplementation may be the answer to sagging libido and muscles. Since hitting the public airwaves on the Oprah Winfrey show in January, 1999, testosterone supplementation for women has become quite popular. Of course, the dose is much lower than would be used for men. It is always best to have saliva testing to determine if your testosterone level is low. Natural, human identical testosterone can be ordered by your doctor at compounding pharmacies in cream, ointment, gel, and capsule forms. The older, synthetic form called methyl testosterone caused many side effects including growth of facial hair, weight gain, deepening voice, and possibly tumors. Natural HIH testosterone is believed to be safer and just as effective (Wright & Morgenthaler, 1997).

OTHER THOUGHTS ON LIBIDO

Perhaps the difficulty with sex is not your hormones, but areas in your life that need clearing or healing. It certainly is harder to enjoy pleasure and have orgasms if you are stressed out from working too hard, or when you feel anger or sadness at being unappreciated by your partner. There are many things that can rob you of vitality and joy. It may be time to take stock and, perhaps, make some changes.

Fuzzy Brain

"Excuse me, I must be having a senior moment." Have you or your friends made this remark when a thought that was just on the tip of the tongue eluded you? Perhaps you had lost your keys for the umpteenth time. Or you found yourself staring at the quarterly report in a panic that you just cannot extract meaning from the numbers. No, you are not experiencing early Alzheimer's disease. Indeed, having episodes of poor concentration, fuzzy thinking, or memory lapses is not an unusual phenomenon on the menopausal journey.

Changes in brain functioning seem to be a combination of biochemistry and something more ineffable: the mind and spirit making a shift. This is a central part of the menopause transition. Our brains, after working at a rapid pace for years, are shifting from focus on concentration and performance to more intuitive processes as we make the transition into our wisdom years. While our forgetfulness can be disconcerting, getting too stressed about it only adds to brain difficulties. Become more philosophical about this phenomenon as it leads to new discoveries of self (see Chapter 5 for spiritual aspects).

WHAT TO DO

- Relax. Breathe deeply to calm and center yourself. Panic or anxiety will exacerbate brain dysfunction.
- Meditate. Pray. Take a seclusion or retreat (see Appendix D).

- Supply the brain with oxygen by exercising, which brings more circulation to the brain, as well as the rest of your body. Do yoga, especially some inverted poses that help oxygenate the brain (see Appendix A).

- Feed the brain with a good diet and with supplements that provide antioxidants and the full complement of vitamins (especially vitamin E) and minerals. Also supplement with lecithin (standardized to contain 30–55 percent of phosphatidyl choline, 1500 mg/day), and with Omega-3 essential fatty acids (or eat cold-water fatty fish, such as ocean salmon).

- Feed the brain with positive, uplifting thoughts. Laugh. Take pleasure.

- Sleep enough. Try to get a full 8 hours every night for a week. How do you feel?

- Take herbs. Ginkgo (*Ginkgo biloba*) improves circulation to the brain. Ginkgo has been demonstrated to improve concentration and memory deficits caused by peripheral arterial occlusive disease (*PDR for Herbal Medicines,* 1999). Take 120 mg of dried standardized extract for at least 12 weeks. Ginkgo is contraindicated if you take anticoagulants or have a bleeding disorder. Siberian ginseng also may improve cognitive function.

- Consider natural HRT.

- Check your thyroid.

Body Image

For many women, there is a correlation between how content they feel about life and how happy they are with how they look. Body image is tied closely to emotions. It is a sensitive subject, filled with fear for many. Body changes are inevitable as we grow into menopause. We have witnessed changes in our mothers, aunts, and grandmothers, such as rounding out, sagging muscles, wrinkling and dimpling skin. Even in women who maintain steady weight, body contours and skin undergo changes. Why is it so difficult to accept this as natural and normal? Primarily this is because of cultural abhorrence and denial of aging, which portends death, and translates into loss, weakness, and powerlessness. This fear is so strong and all-pervading that we strive to be forever young. Media images of rail-thin haute coture models, and pearly faced sex-pots convey powerful messages that women must be young and slender to be valuable. The facts about the bodies and appearance of most women belie these values, however.

We can choose to think differently, if we like. This is not to suggest embracing becoming obese or looking old before our time. Rather, the emphasis is on taking good care of yourself and, then, accepting bodily changes with respect and good humor. All things in nature go through cycles, and these bring changes integral to growth. Dr. Christiane Northrup (2001) uses a beautiful analogy to the cycles of a rose: Perimenopausal women are like the full-blown rose of late summer, just before it transforms into a bright, juicy rose hip in the fall containing seeds from which hundreds of new roses can be born. The rose hip cannot go backward to being the dewy rosebud of early spring. When you are a rose hip, attempting to look like a rosebud is both impossible and ridiculous.

Probably most women would not want to return to their youth and struggle through all those lessons again. It is much healthier to appreciate the present stage of life, and find its special beauty and power. Women face an uphill challenge, however, because our culture worships youthful beauty to the extent that it largely renders invisible the beauty of other stages. The baby-boomer generation of midlife women is changing cultural attitudes by projecting new images of the vibrantly alive, attractive, and talented aging woman.

Did You Know . . .

- If shop mannequins were real women, they'd be too thin to menstruate.
- Marilyn Monroe wore a size 14.
- If Barbie was a real woman, she'd have to walk on all fours because of her proportions. She would also have to have her bottom four ribs removed and carry her kidneys in her purse.
- The average American woman weighs 144 lbs. and wears size 12–14.
- A psychological study in 1995 found that three minutes spent looking at models in a fashion magazine caused 70 percent of women to feel depressed, guilty, and shameful.
- Models twenty years ago weighed 8 percent less than the average woman; today they weigh 23 percent less.

—Anonymous. In Marilyn Nyborg, *Through Women's Eyes*

WHAT TO DO ABOUT BODY IMAGE

How you relate to your body and how you "talk" to it can make a big difference in overall self acceptance. What are the tapes that run in your head? If they are insulting or devaluing, such as "I'm getting old and ugly" or "I hate my thighs," imagine what effect that has on your peace of mind, not to mention your health. Practicing respect and gratitude for your body makes good sense in many ways. Change those mental tapes. Dr. Christiane Northrup (1998) includes in her 12 steps for healing these three aspects of body awareness: listening to, respecting, and working with the body. She recommends becoming aware of what parts of your

What actually is the norm for the American female? An ad in a fashion magazine that celebrates the big and the bold presents this view: "I am not 100 pounds. I am not one-size-fits-all. I am a size 14. 18. 22. I am beautiful. I am half the women in this country. I am not outside the norm. I am the norm. And I am not invisible.

—*MODE,* January, 1999

body you have disowned and the fears you hold about your body. She suggests standing in front of a mirror, thanking your body for all it has done for you, and, while looking into your own eyes, saying "I accept myself unconditionally right now." Do this for 30 days and see if something shifts inside you, allowing for more acceptance of what you see as imperfections.

When the ovaries start diminishing their production of estrogen as women approach menopause, the fat cells in their bodies become the main producers of estrogen. Thus, being a little *zoftig* (soft) in middle age can be a good thing, since women with more body fat often do not experience the menopausal challenges of decreasing estrogen, such as hot flashes and thinning bones, that their thin sisters do (Angier, 1999). Being heavier does not guarantee a smoother menopause, however, since the balance between estrogen and progesterone and their neuro-transmitter effects play important roles in causing symptoms. Because it becomes easier and easier to add pounds as we age, and because obesity can damage our health, slowing this process down is a good thing.

Exercise, Diet, and Attitude   The most simple way to control weight is to lower overall caloric intake and increase exercise. According to Dr. Ojeda (2000), the basal metabolic rate (BMR, the rate at which calories are burned) decreases about 2 percent each decade. Lower caloric intake becomes necessary as people age, unless their level of activity goes up. Lowering calories, however, does not mean dieting. Most weight loss diets result in the yo-yo effect, which resets the BMR lower, so it is even easier to gain back pounds. The most effective approach is making lifestyle changes; eating less and exercising more. Though it sounds almost too simple, it works for most people.

Did you know it pays to be zoftig after menopause? . . . Our fatty tissues make estrogen for us, helping to fill in the void after our ovaries quit. Not only are those rounded contours a comfort to the grandchild on your lap (or the man in your arms), they actually make you more womanly! And help to keep your bones strong.

—Clara Felix, "It's Turning Out Okay," in *Women of the 14th Moon*

Much has been written about weight, and our culture appears obsessed by poundage. Obesity is a chronic, increasing problem in the United States with 61 percent of Americans over 20 in the categories of overweight or obese. This has increased from 47 percent in the 1970s and 56 percent in the 1980s (*UCB Wellness Letter,* 2001). Many health risks are associated with obesity, including heart disease, diabetes, high blood pressure, joint disease, circulatory disorders, and digestive problems. A national initiative is underway to develop strategies for reducing obesity and overweight (see Resources). Analysis of the literature on popular weight loss diets found that a diet with 1,400–1,500 calories daily results in weight loss, regardless of the amount of protein, fat, and carbohydrate consumed, and even in the absence of physical activity (Medicine in the News, 2001).

During the menopause transition, healthy nutrition provides much needed support as the body undergoes significant changes. Women may also need to adjust caloric intake downward to maintain normal weight. Special needs of midlife women for foods and supplements are discussed in Chapter 3.

Here are other suggestions for supporting a positive body image:

- Instead of admiration, feel pity for emaciated movie stars and models. Their lives often are full of pain. Simply stop looking at, listening to, and reading "the perfect body" commercials that urge you to be other than you are and promise success and happiness by using their products.

- Go to your local gym and take notice of the various body types in the locker room. This is undiluted, non–Madison Avenue reality. You might even start taking delight in the incredible variety.

- Replace the fear of change with as much love and acceptance as you can muster. It takes practice, so just keep trying. Affirm: "I accept and love who I am at this moment." Say this while you look deeply into your eyes in a mirror.

- Exercise for the pure joy of it. Get those mood-enhancing endorphins going.

- Explore spirituality. You will learn not to identify so strongly with the body, and come to see it more as a temple for the soul.

When I was a young woman I thought aging meant loss and limitation, but I've learned that it's really about freedom, especially freedom from fear. But also free to be uniquely myself, free to say what I mean and mean what I say, free to genuinely enjoy and celebrate life.

—Sue Patton Thoele, *Freedom After 50*

OLDER WOMEN

Many people fear that to grow older is to lose power, become invisible, disintegrate. Older women have been especially disempowered by Western culture, which has no place of honor for their wisdom and perspective. These conditions are being challenged by contemporary women, who no longer accept this social negativity. Women everywhere have stopped asking permission and, instead, are formulating a culture within a culture that nurtures, supports, and sustains them. This work to change negative perceptions actually begins within. Like a mirror, the inner change will be reflected in the outer world. By deeply accepting ourselves, we are modeling to our whole culture a glimpse of true wisdom.

Many have written about the power of elder women to set the tone of society, but none more eloquently than Joan Borysenko in *A Woman's Book of Life* (1996). She makes a compelling case for mature women taking on the role of "Guardians of Life." Her book is well worth reading.

What to Do When Becoming an Older Woman

- Celebrate your maturity with rites of passages; do not let important birthdays slide quietly by (see Appendix C: A Rite of Passage Celebration). Have a "Croning Ceremony" with friends to celebrate your growing into even greater wisdom.

- Read candid, irreverent books such as The Hen Co-op's *Growing Old Disgracefully* (1994), written by a group of women who have a sense of humor.

- Befriend women who are comfortable about themselves growing older. Have an elder mentor who can illustrate the way.

- Avoid involvement with men or women partners who cannot accept you as you are. Of course, you can take on the task of educating them about how to treat you with respect. If, however, they will not or cannot learn, you are probably better off without them.

- Take on a new challenge to nourish your sense of adventure, to push the envelope and not get too comfortable.

- Nurture your spiritual nature and grow in wisdom by meditating, praying, seeking out and spending time with spiritually mature people.

- Live with like-minded people. Work and create with like-minded people. A Hindu sage said, "Environment is stronger than will" (P. Yogananda). It pays to be in an environment that nurtures and teaches you and brings out your best.

> The stereotype of aging as a progressive loss of function is generally true only for people who stop functioning.
>
> —Joan Borysenko, *A Woman's Book of Life*

TAKING CHARGE OF EMOTIONAL AND MENTAL TRANSITIONS

The inner world of emotions, thoughts, and feelings goes through a profound transition during perimenopause and menopause. Menopause has a grand purpose, once we open ourselves to seeing the bigger picture. The tumultuous hormone shifts re-program women's brains for a different way of thinking, and set up the biochemistry for intuition to flower. This step in women's psychological development leads to expanded creativity, self-discovery, humanitarianism, and new depths of loving. As you move toward thinking of yourself as a "wise woman visionary," these self-care practices will support the process:

- Learn about the mental and emotional changes you can expect during perimenopause and menopause. This lets you be prepared and better able to deal with symptoms.

- Develop plans for managing stress in your life. Simply going through perimenopause is stressful for your body, and most women also have family and career challenges during this time.

- If you are significantly depressed, seek professional help and remain open to all treatment possibilities until you arrive at the best one for you. Perimenopause intensifies the tendency toward depression. After a few years, when hormones become stable, depression usually improves or resolves.

- Support the health of your body-mind with good nutrition, pure water, and supplements according to your unique needs.

- Have a physical examination and laboratory tests if your symptoms point toward such problems as hypothyroid, diabetes, heart disease, or immune disorders.

- Use nutritional, nutraceutical, and lifestyle approaches to support your skin, hair, vital energy, and libido.

- Examine your attitudes and beliefs about body image and aging. Make adjustments to eliminate negativity and promote a positive, self-affirming outlook.

- Connect with other women whose character and abilities you admire, associate with groups that give you uplifting experiences, and learn to avoid others who sap your energy and positivity.

> Becoming a mature female is a natural—and, yes—even pleasurable
> experience. This universal adventure is to be welcomed, not feared.
>
> —Martha Sacks, *Menopaws, The Silent Meow*

- Remind yourself that this process of transition is directional. It is a great start to simply express the intention to gain peace of mind, self-acceptance, inner strength, and a harmonious life.
- Remember that "this too shall pass." You might even laugh about it in years to come.

REFERENCES

Ahlgrimm, M., & Kells, J.M. (1999). *The HRT solution: Optimizing your hormone potential.* Garden City Park, NY: Avery Publishing Group.

Allison, T.G., Williams, D.F., Miller, T.D., et al. (1995). Medical and economic costs of psychologic distress in patients with coronary artery disease. *Mayo Clinic Proceedings, 70,* 734–742.

American Psychiatric Association. (1994). *Diagnostic and statistical manual of mental disorders* (4th Ed.). Washington, D.C.: American Psychiatric Press.

Angier, N. (1999). *Woman: An intimate geography.* Boston: Houghton Mifflin.

Anonymous. In Nyborg, M. (November, 1998). *Seeing the world through women's eyes.* Grass Valley, CA: Nyborg-Dow Associates.

Anonymous. In Nyborg, M. (June, 1999). *Seeing the world through women's eyes.* Grass Valley, CA: Nyborg-Dow Associates.

Askew, J. (1998). Menopause "emotions" more precisely defined. *Menopause News,* July/August, 1–2.

Austin, J. (1999). *Towards an understanding of meditation and consciousness.* Boston: MIT Press.

Balch, J., & Balch, P. (2000). *Prescription for nutritional healing* (2nd Ed.). Garden City Park, NY: Avery Publishing Group.

Ballentine, R. (1999). *Radical healing: Integrating the world's great therapeutic traditions to create a new transformative medicine.* New York: Harmony Books.

Batmanghelidj, F. (1995). *Your body's many cries for water.* Falls Church, VA: Global Health Solutions.

Batten, C. (1991). A journey homeward. In D. Taylor & A.C. Sumrall (Eds.). *Women of the 14th Moon.* Freedom, CA: The Crossing Press.

Bender, S.D. (1998). *The power of perimenopause: A woman's guide to physical and emotional health during the transitional decade.* New York: Three Rivers Press.

Benson, H., & Stark, M. (1996). *Timeless healing: The power and biology of belief.* New York: Scribner.

Berry, C.R., & Traeder, T. (1995). *Girlfriends: Invisible bonds, enduring ties.* Berkeley, CA: Wildcat Canyon Press.

Block, D. (November/December, 2000). Heavenly helpers. *Psychology Today, 33,* 30.

Borysenko, J. (1996). *A woman's book of life: The biology, psychology, and spirituality of the feminine life cycle.* New York: Riverhead Books.

Bourne, E. (1995). *The anxiety & phobia workbook* (2nd Ed.). Oakland, CA: New Harbinger.

Braden, G. (1997). *Awakening to zero point: The collective initiation.* Bellevue, WA: Radio Bookstore Press.

Braden, G. (2000). *The Isaiah effect: Decoding the lost science of prayer and prophecy.* New York: Harmony Books.

Brody, H. (July/August, 2000). Mind over medicine. *Psychology Today, 32,* 60–67

Brown, R. (1999). *Stop depression now.* New York: G.P. Putnam & Sons.

Carlin, P., & Biddle, N. (August 14, 2000). Mercy missionary. *People Weekly, 54,* 149–152.

Carlson, L.E., Sherwin, B.B., Chertkow, H.M. (2000). Relationships between mood and estradiol (E2) levels in Alzheimer's disease (AD) patients. *Journal of Gerontological & Psychological Science in Social Sciences, 55,* P47–53.

Childre, D., & Martin, H. (1999). *The HeartMath solution.* San Francisco: Harper-Collins.

Col, N.F., Legato, M., & Schiff, I. (1998). HRT: New data, continuing controversies. *Patient Care Nurse Practitioner, 1,* 18–34.

Copeland, M. (1992). *The depression workbook: A guide for living with depression and manic depression.* Oakland, CA: New Harbinger.

Cousens, G. (2000). *Depression-free for life: An all-natural, 5-step plan to reclaim your zest for living.* New York: William Morrow.

Dardick, G. (1991). Opening Pandora's box. In D. Taylor & A.C. Sumrall (Eds.). *Women of the 14th Moon.* Freedom, CA: The Crossing Press.

Davidson, J. & Connor, K. (2000). *Herbs for the mind.* New York: The Guilford Press.

DeRosis, H. (1998). *Women & anxiety: A step-by-step program for managing anxiety and depression.* New York: Hatherleigh Press.

Dess, N.K. (September/October, 2000). Tend and befriend. *Psychology Today, 33,* 22–23.

Dossey, L. (1997). *Prayer is good medicine: How to reap the healing benefits of prayer.* New York: HarperCollins.

Drake, E.B., Henderson, V.W., Stanczyk, F.Z., et al. (2000). Associations between circulating sex steroid hormones and cognition in normal elderly women. *Neurology, 8,* 599–603.

Duerk, J. (1989). *Circle of Stones: Woman's journey to herself.* San Diego, CA: LuraMedia.

Epstein, R. (March/April, 2000). Stress busters. *Psychology Today, 33,* 30–36.

Felix, C. (1991). It's turning out okay. In D. Taylor & A.C. Sumrall (Eds.). *Women of the 14th Moon.* Freedom, CA: The Crossing Press.

Firshein, R. (1998). *The nutraceutical revolution: 20 cutting-edge nutrients to help you design your own perfect whole-life program.* New York: Riverhead Books.

Gerber, M. (November, 2000). Maca mania. *Alternative Health.* 100–103.

Gerber, M. (January, 2001). Acupuncture or "aquapressure" for sexual health. *Alternative Health, 90*–94.

Ginghofer, J. (1991). Sex, sighs, and media-hype. In D. Taylor & A.C. Sumrall (Eds.). *Women of the 14th Moon.* Freedom, CA: The Crossing Press.

Gittleman, A.L. (1998). *Before the change: Taking charge of your perimenopause.* New York: HarperSanFrancisco.

Grodstein, F., Chen, J., Pollen, D.A., et al. (2000). Postmenopausal hormone therapy and cognitive function in healthy older women. *Journal of the American Geriatric Society, 48,* 746–752.

Hafen, B.Q., Frandsen, K.J., Karren, K.J., & Hooker, K.R. (1992). *The health effects of attitudes, emotions, relationships.* Provo, Utah: EMS Associates.

Heim, C., Newport, D.J., & Heit, S. (2000). Pituitary-adrenal and autonomic responses to stress in women after sexual and physical abuse in childhood. *Journal of the American Medical Association, 284,* 592–597.

Hen Co-op. (1994). *Growing old disgracefully: New ideas for getting the most out of life.* Freedom, CA: The Crossing Press.

Kabat-Zinn, J. (1990). *Full catastrophe living: Using the wisdom of the body and mind to face stress, pain, and illness.* New York: Delta Books, Dell Publishing.

Kampen, D.L., & Sherwin, B.B. (1994). Estrogen use and verbal memory in healthy postmenopausal women. *Obstetrics & Gynecology, 83,* 979–983.

Karpen, M. (1996). Managing stress: Natural approaches to a modern disorder. *Alternative & Complementary Therapies, 2,* 207–216.

Kelsea, M. (1991). Beyond the stethoscope: A nurse practitioner looks at menopause and midlife. In D. Taylor & A.C. Sumrall (Eds.). *Women of the 14th Moon.* Freedom, CA: The Crossing Press.

Laakmann G., Schule C., Baghai T., & Kieser M. (1998). *Pharmacopsychiatry, 31,* S54–S59.

Le Sueur, M. (1991). Indian Summer. In D. Taylor & A.C. Sumrall (Eds.). *Women of the 14th Moon.* Freedom, CA: The Crossing Press.

Lee, J. (1999). *What your doctor may not tell you about premenopause.* New York: Warner Books.

Lesser, E. (1999). *The new American spirituality.* New York: Random House.

Lindbergh, A.M. (1991). *A gift from the sea.* New York: Vintage Books.

Mandela, N. (1994). Inaugural address on being sworn in as President of South Africa.

Marano, H.E. (April, 1999). Depression: Beyond serotonin. *Psychology Today, 32,* 30–76.

Markowitz, J.C. (1999). Recognizing and treating chronic "mild" depression. *Women's Health in Primary Care, 2,* 855–861.

Matthews, K., Cauley, J., Yaffe, K., & Zmuda, J.M. (1999). Estrogen replacement therapy and cognitive decline in older community women. *Journal of the American Geriatric Society, 47,* 518–523.

McCall, T. (March/April, 2000). Good health: Catch the zzzz's you need. *New Age,* 44–51.

Medicine in the News. (March, 2001). Total calories determine weight loss. *Patient Care for the Nurse Practitioner, 4,* 6.

Mother Earth News (2000). Interview with Richard Firshein, M.D. April/May.

Murphy, M., & Donovan, S. (1997). *The physical and psychological effect of meditation— a review of contemporary research with a comprehensive bibliography from 1931–1996* (2nd Ed.). Sausalito, CA: Institute of Noetic Sciences.

Northrup, C. (1998). *Women's bodies, women's wisdom. Creating physical and emotional health and healing.* New York: Bantam Books.

Northrup, C. (May, 1999). Heart palpitations at menopause: Your heart's wake-up call! *Dr. Christiane Northrup's Health Wisdom for Women, 6,* 2–4.

Northrup, C. (2001). *The wisdom of menopause: Creating physical and emotional health and healing during the change.* New York: Bantam Books.

Notelovitz, M., & Tonnessen, D. (1993). *Menopause and midlife health.* New York: St. Martin's Press.

Novaes, C., & Almeida, O.P. (1999). Premenstrual syndrome and psychiatric morbidity at the menopause. *Journal of Psychosomatic Obstetrics & Gynecology, 20,* 56–57.

Ojeda, L. (2000). *Menopause without medicine.* Alameda, CA: Hunter House.

Palinkas, L.A., & Barrett-Connor, E. (1992). Estrogen use and depressive symptoms in postmenopausal women. *Obstetrics & Gynecology, 80,* 30–36.

People. (2000) Interview with Jim Gordon, M.D. August 14.

PDR for herbal medicines (1st Ed.). (1999). Montvale, NJ: Medical Economics Co.

Pert, C. (1997). *Molecules of emotion: Why you feel the way you feel.* New York: Scribner.

Rako, S. (1996). *The hormone of desire: The truth about sexuality, menopause, and testosterone.* New York: Harmony Books.

Raskin, B. (1991). These fevered days. In D. Taylor & A.C. Sumrall (Eds.). *Women of the 14th Moon.* Freedom, CA: The Crossing Press.

Sacks, M. (1995). *Menopaws, the silent meow.* Berkeley, CA: Ten Speed Press.

Schmidt, P.J., Nieman, L.K., & Danaceau, M.A. (1998). Differential behavioral effects of gonadal steroids in women with and in those without premenstrual syndrome. *New England Journal of Medicine, 338,* 209–216.

Schultz, M.N. (1998). *Awakening intuition: Using your mind-body network for insight and healing.* New York: Harmony Books.

Science Daily. (2000). Estrogen therapy may help prevent memory decline in elderly women. Accessed 10/00: *http://www.sciencedaily.com//releases/2000.*

Shah, A., & Gonsalves, L. (1999). Mood disorders and the reproductive cycle: A brief review. *Women's Health in Primary Care, 2,* 208–224.

Shealy, C.N., & Myss, C. (1993). *The creation of health.* Walpole, NH: Stillpoint Publishing.

Sheehy, G. (1993). *The silent passage: Menopause.* New York: Random House.

Sherwin, B.B. (1998). Estrogen and cognitive functioning in women. *Proceedings of Social and Experimental Biological Medicine, 217,* 17–22.

Sherwin, B.B. (1999). Can estrogen keep you smart? Evidence from clinical studies. *Journal of Psychiatry & Neuroscience, 24,* 315–321.

Sherwin, B.B. (2000). Oestrogen and cognitive function throughout the female lifespan. *Novartis Foundation Symposiums, 230,* 188–196.

Sichel, D., & Driscoll, J.W. (1999). *Women's moods: What every woman must know about hormones, the brain, and emotional health.* New York: William Morrow & Co.

Sovik, R. (1997). Pranayama: Watching the mind, watching the breath. *Yoga International, 37,* 43–47.

Streep, P. (1993). *An awakening spirit: Meditations by women for women.* New York: Viking Study Books.

Taylor, D., & Sumrall, A.C. (1991). *Women of the 14th moon: Writings on menopause.* Freedom, CA: The Crossing Press.

UCB Wellness Letter. (April, 2001). Wellness facts. *17,* 1.

Thoele, S. (1998). *Freedom after 50.* Berkeley, CA: Conari Press.

Tierra, M. (1990). *Planetary herbology.* D. Frawley (Ed.). Twin Lakes, WI: Lotus Press.

Wall, S. (1993). *Wisdom's daughters: Conversations with women elders of native America.* New York: Harper Perennial.

Warga, C. (1999). *Menopause and the mind: The complete guide to coping with memory loss, foggy thinking, verbal slips and other cognitive effects of perimenopause and menopause.* New York: The Free Press/Simon and Schuster.

Weed, S. (1992). *Menopausal years: The wise woman way.* Woodstock, NY: Ash Tree.

Weintraub, A. (November/December, 2000). Yoga: It's not just an exercise. *Psychology Today, 33,* 22–23

Wellner, A.S., & Adox, D. (May/June, 2000). Happy days. *Psychology Today, 32,* 32–37

Whooley, M.A., Grady, D., & Cauley, J.A. (2000). Postmenopausal estrogen therapy and depressive symptoms in older women. *Journal of General Internal Medicine, 15,* 535–541.

Williams, D. (October, 2000). *Alternatives, 8*(16), 124–126.

Wright, J.V., & Morgenthaler, J. (1997). *Natural hormone replacement for women over 45.* Petaluma, CA: Smart Publications.

Wurtman, J, (1986). *Managing your mind and mood through food.* New York: Harper & Row.

Yaffe, K., Grady, D., Pressman, A., et al. (1998). Serum estrogen levels, cognitive performance, and risk of cognitive decline in older community women. *Journal of the American Geriatric Society, 46,* 816–821.

Yogananda, P. (1982). *How to be a smile millionaire. Man's eternal quest.* Los Angeles, CA: Self-Realization Fellowship.

SUGGESTED READING

Bloomfield, H.H. (1998). *Healing anxiety with herbs.* New York: HarperCollins.

Haas, Elson M. (1996). *The detox diet.* Berkeley, CA: Celestial Arts.

Holstein, Lana L. (2001). *How to have magnificent sex: The seven dimensions of a vital sexual connection.* New York: Harmony Books.

Root, B. (2000). *Understanding panic and other anxiety disorders.* Jackson, MS: University Press of Mississippi.

Worksheet 4–1

Depression Checklist

Use this checklist of depression symptoms to gain an idea of whether or not you are significantly depressed. If you check several symptoms "some of the time" or a few symptoms "most of the time" you should discuss depression with your health practitioner.

	Seldom/Never	*Some of the Time*	*Most of the Time*
I feel sad or moody	☐	☐	☐
I have feelings of hopelessness	☐	☐	☐
I feel worthless or guilty	☐	☐	☐
I don't have much energy	☐	☐	☐
I have trouble concentrating	☐	☐	☐
I have insomnia, or sleep too much	☐	☐	☐
I've lost interest in people or things	☐	☐	☐
I criticize or blame myself for things	☐	☐	☐
I dislike myself	☐	☐	☐
I feel that life is too hard to cope with	☐	☐	☐
I think about killing myself	☐	☐	☐

Progressive Relaxation Technique

Progressively relaxing the muscles in a systematic way counteracts the effects of stress. Practicing 10 to 15 minutes per day will bring you results within 1–2 weeks. Results include less muscle tension, reduced anxiety, greater sense of well-being, and decreased effects of stress on your heart, digestive system, brain, kidneys, and endocrine glands.

Method

Check off each step once you have memorized it.

☐ Take several deep, slow breaths, fully expanding your lungs and moving your abdomen out and in.

☐ Tense feet and curl toes inward, hold briefly (5–10 seconds), then relax. Tense calves and relax, then tense thighs and relax. Continue to tense then relax muscles, progressing from the genitals, buttocks, and abdomen, to the lower back, upper chest, and upper back. Next clench the fists, tense the forearms, then upper arms, then shoulder muscles, following each group with relaxation. Tense then relax the neck, jaws, and face (frown, squeeze eyes closed, purse lips, press tongue against roof of mouth.) Even try tensing and relaxing the scalp.

☐ Take several deep, slow breaths. Then tense the entire body with a double breath inward, hold the tension and vibrate the muscles for a few seconds, then relax all at once, throwing the breath outward in two short exhalations. Repeat 1–2 times more.

☐ Return your attention to the toes and feet. Notice how they feel, identifying looseness, warmth, relaxation, softness, heaviness or continued tension. Scan your body systematically, feet to head. Tense then relax any muscle group that is still retaining tension or discomfort.

☐ Using background music or sounds, imagine your body progressively dissolving or melting, starting at the feet and moving upward. You can imagine (1) Lying on a beach, with warm azure waves gradually washing over you from feet to head, dissolving your body. (2) Blue or golden light, or a rainbow of colors gradually absorbing or melting your body from feet to head.

Worksheet 4–3

Therapy History: The Mental-Emotional Experience

This history can serve as your therapy profile to take with you on visits to health practitioners. Record when you start (and end) taking a drug or herb, for example; or when you start and complete a series of visits to the acupuncturist or masseuse. It is important to record the results. Over time you will get a clear picture of what is working for you and what is not.

Symptom Treated	Kind of Therapy	Date Started	Date Stopped	Results

CHAPTER 5

Women's Spiritual Journey

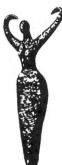

Nile Goddess.
Reproduced with permission.
Copyright © Kate Cartwright.

The process of going through menopause signifies a spiritual passage for women. It is a major step in the journey of spiritual unfolding in women's lives. Whether grounded in a religious tradition or not, women sense that deep within, their essential self is changing. The direction of change seems to move women toward expanding awareness, broadening views, and deepening connections. Many think of this as emergence of soul qualities, or from a secular perspective, as expression of the highest potential for the self.

The menopausal years are a time of great transitions in women's lives. This may be the truest meaning of the term "change of life." Biologically, menopause marks the end of childbearing; socially, it brings to completion the phase of family life focused on launching young adult children; and for many women it means careers are drawing toward a close. Women face the next phase of life, one that signifies birthing and nurturing the essential self, and exploring its nature. To the spiritually minded, the essential self is the soul, or higher self, that reflects the expression of our innate Divine nature.

Spirituality is a very personal thing. This chapter draws from several spiritual traditions, but cannot include every religious perspective. Some women are deeply connected with a particular tradition, while others do not relate to any

Your life is your spiritual journey.

—Caroline Myss, Intuitive Training Seminar II

religious traditions, spiritual images, or concepts of Goddess or God. If you do not resonate with the ideas expressed here, simply read no more. You will still find the earlier chapters useful in managing your menopause transition. Most people do connect with seeking the highest, most expansive, most perfect expression of ourselves of which we are capable. This chapter is an invitation to a process of inner growth which promotes this expression.

MENOPAUSE AS A SPIRITUAL PASSAGE

The menopausal process is a gateway into the second half of life. Most women can expect to live another 30 to 40 years, remaining healthy and functional. In legend and myth, a gateway symbolizes both a special time and a special place. Once at the gateway, a woman must choose whether to step through and go beyond her known world, mustering the courage to face uncertainty and drawing upon faith that she will be guided to do what is needed. When she has passed through the gateway, the woman can no longer be the same person she was before. She will be changed in some permanent, unavoidable ways. Menopause, with its physical and emotional changes, appears to be an inevitable gateway for women. Their bodies, minds, and emotions will never be quite the same again. The element of choice for women at the menopause gateway involves whether they will embrace the new self, or try to cling to identities from earlier life.

Midlife transitions are described by Jungian analyst Murray Stein (1983) as periods of liminality (from the Latin word for threshold), a time in life when we are in an "in-between zone." We are neither who we were before, nor completely who we are becoming. During this phase, we feel more sensitive and vulnerable, which often goes along with being more psychologically receptive and open to new growth. We may experience more synchronicities, which Carl Jung described as coincidences between our inner subjective world and outer events. In the liminal psychological state that typifies these passages, we often have glimpses of the eternal overlapping with our ordinary perception. The invisible spiritual world and visible outer reality often come together. The instability of this time provides an impetus for us to respond to opportunities for spiritual growth. Our inner readiness often draws to us the outer events that catalyze deep transformations (Bolen, 1994).

The physical and emotional experiences women go through during perimenopause and menopause have been reframed by Dr. Joan Borysenko (1996) as "psychospiritual opportunities." They can serve as motivators for women to enter new relationships with their bodies, minds, energy systems, and spirits. By midlife, most women come to an appreciation of the feminine values triad composed of love, authenticity, and service. Through loving relationships women help bring an expanded state of creativity and happiness to themselves and others. Living as one's authentic self leads to a sense of serenity. Being of service to others brings

> From a spiritual perspective, service is a good working definition of spirituality in action. The Jewish faith is firmly based in the practice of mitzvot, acts of kindness, compassion, and service to others. These are considered the highest forms of prayer.
>
> —Joan Borysenko, *A Woman's Book of Life*

satisfaction and positive energy to one's own system, since all things are interconnected. For midlife women, service often focuses on the environment and preservation of the planet for future generations.

With the childrearing years behind them, women often feel a new urgency in their search for life's meanings. A vast storehouse of creative energy is opened through shifts in the body's energy systems. Midlife seems to be a time associated with the serious pursuit of the spiritual dimensions of life. Dr. Christiane Northrup (2001) observes that the great majority of attendees at conferences on the body-mind-soul connection are midlife women. She believes that people's lives are directed by a force (that she thinks of as God) that is much bigger than their intellects and self-definitions. It always moves a woman toward her highest purpose, working through the unique characteristics that each woman possesses. Each woman goes through several key life passages in order to reach her full wisdom, with specific shifts in consciousness which, if given expression, open her to her full potential. The decade of the 40s leads to transformation, and the 50s to transmutation.

In describing the seven steps in women's spirituality, Maria Harris (1991) notes special times of spiritual receptivity. For postmenopausal women, this occurs at the time of the new moon. As the moon moves into this phase, women are reminded to be still, to listen, and to rest in their bodies so that spirituality will have time to flourish. The cycles of spiritual growth include both awakening times and resting times. After resting and receiving, mature women's spirituality turns to engagement with life, new beginnings, and caring for others in a broader sense. In the last step of spiritual growth, transforming, women find and renew themselves. They rejoice because they have faced brokenness and come through, and recognize that the past is alive in the present. Postmenopausal women are the

> We *form* at age 30, we *transform* at age 40, and we *transmute* at age 50.
>
> —Barbara Hand Clow, *The Liquid Light of Sex: Kundalini Rising at Midlife Crisis*

messengers of good news, offering the richness of their life experiences to the world.

Harvard theologian James Fowler (1981), in his penetrating study of how faith develops, describes six stages of psychospiritual growth. By midlife, at the fifth stage, we have become aware of life's paradoxes, experienced that life is not easy, and seen that there are no simple prescriptions for happiness. We have tasted the "sacrament of defeat" and the apparent injustices of life. We can perceive powerful truths and at the same time appreciate the relativity of how these are expressed in the material world. Often we feel simultaneously alone and all one, living with internal tension as we are caught between "an untransformed world and a transforming vision" (Fowler, 1981). The sixth stage, universalizing faith, is expressed in mysticism and union with the greater Whole, and can have a world-changing impact. It is considered relatively rare by Fowler.

Among Native Americans, postmenopausal and elder women hold positions of special importance to traditional tribal life. In most tribes, certain ceremonies cannot be held without the empowerment brought by postmenopausal women. Medicine women among the Pomo of California are not able to practice until they reach sufficient maturity. Until then, their power is diffuse and might interfere with their healing practices; adequate time and experience enable them to bring this power under conscious control. Creation myths of many tribes say that the Grandmother spirit created the firmament, earth, and all the beings in it. The peoples knew that their power to live came from the Grandmother spirit, not only originally but continuously to the present. The spiritual power of elder women gave them a key position in tribal decision-making. Among the Mohawks (and other tribes) the clan mothers would make the decisions and advise the chiefs on what to do (Allen, 1986).

Menopause is women's call to integration, wisdom, and spiritual expansion. It is the gateway to discovering inner spiritual riches, seeking deeper connection with higher purpose and the greater Whole, and sharing gifts from our wisdom and abundance with our societies and the world.

SPIRIT, BODY-MIND, AND ENERGY

From the holistic view, all aspects of being are woven into a unity. This wholeness transcends any of these aspects and includes them all: body, mind, emotions, energy, and spirit. Different systems are used to describe the links and interconnections, some more comprehensive, such as Eastern and native metaphysical philosophies, and others more limited, notably the Western view that historically separates body and mind, and often denies spirit. Quantum physics and neurotheology are causing radical shifts in Western understanding of reality, however, suggesting a movement in the direction of mystical perceptions.

The new American spirituality is more open to metaphysical perspectives than ever before. People are seeking a direct relationship with Source, the Divine Spirit, or God, however that infinite essence is conceptualized. They want to understand how the forces of Spirit work through them and manifest in the world. They are turning their attention to the mysteries of consciousness as a glimpse of Spirit expressing within self (Smith, 2001). The major characteristics of the new American spirituality include (Lesser, 1999):

- Your inner guidance is the best authority to follow; as you come to know and love yourself you discover ways to live a spiritual life.
- Your deepest yearnings are your compass on the search for spiritual definitions.
- There are many paths to spiritual freedom and peace, and you can draw illumination from religious traditions, mythology, philosophy, psychology, science, healing methods, and your own experience.
- Everything is sacred in the world, including your body, mind, psyche, heart, and soul. Seek to unite all parts, darkness and lightness, into your whole self.
- Truth unfolds according to your spiritual growth.

Many people are using meditation techniques and other spiritual disciplines to deepen their relationship with the Infinite and to provide support for spiritual experiences. The widespread use of yoga methods to integrate body-mind-breath and bring the soul to peace was noted by *Time* (Corliss, April 23, 2001), and the emerging interest in the biological basis of spirituality was reported in *Newsweek* (Begley, May 7, 2001).

The concept of energy fields and flows through the body is ancient, probably originating in India and the Far East. The physical body is understood as the most dense, material manifestation of Infinite Consciousness. Permeating and surrounding the physical body are several layers of subtle energy fields, some corresponding to electromagnetic fields which scientists can measure emanating from various body structures, for example, electrocardiograms (ECG), electro-encephalograms (EEG), and skin conductance of electrical current (galvanic skin response).

The HeartMath Institute has used sensitive magnetometers to measure the heart's electromagnetic field (EMF). Shaped like a taurus, this field projects 8–10 feet away from the body. The heart's EMF is the strongest in the body, 5,000 times greater than the field produced by the brain. It also permeates every cell in the body, and pulls other body systems into entrainment with the heart's rhythms. By measuring heart rate variability, patterns of coherence or incoherence can be observed. Coherence in heart rhythm occurs when people experience positive emotional states such as love and appreciation, or when they are meditative or centered. Incoherence in heart rhythm occurs with anger, stress, or fear. Groups of people can bring their heart rhythms into coherence by projecting positive thoughts, meditating, or praying (Childre & Martin, 1999).

In the Eastern model, beyond this energy field, which occurs closest to the body, are emotional, mental, and consciousness fields that vibrate at increasing frequencies as they move farther from the physical form and closer to Infinite Consciousness. These fields provide connections for energy that flows from the Source, and gives life to physical forms. This model provides an understanding of how spirit and body-mind are connected, and how our life experiences and physical or emotional symptoms are related to our spiritual journey.

Energy Centers and Quantum Physics

One way of thinking about how spirit and body-mind work together is based on Eastern theories of energy flows. According to these models, the physical body is maintained and energized by seven energy centers (called "chakras" or wheels in eastern spiritual tradition) which act as transformers of universal-cosmic energy (life force, prana, chi) into frequencies that enliven body cells and organs. Flows of energy through body structures follow nadis (Indian) or meridians (Chinese), channels that run to every body part. Acupuncture research has demonstrated this flow through acu-points located on the skin surface (Gypson, 1997; Darras, 1989). There are associated energy fields that surround and interpenetrate the physical body. These fields have several layers that radiate outward, reflecting our physical vitality and emotional and mental states. Some fields and energy centers are electromagnetic, some are light, and some are vibrations of consciousness (Yogananda, 1994; Brennan, 1987; Johari, 1987). The energy centers, or chakras, are located near the spinal column, close to the major autonomic nervous system ganglion plexes (Kriyananda, 1988). Each center relates to specific body structures as well as to particular mental/emotional issues. Physical and emotional problems can result if there are blocks in the flow or leaks of energy from these centers. When the energy centers are functioning in balance, our body-mind-spirit comes into harmony, we can heal diseases, and the pathway to higher consciousness is opened (Myss, 1996).

Although this theory has ancient origins in Far Eastern, mystical Christian, Kabbalistic, and native cultures, the realm of theoretical physics takes us to similar conclusions. Quantum physics' understanding of the nature of reality points to an interrelated universe in which energy and matter are simply two expressions of the same essence (Zukov, 1980; Hawking, 1998; Heisenberg, 1971; Kaku, 1994). Quantum physics reports the radical effects that our consciousness has on the behavior of the physical universe. It also dismantles our ideas about time, and implies multiple simultaneously existing universes waiting for us to call them into

> Anyone who is not shocked by quantum theory does not understand it.
>
> —Neils Bohr, 1927, in W.R. McWayne, *Radical Reality*
>
> Neils Bohr wrote that quantum mechanics, by its essence, entails ". . . the necessity of a final renunciation of the classical ideal of causality and a radical revision of our attitude toward the problem of physical reality."
>
> —Gary Zukov, *The Dancing Wu Li Masters*

manifestation (McWayne, 1998). This understanding of the nature of reality is similar to that described by mystics from all religious traditions, who could envision energy, matter, and consciousness working according to "Divine laws" that now seem expressed in quantum mechanics.

In our spiritual quest, we will encounter the laws of quantum reality. Working with these brings us to realize that whatever we can dream (re-image) can be created (manifested). Robynne McWayne, a physician and science teacher, explains quantum reality in clear everyday terms in her book *Radical Reality* (1998). Here are the basics:

- Nothing, no thing, is physically there until it is observed, or perceived, or looked for, or expected. The act of observing quantum particles affected how they behaved in experiments. *We create our own reality.*

- The particles themselves had some type of awareness, and were capable of making some type of self-determining choice, apparently based on awareness of the experimenter's expectations. *All matter has intelligence.*

- Energy and matter are one ($E = mc^2$). Matter is made of energy, and energy can condense into matter. The amount of energy contained within a tiny bit of mass is enormous, because it becomes multiplied by 34½ billion, according to Einstein's special relativity equation. *Existence is eternal, changing in form and expression, full of limitless power.*

- Energy comes from consciousness; so consciousness, energy, and matter are one. Energy comes from your consciousness, because in everything you experience, you are the only observer that you can sense directly. *Truth lies within you.*

- Your consciousness presents itself in states, most prominently as your thinking awareness, then as your physical body and surroundings, and finally as your experiences. *We exist on many levels, all permeated by Spirit.*

- Everything has both wave and particle properties, and two particles that have been associated (such as electrons) will continue to affect each other, no matter how far apart they may later travel. Repeated phase entanglement, as this is called, leads to an entire universe that is connected and can communicate instantly. *All is one.*

- All physical matter, though non-local (not being perceived in your universe), still exists as a probability in some state of suspended animation, ready to pop into manifestation when you call it forth. This is the theory of parallel universes. *Everything that ever was or will be exists simultaneously on some level of reality.*

Bringing quantum physics and energy field theory to our spiritual journey as mid-life women, we look afresh at our menopausal symptoms and life issues. There are communications in each physical, mental, and emotional experience. These are opportunities to learn more about our shadow, to see where energy is stuck or leaking, and to discover what part of ourself is keeping this problem going. When we really come to know the power that our choices have on our physical reality, we can learn to use the many levels of choice to focus our energy toward our most deeply held goals. Table 5–1 outlines the issues and symptoms (physical and emotional) that are connected with each energy center (chakra), which have particular importance for midlife and menopausal women. Figure 5–1 shows the location of each energy center (chakra) and the areas of empowerment which each brings into focus. Worksheet 5-1 on page 228 offers an exercise for awareness and energizing of the chakras. Our spiritual journey brings us through challenges associated with each area of empowerment, so we may learn lessons in how to manage this power for our own and others' highest good.

ENERGY DYNAMICS OF MENOPAUSE SYMPTOMS

The word menopause has symbolic meaning for women's energy dynamics:

"Meno" = menstruation

"pause" = holding in place, stopping movement

The movement and flow of the menstrual cycle stops at menopause. Think of it as "holding the pause after menstruation," holding space for something new to emerge. A period of confusion, uncertainty, and loss of bearings often occurs. You are changing, but into what? The many physical and emotional symptoms women experience at this time can be unsettling. What are our bodies up to? What surprises hide in our inner thoughts and feelings?

This is a time for inner exploration. We need to know ourselves, with an urgency that makes it hard to put things off with distractions such as "the children need me" or "I'm just too busy" or "I can't take time from my job." But, the

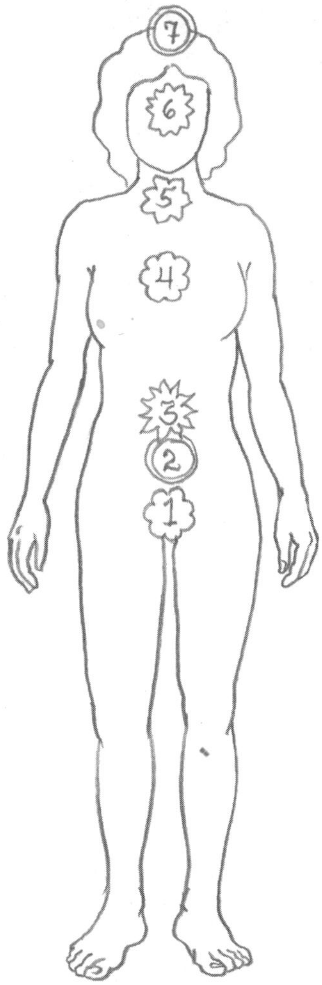

	Center/Chakra	Location	Issues
7	Crown	Top of head	Connecting to source Knowing Trusting
6	Brow	Forehead	Intuition Imagining Psychic perception
5	Throat	Neck	Communicating Self-expression Truthfulness
4	Heart	Chest	Emotions, love Compassion Connecting to others
3	Navel	Solar plexus	Self-esteem Willpower Responsibility Sense of purpose
2	Pelvic	Pelvic	Creativity Sexuality, pleasure Boundaries Control/dependency
1	Root	Base of spine	Physical health Right livelihood Prosperity Security, survival Grounding

Figure 5–1 Energy Centers (Chakras) and Areas of Empowerment. The seven energy centers (chakras) located near the spine distribute life force energy to all the organs and tissues of the body. They connect emotions and mind forms with physical anatomy. Each chakra relates to certain body areas and life issues.

realities of many midlife women's circumstances pull at their energy and attention. As the "sandwich generation" we cope with many pressures. Aging parents may need our help, adult children may cycle back home to work out crises, and careers may reach heights of responsibility. But another pressure comes from the soul, with the mandate to give attention to our spiritual self. The ego-self often resists this call for change, using many tactics to delay the spiritual quest, for this would mean your Higher Self and not the ego-self is in charge.

TABLE 5–1	**Energy Meanings of Menopause Issues and Symptoms**

The Energy Center, Menopause Issues, and the Menopause Symptoms are grouped according to the chakra to which they are energetically connected. There is not a direct one-on-one relationship between each issue and specific symptom. For an individual woman, a unique relationship exists between issues and symptoms within each chakra, and multiple symptoms can relate to a given issue.

ENERGY CENTER (CHAKRA)	MENOPAUSE ISSUES	MENOPAUSE SYMPTOMS

1st	Security
	  Cannot trust body
	  Illusion of safety
	Tribal belonging
	Self vs. group/family
	Stand up for self
	Trusting life vs. fear
		Multiple symptoms
		  Cycles change
		  Symptoms worsen
		Energy and reserve less
		Leg and foot problems
		Cramps, restless legs
		Depression, insomnia

2nd	Creativity Shedding limitations Joy running out Control, ethics in relationships Blame, guilt in relationships	Fibroids (uterine tumors) Ovarian cysts, tumors Heavy, irregular bleeding Pelvic congestion, pain Sexual, libido problems
3rd	Self-esteem, worth Personal honor code Fear vs. trust Self-caring, nurturing	Adrenal depletion, fatigue Digestive problems (stomach, bowels) Overeating, cravings Hypoglycemia (metabolic problems, pancreas)
4th	Capacity for love (self, others) Accepting self, others Forgiveness Grief, loss Anger, resentment, bitterness	Breast problems, cancer Lung problems, asthma, bronchitis Heart problems (blood pressure, palpitations, heart disease) Shoulder, arm problems Hot flashes
5th	Expressing self, finding voice Speaking your truth Manifesting your dreams Choice and decisions Judging, criticizing	Thyroid gland problems Teeth, gum problems Cervical spine problems Neck pain Throat pain, esophageal spasm

(Continued on next page)

ENERGY CENTER (CHAKRA)	MENOPAUSE ISSUES	MENOPAUSE SYMPTOMS
6th	Expanding inner vision, knowing Listening to voice of wisdom, truth from within Intuition expansion	Memory disturbances, brain fog Concentration problems Confusion, not understanding Mental blocks
7th	Spiritual connections Faith, inspiration Selfless service Seeing greater patterns Attuning to Divine, your higher purpose in life	Joint and muscle aches, pains Osteoporosis, osteopenia Skin problems Despair (mystical depression) Energy disorders (chronic fatigue syndrome, fibromyalgia) Environmental sensitivities

HOW WOMEN'S ENERGY GETS BLOCKED AND STUCK

The most powerful energy block is fear of change. Because of negative societal images, the changes we face around menopause can be especially frightening. Deeply embedded in this is the fear of aging, disability, and death. As long as these fears have a strong grip on you, even if acting at the unconscious level, you resist movement. This leads to avoidance and may underlie physical-emotional symptoms.

From an energetic view, symptoms serve as metaphors for your psycho-spiritual processes. They are messengers bringing you symbolic communications about the status of your biologic-conscious being. When you listen to these communications, seeking to understand their message, you can use them to guide choices and actions. The underlying theory proposes that our physical structures come to hold our memories, experiences, and habitual thought forms (Myss, 1996; Shealy & Myss, 1993). Organs and tissues actually change over time as a result of our mind's activities. The good news is that if cells can change in one direction (toward illness) then they can also change in the other (toward health).

Menopause-related symptoms can signify certain energetic patterns that are being held in the body or emotions. In general, menopausal problems may reflect fear of aging, self-rejection, fear of no longer being wanted, or not feeling good enough as a woman. Or, they may symbolize deeper levels of change that are transforming consciousness and vibrational frequencies. Symptoms are not "bad" and may simply be an integral part of the vast body-mind-consciousness changes that are happening for menopausal women.

> Perhaps middle age is, or should be, a period of shedding shells; the shell of ambition, the shell of material accumulations and possessions, the shell of the ego.
>
> —Anne Morrow Lindbergh, *A Gift From the Sea*

SPIRITUAL PURPOSES OF MENOPAUSE SYMPTOMS

The physical and emotional symptoms of menopause present an opportunity to discover our bodies as sacred. Going into these bodily events, learning from their symbolism, helps us realize that spiritual meaning is found within the physical experience itself. Menopause brings forth the soul of the body. The body becomes the sacred vessel of transformation, the crucible of fire which clears out what no longer serves us and makes way for what has not yet found its expression.

The following interpretations of common menopause symptoms are drawn from Louise Hay (1999), Caroline Myss (1996), and reflections on the authors' own menopausal journeys. This is one way of interpreting menopausal symptoms which looks at deeper meanings, and may not apply to every situation. The first level expresses symbolic meanings of symptoms, while the second level suggests metaphysical or spiritual meanings. Both levels may be operating simultaneously, and both have their own lessons to assist our spiritual journey.

Hot flashes   Surges of inner heat make women feel as though something is burning up inside. This heat resembles fever, which symbolically stands for anger or irritation. Hot flashes represent the fire of kundalini (feminine creative force) rising into higher chakras (energy centers within the body). According to Caroline Myss, kundalini naturally awakens more powerfully in women after age 40. Yogis spend years learning techniques to awaken this dormant power, which seems to rise naturally in menopausal women. This inner fire burns off impurities and limitations in consciousness. It symbolizes burning away the dross, the unnecessary, all that limits women from expressing our higher spiritual nature.

Fever = burning up, anger or irritation at limitations

Inner heat = kundalini rising, fiery fierceness of protectress-guardian

Tumo Yoga and Hot Flashes

At age 47, Alexandra David-Neel left her privileged life in Paris, her husband, and everything familiar, to seek enlightenment in Tibet. She shaved her head, donned saffron robes, and impersonated a male lama, sneaking

(Continued on next page)

into a forbidden mountain monastery. There she was one of the first Westerners to witness ancient Tibetan sacred rituals and personally learn their meditation practices. On a freezing full-moon night in a Himalayan cave, she watched a ritual called *tumo* (Tibetan for "fierce woman"), in which monks stripped naked then wrapped themselves in wet sheets. The monks raised their body temperatures to dry the sheets; the one who dried the most sheets was considered the highest adept. Through visualizations and sacred sounds, the monks raised life force energy through the chakras and radiated it out as heat. Monks have melted snow for several feet around their bodies with *tumo*. Dr. Herbert Benson, who has extensively studied *tumo* practices, verified that the monks could raise their body temperature more than 10 degrees Fahrenheit.

Used as a spiritual practice, *tumo* is meant to burn away mistakes, false beliefs, and ego attachments that keep the monks from realizing the nature of their True Self, called *rigpa* in Tibetan. Dr. Joan Borysenko suggests that menopausal women can use their hot flashes in this same way, consciously thinking of stresses, worries, and issues, then offering these into the inner fires of transformation to be burned away. She believes that "hot flashes represent a rising and rebalancing of the life-force energy that can help women burn off stress, rather than adding to it."

As this fiery energy first begins to rise in perimenopausal women, it moves through energy channels in erratic, jerky ways. This gives rise to hot flashes. As the energy channels become more open, the flow stabilizes and hot flashes subside. When women have persistent stress, however, energy flows remain erratic and hot flashes persist. Using stress reduction techniques, meditation, relaxation, and breathing can reduce hot flashes by increasing the flow of life energy and opening the channels. Women can use their hot flashes to clear up or release memories, issues and beliefs that are holding back their spiritual process (Borysenko, 1996).

Insomnia Sleep patterns change, with regular awakenings two or three times a night. This may symbolize the accumulated energy consequences of chronic stress, which keeps our sympathetic nervous system alert. We are reaping the results of underlying fears and the inability to trust the process of life. Sometimes the lesson is simply endurance and learning to take better care of yourself. From a mystical perspective, during the early morning hours, the veil between ordinary awareness and other dimensions of reality becomes thinner. Spirit forms or consciousness from other dimensions may be contacting women during these nightly awakenings, particularly between 2 and 4 A.M. We can re-frame middle of the night awakenings as opportunities to receive other-dimensional messages, to meditate, or to tune into deep relaxation that rejuvenates the body.

Insomnia = fear, not trusting life; or the call to trust all life more fully

Midnight awakenings = being touched by the other dimensions

Memory disturbances   Brain fog, forgetfulness, and less concentration are shifts in mental processes that signal a change for midlife women from more left brain, linear-rational functions to right brain intuitive functions. Women's brains are being re-configured to access different ways of knowing, to become more intuitive and synchronistic, and to depend less upon rational and logical thinking. Information is being obtained in other ways from higher levels of consciousness. If, however, women become overwhelmed by life, or feel hopeless and unable to cope, their brain-mind may withdraw from life and lose reasoning power and memory, leading to decreased mental function or possibly dementia.

Dementia = refusing to deal with the world as it is; hopelessness, anger

Synchronistic-intuitive thought = sourcing information from higher consciousness

Depression/anxiety   Fears over the vastness of changes, confusion about the process, and feeling unclear about what's happening underlie these emotional states. Women feel frightened about the impact of menopause on their lives. Anger is the mirror image of depression, but we feel no right to express it, so it turns inward, contracting us into depression and hopelessness. The lesson is to trust the process of our lives and attune to our higher purpose in life, to make the choice of love instead of fear, and to expand outward in service to others.

Depression = anger turned inward, no right to express it, hopelessness, contraction

Trusting the process = being connected with Spirit, knowing change as expansion

Joint/muscle aches   Joint and muscle aches can symbolize body resistance to change. Joints represent changes in direction in life, and the ease with which we flow with these movements. Muscles represent our ability to actively move in life. At menopause women are moving into the spiritual phase of life. The vast changes ahead are frightening, and the body develops "armor" by tensing and stiffening to ward off change or to hold back movement. As we learn to deeply trust our spiritual guidance, inner relaxation takes place. Our joints and muscles become flexible and limber, and we are able to flow into the new directions of our lives.

Joints = resisting changes in life directions

Muscles = resisting new experiences and unable to move forward in life

Inner relaxation = dissipating the fears, opening to spiritual growth

Decreased libido   Less interest in sex is usually attributed to decreased hormones during menopause. It may symbolize issues with our changing bodies feeling less sexual or pleasurable. On the spiritual journey, a time of "celibacy" is required during which the seeker's attention and energy are focused on inner processes and relating to the Divine. This has been part of spiritual initiation, and was built into monastic traditions. A withdrawal of vital life energy appears to be necessary for transformations in consciousness. While women may not actually become celibate, interest in and enjoyment of sex decreases during this phase. It usually returns but often in transmuted forms.

> *Lack of sex drive = issues with changing bodies, feel less pleasure in sexuality*
>
> *Symbolic celibacy = transformative re-direction of energy for spiritual growth*

Fatigue (increased need for sleep)   Feeling fatigued symbolizes resistance to our life processes, or lack of enthusiasm about our lives. We may no longer love what we do, or feel drawn to put energy into our activities. We may not be taking time to restore ourselves, to keep our inner balance in light of our accumulated life stresses. Increased sleep needs often serve the process of spiritual growth. When the conscious, rational mind relaxes its control during sleep, deeper levels of consciousness become active and process buried material in symbolic dreams. Menopausal women often have vivid dreams. The Higher Self or Spirit dimension has greater ability to communicate with us during sleep states, and help us resolve problems or expand our consciousness.

> *Fatigue = resistance, lack of enthusiasm about life, not restoring ourselves*
>
> *Sleep need = deeper levels of consciousness doing symbolic processing for spiritual growth*

Neurotheology: The Brain Is Wired for God

Neurotheology, an emerging field of scientific research, uses advanced brain imaging techniques to uncover the neurological basis for spiritual and mystical experiences. It detects what happens in our brains when we experience a reality different from, and in a crucial sense higher than, our everyday reality. Certain regions of the brain turn on, and others turn off, during experiences that seem to exist outside time and space. When we think we have encountered Spirit, and when we feel transported by prayer, ritual, or sacred music, certain brain circuits surge with activity while others go quiescent. Spiritual experiences are so consistent across cultures, time, and faiths that scientists believe this points to "a common core that is likely a reflection of structures and processes in the human brain" (Begley, 2001).

Dr. Andrew Newberg of the Division of Nuclear Medicine at the University of Pennsylvania describes the neurobiology of mystical experiences in his book, *Why*

God Won't Go Away: Brain Science & the Biology of Belief (Newberg, D'Aquili, & Rause, 2001). Using a SPECT (single photon emission computed tomography) machine, brain activity at the peak of meditation and contemplative prayer was mapped, using experienced Tibetan Buddhists and Catholic nuns. Intense, deep meditation or concentration, regardless of the technique used, eventually causes quieting of activity in the neurons in brain regions that orient people in space, and those that mark the distinction between self and world. This leads to the vast, expansive feeling of unity in which one merges into the infinite. According to Newberg and colleagues, the following brain processes occur:

- The *autonomic nervous system,* responsible for the body's fight-or-flight response and for quieting afterwards, is fundamental to religious experience. The arousal and quiescent parts of this system operate inversely; when one increases, activity in the other decreases.

- *Hyperquiescence,* a state of extraordinary relaxation, is evoked through meditation and slow, quiet rituals such as chanting and prayer. At intense levels, body and mind enter a sense of oceanic tranquility and bliss in which no thoughts, feelings, or body sensations are present.

- *Hyperarousal,* a state of unblocked excitation, is produced through continuous, rhythmic motor activity, such as rapid Sufi ritual dancing, marathon running, and long-distance swimming. In this state people feel keen alertness, intense concentration, and effortless flow of vast amounts of energy through their consciousness.

- *Breakthrough states* occur when either hyperquiescence or hyperarousal go so far that the normal balancing of the autonomic nervous system is overwhelmed. This neurological spillover leads to intensely altered states of consciousness.

- In *deep meditation,* when quiescent levels reach maximum, the arousal system erupts causing an exhilarating rush of energy that makes one feel absorbed into the object of concentration: a candle, lotus, cross, or religious figure, for example. When the technique of clearing the mind is used, this process results in a sense of limitless self and oneness with the universe.

- With *intense, rhythmic activity,* after maximum arousal occurs, the quiescent system surges forth to produce a trance-like state, which often is experienced as an ecstatic rush of orgasmic-like energy.

- In *SPECT images* of meditators, the prefrontal cortex of the brain (seat of attention) lights up as focus deepens (Figure 5–2). The orientation association area goes dark, showing little activity as intense concentration blocks sensory inputs to this region. The function of this region is to process information about where the body ends and the rest of the world begins. The left orientation area creates the sensation of a physically delimited body, and the right orientation area creates the sense of physical space around the body.

- When *sensory inputs are blocked* to these regions (called *deafferentation*), the brain cannot distinguish between self and not-self. With no incoming information, the left orientation area cannot find a boundary between self and world. The brain then must perceive the self as endless and interwoven with everything. The right orientation area deprived of information cannot locate the body in space. The brain perceives a feeling of infinite space, an expansion of self into infinity.

- The *limbic system* (refer to Figure 5–2) is involved in this process. The two basic pathways are *passive* (clearing the mind) and *active* (focusing on object):

    Passive: As deafferentation progresses, the hippocampus (which regulates arousal and quiescent autonomic functions) blocks neural flow to the orientation association area. The hypothalamus (which links limbic and autonomic systems to the cortex) creates strong quiescent sensations. This causes bursts of neural impulses back through the limbic system to the attention association area, which registers calming impulses and

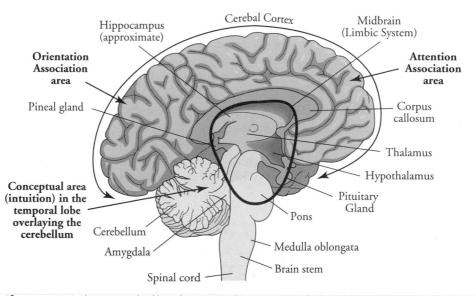

Figure 5–2 Brain Areas Involved in Unitary States of Consciousness. The Attention Association area, located in the frontal lobe activates as focus deepens in meditation. When concentration becomes intense, sensory inputs are blocked to the Orientation Association areas, which go dark on brain scan resulting in expanded or unitary states. The temporal lobe, overlaying part of the cerebellum, is related to conceptual function and intuition, important for spiritual experiences. It connects with limbic system structures (seat of emotions) which lie underneath it.

relays them back through the same circuit. This reverberating circuit continues until the hypothalamus is pushed to its calming limits. Then neurological spillover occurs, triggering an instantaneous maximal arousal response. This supercharges the orientation association area, causing total shutdown of neural input, resulting in mystical experiences of absolute spacelessness and oneness with all.

Active: Increased neural flow causes the right orientation area to fix on the object (actual or imagined). Discharges from this area travel down through the limbic system to the hypothalamus and trigger arousal. As contemplation deepens, discharges flow more intensely until the arousal function reaches maximal levels. Then spillover occurs, causing immediate maximal activation of the hypothalamus' quiescent function. These impulses flood back through the limbic structures to the attention association area, pushing it to maximal levels. This profoundly affects the orientation areas. The left orientation area becomes deafferented, causing blurring of the sense of self. The right orientation area focuses more sharply on the object, and is deprived of all neural input not originating from this focus. The image of the object (lotus, Christ) becomes the spatial matrix in which the self exists, leading to mystical absorption into the transcendent reality of the object.

These neurological processes and their accompanying spiritual experiences are fundamental to being human. The intensity of these states of unity depends upon the degree of neural blockage, and occur along a continuum. The most profound experiences of the mystics of all religions, and the smaller transcendent moments that are common in many people's lives, are different essentially by degree. Mystical spiritual experiences are surprisingly prevalent. Sociologist Andrew Greeley (1987) conducted a landmark study for the National Opinion Research Center asking the question: "Have you ever felt as though you were very close to a spiritual force that seemed to lift you out of yourself?" More than 35 percent of the people surveyed said that they had. Of that number, 18 percent had one

---

Humans, in fact, are natural mystics blessed with an inborn genius for effortless self-transcendence. If you ever "lost yourself" in a beautiful piece of music . . . or felt "swept away" by a rousing patriotic speech, you have tasted in a small but revealing way the essence of mystical union. If you have . . . been wonder-struck by the beauty of nature, you know how it feels when the ego slips away and for a dazzling moment . . . you vividly understand that you are a part of something larger.

—Andrew Newberg, *Why God Won't Go Away*

or two experiences, 12 percent had several, and 5 percent had experienced this often.

Midlife women seem especially open to entering expanded states of consciousness, and exploring processes that lead to feelings of unity and oneness. Perhaps the hormonal changes of perimenopause and menopause, with their effects on the limbic system and intuitive brain structures, are priming them for spiritual and mystical experiences. Many of the activities to which midlife women are drawn, such as meditation, contemplation, women's groups, drumming, chanting, and healing prayers or circles, act as catalysts for the mental and neurobiological events that create these unitary states.

Worksheets 5–2 (page 229) and 5–3 (page 230) offer exercises for relaxation, enhancing intuition, and meditation.

Ways that Women Experience Unitary States

Unitary states include the sense of softened self-boundaries, expansive awareness, opening the heart to universal love, deep tranquility, bliss, ecstasy, and being connected with all. These occur along a continuum from absorption in music or nature, to shared inspiration during a religious service, to heart-coherent rhythms during singing or drumming, to spiritual awe and rapture, to ecstasy and hyperlucid visions, and finally to profound states of mystical union. Here are a few examples of how women experience unitary states.

Drumming

The repeated rhythmic beats of drumming entrains heart rhythms into coherence, and drives brain pathways that produce intense pleasurable feelings, the sense of being connected with ancient patterns, and feelings of unity with others.

> Drumming connects me with the heartbeat of Mother Earth, it leads to entrainment of the heart. I lose self-consciousness and become one with the drum and the other people. It takes me out of myself, into my center and removes me from the ego; it's almost ecstatic. It's a powerful way to be connected with something bigger than the self—something very primal.
>
> —Harmony Rose, medical technician

(Continued on next page)

Chanting

The repeated auditory and rhythmic stimulation from singing or chanting activates the limbic and autonomic systems, creating the sensation of being out of yourself and merging into a larger, exhilarating state of being, or creating a state of deep inner calmness.

> I particularly like chanting in groups. At the deepest moments, it's as if I am floating above the body, watching myself. My voice is unusually beautiful—it must be someone else's voice! The devotional chant seems to be playing itself through me, as I sing and sway to the rhythm. As the heart rejoices, there's an elevation of my energy until I am swept into the current of Divine grace. Those times are magical, yet familiar, for I am but touching my own higher Self.
>
> —Nalini Graeber, accountant

Healing Prayers

The intense focus and direction of healing energy to others activates the brain's arousal and quiescent systems, resulting in states of expanded awareness, feeling out of yourself, and being connected to a greater power. This enhances immune system function, reduces stress responses, and generates feelings of calmness and well-being.

> First I light a candle and focus on the flame. I burn incense of a healing herb, like sandalwood or cinnamon, and visualize healing energy going out on the smoke to the person I'm doing healing for. Sometimes I put their picture on my altar. I'm in a light trance state, feeling expanded beyond myself, and less aware of my physical boundaries.
>
> —Kathi deAnda, co-op herbal and mercantile buyer

Meditation

Regardless of method, the purpose of meditation is to silence the conscious mind and free its awareness from the limits of ego or the material world. It triggers the process of deafferentation (neural blocking that deprives brain areas of information) and related brain functions to

(Continued on next page)

create states of inner stillness, expanding beyond self, merging into the infinite, or pure awareness.

> I practice meditation gratefully, knowing it is the door to my Higher Self. I sit, take a deep breath, and feel like I've come home. I get very quiet inside, a familiar place, it feels like where I want to be. If anything will get me to union with God, meditation will.
>
> —Nancy Hill, musician and teacher

BALANCING ENERGY AND AWARENESS FOR SPIRITUAL EXPANSION

When vital energy flow is blocked or when it leaks out of organs and tissues, the body is unable to function properly. To re-energize depleted cells, or to open blocked energy flows, you can use a combination of physical, mental and spiritual techniques. Many of the physical approaches are covered in Chapter 3. While these are useful tools, and often provide great relief of menopause-related symptoms, they do not restore energetic balance by themselves. Women also need healing, integration and harmony in the mental/emotional and spiritual aspects of their being.

Following are some major areas to help with energy integration and awareness.

Shaping Our Attitudes

- *Develop positive attitudes toward older women.* Find ways to have positive, self-affirming attitudes about menopause, the wise woman and crone stages, and growing into very old age. Avoid being influenced by cultural negativity about older women. New models of vital mature women are all

. . . Think of yourself at all times as an energy being as well as a physical one. . . . Spiritual instruction teaches us to keep our focus on ourselves—not in an egocentric way but as a way of consciously managing our energy and power. . . . Our spirits, our energy, and our personal power are all one and the same force.

—Caroline Myss, *Anatomy of the Spirit*

around. Growing older can be viewed as the ultimate adventure. Nearly all religions teach that *we are infinite spirit* beyond the temporary body, that our essential being always continues to exist in some form. Physical death is seen as a transition into another state of being (soul, spirit, infinite consciousness, astral self).

- *Replace negative tapes running in your mind.* These usually keep repeating how inadequate, worthless, undeserving, inept, dumb, ugly, or miserable you are. Anything you repeat often enough in your mind, it will come to believe. You can effectively replace negative tapes with positive ones, even if you find it hard to "believe" in the beginning. Keep at it, use affirmations that support new attitudes, and you will see new grooves cut in your habitual mental processes.

- *Understand how reality is shaped by your perceptions.* What you see "out there" in the world is a projection of your inner consciousness, the creator of your perceptions. Those who see love and goodness in others are expressing those qualities within themselves. Watch what you criticize in others, for that very quality lives within you and your critique actually is aimed at yourself. Refrain from envy and jealousy; these are caustic to the soul. Every being is given exactly what is right for her or his life journey. Recognize and celebrate what you have been given, even if it seems more humble or challenging than the lot of others.

- *Cultivate a sense of being empowered in your life.* Only you can assign meanings to the events of life (unless you give this over to society, your mother, a church, friends, and so on). Find your own meanings, always seeing things from the highest viewpoint. We are in truth co-creators of our lives. Although you cannot control many events and situations, you *always have the choice* of how to react to them—and the meanings you give them.

> Fish cannot drown in water,
> Birds cannot sink in air,
> Gold cannot perish
> In the refiner's fire.
> This has God given to all creatures,
> To foster and seek their own nature,
> How then can I withstand mine?
>
> —Mechthild of Magdeburg
> (1210–1297?) in Carol Lee
> Flinders, *Enduring Grace: Living
> Portraits of Seven Women Mystics*

- *Develop the qualities of compassion and acceptance.* These have the power to transform yourself and others. Have compassion for yourself; love all parts of the self, even the apparently "negative" ones. From this it follows that you will have compassion, forgiveness, and acceptance for others.

The process of working with our energy anatomy, using the forces of attention and intention, is described by Caroline Myss (2000) as "spiritual alchemy." The principle of spiritual alchemy is that our habitual thoughts convert into forms that find expression in our lives. Our challenge is to become alchemists in our own lives, by changing the "lead" of our wounds into the "gold" of wisdom. It requires an enormous amount of focused energy to actually create physical manifestations of our thought forms. For most of us, the outside world largely shapes our thought forms, and we are plugged into the commonly held social views of life's realities. Every thought form that we hold takes energy from our electromagnetic system. This energy from thousands of people keeps these limiting thought forms alive and powerful in our culture: Money equals power; success means having power over others; resources are limited, so look out for No. 1; men are better than women; you are either in control or being controlled; happiness equals having a new BMW, big house, and diversified portfolio . . . and so on.

Other thought forms with a more expansive outlook simultaneously exist in our culture. Concern for the environment, service to those in need, the power of unconditional love, the interconnection of all life, and happiness as an inner state of being are commonly held ideas. Dr. Beatrice Bruteau, religious scholar, believes that mysticism provides the world with its best hope for overcoming the greed, mistrust, and self-protective fears that have led to so much strife and suffering. Expanded awareness and experiences of mystical wholeness show us that we are fundamentally connected with each other, and actually do have what we need to be happy. According to Brutreau, from the preface in Teasdale (1999), "This oneness—this freedom from alienation and insecurity—is the sure foundation for a better world. It means that we will try to help each other rather than hurt each other."

We animate these various societal thought forms with the energy of our body-mind-spirit system. Since parts of our personal energy and consciousness are given to these ideas, it is important to choose carefully where we want to invest our self. If we give too much energy to thought forms that are limiting, negative, or draining, then our energetic systems are not being fed and nurtured. This diminishes the total energy we have available to work our own spiritual alchemy, and we then lack enough magnetic force to attract to ourselves the people and circumstances necessary to make the changes we want in our lives. The key questions to ask yourself about investing your life force energy are:

1. Do I want my energy to animate that particular vision of the world?
2. What world vision, belief system, and actions do I really want to invest with my life force energy?

The steps in spiritual alchemy of making your life change are, according to Myss (2000):

- *Evaluate where your energy is,* sense when energy is leaving your system (it may be drawn out by other people, sapped by societal thought forms, or invested in negative beliefs).

- *Complete "unfinished business"* that is influencing your physical life. This often requires letting go of painful memories, forgiving and accepting betrayals, giving up judgments, and living by your honor code.

- *Identify and put into language* what you want to manifest in your life, and get your mind, willpower, and heart in line with your vision.

- *Activate the archetypes* connected with this aspect of yourself. These universal thought forms activate your inner magnetic patterns through imagery, myth and dreams, as described by Carl Jung (Pascal, 1992). The patterns of these archetypes guide you in the process of converting energy into matter. You tap into tremendous power to animate your vision through using archetypal energies. (Chapter 6 describes archetypes and myth, and focuses on important archetypes for midlife and menopausal women).

Many techniques can be used to activate and balance our energy centers. These can be learned from spiritual teachers, holistic counselors, energy practitioners, and many self-help books and workshops. Methods include these categories:

- *Breath techniques* such as consciously directing breath and energy into areas of the body (pranayama, shamanic breath work, kahuna breathing).

- *Visualization* of light, space, or colors flowing into areas of the body.

- *Meditation techniques* which usually include quieting the body-mind, focus and concentration, creating a state of inner stillness, then feeling expansiveness.

- *Integration work* in which we finish any unfinished business with self and others, bring issues or processes to closure, face and explore our fears and the shadow side, and accept and integrate what we find there. Ultimately the purpose is to recognize, come to know, accept, and integrate all parts of ourselves, even those we dislike, loathe, or fear. Every experience, thought, attitude, and intention we have had is part of our life journey. We must see the role each plays, and choose which to keep current and which to acknowledge and put aside.

- *Physical self-care* affects energy patterns in the body-mind. We need nutritious foods, pure water, moderation in eating, minimal stimulants, avoidance of toxic substances, clean air, toning and limbering exercises, adequate sleep, relationships that support our growth, peaceful home environments, and avoidance of "mind-stealers" such as excess television, movies, and videos.

Place your mind before the mirror of eternity!
Place your soul in the brilliance of glory!
Place your heart in the figure of the divine substance!
And transform your entire being into the image
Of the Godhead Itself through contemplation.

—Saint Clare of Assisi (1195–1253), in Carol Lee
Flinders, *Enduring Grace: Living Portraits of Seven
Women Mystics*

From Being Stuck to Flowing with Life

I had not met Anika until she came to see me at the medical clinic, although we lived in the same Sierra Foothills community and were both in the alternative healing field. A usually healthy 53-year-old woman who had passed through menopause with few symptoms, Anika was now experiencing severe constipation. She had already tried self-care such as more water, fruits, and vegetables, psyllium seed drinks, and herbal laxatives. However, she felt bloated and toxic and experienced hard painful bowel movements only once a week. I prescribed maximum-strength stool hydrators, but we quickly agreed that the problem was deeper and began working together in my private consulting practice on the symbolic energy-body meanings that constipation held for her.

Constipation is a malfunction of the colon and rectum. Rectal problems are energetically connected with the first chakra, and colon problems with the third chakra. Associated issues include security/safety, feelings of belonging, being able to stand up for yourself, self-respect, caring for yourself, and facing fear or intimidation. Being constipated is a metaphor for being stuck in old ideas or ways of doing things, and having trouble releasing things of the past.

This exactly described the issues that Anika was grappling with in her life. She felt stuck in a joint business venture with her husband and his partner, which she did not have much voice in shaping. They were running a retreat on an isolated property in the mountains that was minimally developed. To her mind, the land was dry and harsh. The earth was red clay with many gray-brown rocks, and the ground was like cement in the arid summers. She yearned for the moist, gentle coastal breezes and the cool greens and blues near the ocean. Everything at the retreat was difficult,

(Continued on next page)

even getting drinking water and food and coaxing plants to grow. There were financial issues and it was a struggle to make ends meet.

Anika realized she had not stood up for her beliefs in this business venture. She had felt intimidated by the two powerful men shaping the project. Because of this, she harbored resentment and found herself stuck in old patterns of relating to her husband. She had not been taking care of herself or listening to her body's needs. This holding back, being stuck, and not releasing old ways of relating was being expressed in her body as constipation.

Following these insights and some soul-searching, Anika decided to make changes to take care of her own needs. First she took an extended visit with a friend living near the coast. This led to starting a parttime counseling business in that area, with regular visits to the mountain retreat to do programs with her husband. Anika created a home and work for herself in the coastal town, where she felt she belonged. She also re-patterned ways of relating to her husband and the business venture. By making her needs clear and her concerns visible, she regained self-respect, overcame intimidation, and took care of herself. During this process, her constipation gradually resolved.

— Lennie Martin, RN, FNP

Creative Expression

We are all naturally creative. When we create, our Divine or higher nature is being expressed. The need for growth in consciousness, and expressing our creativity, is programmed into our genes. When growth or creativity are blocked, some part of the body-mind structures will symbolically carry out these processes, and this may produce tumors, mental illness, or other health problems. Creativity has a vast range of expression, including but not limited to art, dance, music, drama, and writing.

Consider the suggestions listed below and create:

- Sacred space inside or around your home
- Loving relationships
- Joyful friendships
- Inner wisdom

> Let us imagine that within us is an extremely rich palace, built entirely of gold and precious stones. . . . Within us lies something incomparably more precious than what we see outside ourselves. Let's not imagine that we are hollow inside.
>
> —Saint Teresa of Avila, "Way of Perfection 28.10" in Carol Lee Flinders, *Enduring Grace: Living Portraits of Seven Women Mystics*

- Beauty or harmony in everyday activities
- New hobbies; find your fun/passion
- A new image of the menopausal woman
- Space for growth and transformation
- Songs and rituals to reclaim women's traditions
- The aura of compassion for animals and other creatures
- The consciousness of unity for the planet Earth
- A safe space for someone else's self-expression

Listening to Inner Guidance

The "inner voice" is our intuition speaking to us, providing guidance about choices and directions in life. We have "gut instinct," which is basic survival intuition and can be felt in the solar plexus (third chakra) or pit of the stomach. This informs us of danger, and gives a strong message that things are not right. A higher level of intuition comes from the "spiritual eye" energy center (sixth chakra) located near the forehead. When we tune into this intuition, we receive guidance from our higher self, the indwelling divine spirit, or, we can receive information and communications from spirit guides and angels through this higher center.

We are all naturally intuitive. This process gets blocked for many in early childhood, and we learn to distrust our inner sense of things. Menopause can be the time to reconnect with our innate intuitive capacity, if it has not already happened. If this is new territory for you, many resources can help get you going (see Worksheet 5-2 on page 229 and books in this chapter's references). There are many approaches to expanding intuition. The basic principles usually include:

- Stilling, quieting, and relaxing the mind
- Calming or tuning out fear
- Concentrating deeply in the heart or spiritual eye energy centers

> Yet the Goddess does not merely give us knowledge. She is the knowledge . . . the womb through which we are reborn into the world of truth. . . . Ultimately the Goddess is not merely knowledge but pure consciousness itself. . . . She is the knowledge that puts the mind to rest and returns us to the source.
>
> —David Frawley, *Tantric Yoga and the Wisdom Goddesses*

- Observing your feelings and thoughts carefully
- Tuning into physical sensations (the body never lies about our perceptions)
- Trusting your first responses
- Being patient and open to the unexplainable or unexpected
- Keeping a journal (writing experiences, perceptions, and dreams)
- Using "oracles" (Tarot, pendulum, I Ching, and so on)

Connecting with Spirit

Nearly every human being deeply yearns for connection with her/his Source, that infinite beingness from which we originated, the Divine and Sacred One, or however we may think of it. Most of our desires, goals, ambitions, pursuits, attachments, loves, and passions are expressions of our quest for reunion with this Divine Source. The numerous religious traditions in the world have as their highest purpose finding ways to assist us on this spiritual journey (Smith, 1992). Every person's way is unique, to be discovered during the tests and lessons of life. So, ultimately we must apply what religious traditions offer us in our own particular, unique way to support our path of reconnecting with our Divine essence. Many tools are available to aid this quest. Most religious traditions have some form of these and it is unifying to note the commonalities:

PRAYER

Communicating with Goddess or God.   In prayer, we "talk" to the Divine and may be asking for help, seeking guidance, offering love and devotion, sending prayers to others, examining ourselves and asking forgiveness for faults, and many other purposes. The highest form of prayer seeks union with the Divine and a merging of the self (ego-personality) into the Self (Higher Self, Divine Essence). The main types of prayer are associated with various stages of the spiritual journey (discussed in a later section, Path of Modern Mystics).

MEDITATION

Listening to Goddess or God   After using techniques to quiet the mind, concentrate, become still, and focus attention on expanded states of consciousness, we can enter the true state of meditation which is a form of Divine union. In that state, we often receive communications from spirit or our higher Self. We can experience vastly expanded states of consciousness, feeling oneness with all life, getting the sense of our cosmic reality, or intuitive knowing that gives great insights. Bliss, peace, serenity, and ecstasy are feeling experiences of Divine union.

SERVICE

Giving Our Talents/Energy to the World to Benefit Others   In the Christian tradition, this is called "good works." The Hindus call it "dharma" or right action. The act of selfless giving, whatever its form, opens the heart. It takes us out of self-centered concerns, and keeps us from over-focusing upon our own needs or troubles. Serving others is one of the best ways to "purify" our hearts, to remove veils or clouds that keep our love and light from shining through. As Christ said: "Blessed are the pure of heart, for they shall see God." And, "That which you do unto the least of mine, you do unto me."

INTROSPECTION/CONTEMPLATION

Study of the Inner Process and Eternal Truth   Through these practices we are becoming aware of levels of self, understanding our minds and behaviors, and learning from going into the mystery of life. This "examination of conscience"

> Wouldst thou know my meaning?
> Lie down in the Fire
> See and taste the Flowing
> Godhead through thy being;
> Feel the Holy Spirit
> Moving and compelling
> Thee within the Flowing
> Fire and Light of God.
>
> —Mechthild of Magdeburg (1210–1297?),
> in Carol Lee Flinders, *Enduring Grace:
> Living Portraits of Seven Women Mystics*

brings shortcomings into awareness and puts us at choice. We contemplate the mystery of "who is the observer" of ourselves? Contemplation requires going into the midst of paradox; for we can only know the Mystery by letting go of knowing, and find the course of action within stillness.

PATTERN DISRUPTION

Shifting Our Awareness by Changing Habitual Ways of Being   The practice of fasting or giving something up can lead quickly to altered perceptions. We can "fast" in many ways, such as giving up television, sweets, coffee, driving the car, criticizing, complaining, or worrying for one day. This often enables us to establish a different relationship with our bodies or minds, and it broadens our perspectives on our families, society, or the world. As a discipline, periodic pattern disruption strengthens our will and aids mastery over physical and emotional drives.

RITUALS

Ceremonial Activities with Symbolic Meanings   Rituals include private and communal practices which serve many spiritual purposes. Group rituals bring people together to share and support each other's spiritual life. Group worship, sacraments, singing, eating together, retreats, rites of passage, and ceremonies are common to most religions. Women are developing their own rituals to honor the important stages of life. "Coming of age" ceremonies for girls at menarche recapture the rich tradition of celebrating their entry into womanhood, and its importance to community creativity and regeneration. "Creatrix and Croning" ceremonies are done for midlife and menopausal women, acknowledging their transition to the life stage of abundant creativity, wisdom, clarity of vision, and seed-carrier for the coming generations. These ceremonies are becoming more common, as women reclaim ancient traditions that honor our sisters reaching their wisdom years. Having a ritual for the transition into the wise-woman phase of life, witnessed and supported by friends, is a powerful affirmation. It is one way to invoke the archetypal pattern of the Wise Woman/Sage, and thus activate this pattern into our lives (see Chapter 6).

PATH OF MODERN MYSTICS

- "Why am I here?"
- "For what purpose was I born?"
- "What is the real meaning of life?"

When we begin to ask these questions our spiritual journey really takes off. We will be propelled on the path of mysticism that takes us out of our ordinary lives.

To all of us who seek life's deeper meanings and purposes, Caroline Myss in her audiotape "Spiritual Madness" says: "You're mystics without monasteries . . . everyday mystics and saints" (Myss, 1997). Our entire life is up for examination. Basic assumptions and belief systems may be questioned and upturned. Often we do not fit comfortably in our own lives any more. This can be deeply disturbing and unsettling. We fear that major changes will be needed, and nothing will be the same again. For some it is time to face the truth about an unfulfilling job, unsatisfactory relationship, unexpressed talent, over-committed life, unhealthy lifestyle, or lack of spirituality.

The path for modern mystics is new and uncharted. In earlier times, when a person heard the call to seek spiritual intimacy with God, she or he left society and entered a monastery. In this specially structured setting, issues of the ordinary life were set aside and practices established to support the inner quest for union with Spirit. It was expected that one's self-concept would be dismantled, that a period of chaos or madness would occur, and then an entirely transformed being would emerge who communicated with God and carried out the Divine plan on earth, whether that was a life of prayer and austerities or dedication to humanitarian causes.

Now we are being called to stay in ordinary life and seek to experience the mystical. We must spiritualize everyday life. This means living in the world of families, jobs, activities, pleasures, creativity, and conflicts without losing ourselves to this world. We are being asked to see all these things as aspects of the Divine essence, to be able to enjoy them while keeping our spiritual center and realizing that they do not define us. We need the inner spiritual power to "Be among the jewels but not sell our soul to have them" (Myss, 1997). To arrive at this center, you must attain a degree of mastery in two directions: self-discovery which takes you into yourself, and mysticism which takes you out of yourself. No wonder we enter a time of spiritual madness, as we are pulled in such vastly different directions.

Stages of the Spiritual Journey

The stages on the spiritual journey have been described in many traditions. Following is a blending of contemporary thinking that draws from mystical Christian, Jewish kabbalistic, and eastern (Hindu, Buddhist) sources.

AWAKENING

The Call to the Spiritual Journey   More often that not, a crisis or tragedy provokes our awakening. While this can happen at any time during life, having a major life crisis is quite common around ages 40 to 50. For women, menopause may be this crisis, or it may combine with other events to throw our lives into upheaval. We ask "Why is this happening to me? Where am I going? Who am I?" Sometimes we are provoked not by a crisis, but by the lack of one. Life begins to lose its meaning, we have no sense of direction, or things we enjoyed before just do not engage us anymore. The goals we have been seeking, and to some degree have realized, are failing to bring us lasting satisfaction and happiness. We ask "Is this all there is?"

We question the values of materialism. We yearn for something deeper, purer, and more true. On an intuitive level, we realize we must be more than our physical, material selves. Thus, we revisit spirituality, often taking a fresh approach from some other tradition than the one in which we were raised. Americans and other Westerners have flocked to eastern spiritual paths over the past 2–3 decades, and many Indians and Asians have turned to Christianity.

Whether our intention is clear or not, what we are seeking is to become more conscious of spirit or God/Goddess in our lives. We want to hear the voice of the Divine giving us understanding and guidance. The consequence is that we are asking the Infinite Force to reorder our lives, to strip away every false voice, and to remove distractions so we can hear that higher voice clearly, which propels us into the next stage.

PURIFICATION

Separation and Aloneness   We are taken out of our ordinary lives, sometimes physically and at other times symbolically. We begin to see what we are doing that keeps our lives from working. This self-examination is often painful, but if we can keep a sense of humor about our own and other people's human foibles, we can have plenty of good laughs. We want to clean up our act, and start working on things that keep us from intimacy with God/Goddess, such as food, alcohol, other addictions, meanness, carping, gossiping, selfishness, worries, and fears. This is the stage of "do's and don'ts" on the spiritual path, called by the great Indian sage Patanjali the Yamas (abstentions) and Niyamas (observances) (Prabhavananda & Isherwood, 1953; Johnston, 1993). These are akin to Moses' Ten Commandments and Christ's Beatitudes. Table 5–2 summarizes these principles.

The stage of separation and aloneness can lead to depression. As we shift from accepting the material values of the world, and observe injustices that negate the law of human cause and effect, a sense of alienation sets in. We feel detached, incongruent with the once familiar, strange in what was once comfortable in our lives. We wait for some sign. Are we going crazy? The deep aloneness comes from our sense that no one will understand, that there is no way to fully explain our discomfort. Even when we stay in our relationships, family, or job, we still face the fear of being alone in a soul sense. We wait. Will we ever hear the voice of higher guidance? The classic spiritual lessons of this stage are patience and

TABLE 5–2	The Do's and Don't's on the Spiritual Path

ABSTAIN FROM (DON'T)	OBSERVE (DO)
Injury, violence	Positive thinking
Lying, speaking untruth	Speak kindly, harmoniously
Stealing, coveting	Physical cleanliness, order
Misuse of sexuality	Contentment
Greed, overindulgence	Self-control
Negative thinking	Self-study, introspection
Judging others	Attunement, meditation, devotion

endurance. As we are purified of limitations, we become strong enough to face any challenge without fear.

ILLUMINATION

Filling with Inner Light   Turning inward, we discover something marvelous that lies at our core. What we have been waiting for was inside all the time. Our lives become filled with mystery and wonder, we feel more fully alive than ever before. Each moment, each event takes on incredible meaning and richness. In her own unique way, each woman experiences contact with the Divine essence. These spiritual experiences come through dreams, inner visions, an expanded capacity for love, or a sense of being connected with everything. Some people will discover abilities such as clairvoyance, prophecy, and healing. Some may see or communicate with angels, Masters, or Divine beings. Miraculous things may happen in your life, synchronicities may occur that could only be directed by some higher intelligence.

Spiritual phenomena are a double-edged sword. These experiences explode our minds so that we can perceive the world differently. However, they also can be destructive, and the great Masters warn against getting too caught up in "powers." Yogananda said, "The spiritual path is not a circus" and Jesus Christ said, "Lest ye see signs and wonders, ye believe not." The real shadow side is spiritual pride or elitism, when the ego sneaks in to claim these events as its own and wants us to feel special, better than others. Most spiritual teachers advise us to be careful about how we relate to mystical phenomena. This is one reason why mystics and great spiritual traditions teach the love of neighbor as a core doctrine. Catholic saints are chosen for their charity and service, not their mystical experiences. Bodhisattvas in the Buddhist tradition are noted for their endless compassion, not their spiritual attainments. In the Jewish tradition, the "day of atonement"

Vision of God at Machu Picchu

Sophy Burnham describes how her perceptual abilities were radically changed during a mystical experience she had at Machu Picchu in the Andes. Hearing a hollow, roaring sound in both ears, like listening to a seashell, she realized she needed to be alone, and she left her group to find an isolated spot on a hillside. The roaring sound became overpowering, then she felt a terrible and majestic pressure on her neck. A wordless voice resounded within, "You are mine" and filled her with its intent: that hard work would be required of her. At first she resisted, then thought "If you are God, yes. . . . With your help." Upon surrendering, she was immersed in sweetness that words could not express. She was washed in waves of light, and also was the light, dissolved into the light. She heard the singing of the planets, saw their destruction as in nuclear fires, the passing of millions of years, and the re-growth of life. Seeing into the very structure of the universe, she realized the perfection of all things, and how destruction was simply transmutation of matter into energy, in endless acts of love and creativity, all expressions of pure God-essence. For hours afterward, she perceived light streaming from her hands, flashing in the fields, and flowing out of other people.

The impact of this inner vision changed Sophy's life, and propelled her into difficult times. Her marriage ended, her work changed, many associations ended and others began, and she embarked on a spiritual search that was often filled with pain and loneliness. All her ideas about how God worked in the world were turned upside down. Years later Sophy wryly remarked:

The ecstasies, of course, don't last. You always come back down . . . and continue just what you were doing before, one foot in front of the other. . . . Except that nothing looks the same. For one thing, you see that God is found in the *dailyness* of life. . . . You see that all life is a feast, all right there spread out for us to enjoy.

—Sophy Burnham, *The Ecstatic Journey*

is considered the highest holy day, when people right any wrongs done to their neighbors.

The purpose of mystical phenomena is to let us directly experience that we are more than the body, physical reality, or our usual conceptions of ourselves. This moves us from the realm of believing to that of knowing. We know we are one with Spirit, that the Divine essence resides within. We have entered Saint Teresa's "Interior Castle" and glimpsed its wonders. In experiencing our oneness with all, our hearts open wide with universal love. We become aware of the power of that love.

Now we are prepared for the next stage, the dismantling of our dearest spiritual fantasies and ambitions, so we may peel off the next layer: the Dark Night.

THE DARK NIGHT OF THE SOUL

Much has been written about the Dark Night, first coined by St. John of the Cross. It is the phase of soul despair, of fearing that God/Goddess has deserted us, of confronting our spiritual shadow. We all have spiritual fantasies about how God/Goddess should look, talk to us, come to us, and relate to us. We have spiritual ambitions, perhaps defined as attaining samadhi (God-union), enlightenment, heaven, nirvana, bliss, or various powers as a seer, mystic, or healer. Now we must go through these and let them go, because these mind forms are keeping us from experiencing the Infinite beyond our definitions and conceptions.

People who were having visions or hearing angel voices may lose this ability. Those who felt great peace, joy, and serenity may become restless, disturbed, and discontent. Any remaining seeds of negativity and limitation must be sought out, brought up, and released. The process gets more and more subtle. Whereas before we attained the discipline to refrain from speaking unkindly of another, now we are called to restructure the mental process that would even lead to an unkind thought.

We reverse mental and electromagnetic processes within our body-mind. This is complex and many yogic and esoteric practices are used to rewire our systems. There are yoga postures that integrate body and mind, and balance life energies. Other postures help us attain stillness, quietude, and a solid foundation for sitting in meditation. Yogic techniques for breath control bring vital life force energy into the body-mind and allow us to direct the flow of prana or chi. By learning to withdraw the senses and turn sense attention inward, we attain detachment from our reactions to objects or experiences. This brings us to the "observer" phase of spiritual growth where we watch the play of the mind. Concentration techniques using mantras and breath focus attention on one object, deeply interiorizing our consciousness. As meditation brings absorption in the object of contemplation, an effortless serenity and expansion beyond thoughts occurs. In advanced stages, there is unification of consciousness, at-oneness, and bliss (Kriyananda, 1988).

A few examples of changes in our perspectives that result from these processes are:

- The union of opposites—chaos is as much part of Divine order as is stability; pleasure and pain are equally valuable; all events are neutral.
- Have no expectations—give up the need to know why things happen as they do; stop judging yourself and others.

Hildegard of Bingen, a Medieval Mystic

Born in Germany at the end of the eleventh century, Hildegard of Bingen was clairvoyant and clairaudient from early childhood. When three, she saw "so great a brightness that (her) soul trembled." Her parents gave her as a tithe (she was their tenth child) to the nearby Benedictine monastery of Disibedenberg when she was eight years old. She became a nun in this order when 15 years old, remaining in the monastery for over 40 years and becoming a leader of her community. She left at age 59 to found the famous Rupertsberg convent for her nuns. She had many visions and mystical experiences, and from her inner knowledge she composed exquisite music, painted beautifully, wrote books about spiritual domains and the natural sciences, and corresponded with abbots, popes, and kings. Hildegard was outspoken and scolded church leaders when she felt they were wrong. For the last 12 years of her life, she traveled widely speaking to both clergy and laypeople, a courageous act during a time when women were not allowed to preach by scriptural injunction.

At first she did not reveal her visions, but at age 42 she received a divine command to disclose her experiences and understandings. She describes how this occurred:

> . . . a fiery light, flashing intensely, came from the open vault of heaven and poured through my whole brain. Like a flame that is hot without burning it kindled all my heart and all my breast, just as the sun warms anything on which its rays fall. And suddenly I could understand what such books as the Psalter, the Gospel and the other Catholic volumes both of the Old and New Testament actually set forth . . .

—Hildegard of Bingen, *Scivias,* in *Hildegard of Bingen: Mystical Writings* by Bowie & Davies, 1990

The dark night of the soul comes just before revelation. When everything is lost, and all seems darkness, then comes the new life and all that is needed.

—Joseph Campbell, *The Power of Myth*

> Consider our soul to be like a castle made entirely out of a diamond or of very clear crystal, in which there are many rooms. . . . For if this castle is the soul, clearly one doesn't have to enter it since it is within oneself. How foolish it would seem were we to tell someone to enter a room he is already in. But you must understand that there is a great difference in the ways one may be inside the castle . . .
>
> —Saint Teresa of Avila, *Interior Castle* (1515–1582), in Carol Lee Flinders, *Enduring Grace: Living Portraits of Seven Women Saints*

- There are no wrong choices—every choice serves your life; no matter what you are living it is an expression of your life purpose; you cannot miss your life's calling.
- Rest in the "I Am"—the pure essence of your being is already perfect, cannot be harmed, and is united with the Infinite Source.

MYSTICAL UNION

Living in Gratitude and Appreciation   The end of madness, the Dark Night, may be subtle. Inexplicably, we simply feel better. We may not know where we are going, or what our lives are all about, but somehow we no longer feel lost or disturbed about it. You may find yourself doing fine in situations that would have scared you before. Things that used to set you off, cause strong reactions, or make you lose your center do not have that power over you any more. There is more humor in your life; you can laugh at yourself and with others. Things do not have to be "spiritually right," and it becomes easier to drop judgments and expectations of our spiritual teachers and groups.

Appreciation of life becomes a dominant theme in spiritual outlook after mystical union. Instead of "getting by" or "making the best we can of life" we realize our life is actually perfect, and we are exactly where we are supposed to be. We see the elements inside ourselves that are no longer life-giving, that drain our energy, and we choose not to animate these things. We can say, and really mean it, "Everything is well in my life."

This is the stage of bliss, being "unreasonably happy" and knowing that anything is possible. Miracles are not surprises, but the right understanding of Divine or cosmic laws. It is called transcendence, because we have gone beyond ordinary understanding and experience of life. All is well, regardless of circumstances. We know our connection with God/Goddess through our own experience, and do not need any person's or group's recognition of this. We are able to live our lives fully, with complete openness to having abundance, love, intimacy, material comfort, and pleasures; we also have no expectations, no comparisons to what others have, and no fears about not having these things.

> Let nothing upset you,
> Let nothing disturb you.
> All things are passing;
> Only God never changes.
>
> —Saint Teresa of Avila (1515–1582),
>   in Carol Lee Flinders, *Enduring Grace:*
>   *Living Portraits of Seven Women Saints*

WOMEN'S PROCESS OF SPIRITUAL UNFOLDING

The spiritual journey outlined above certainly has variations, side roads, and replays in women's individual lives. It is a general model for humans seeking to know their Divinity. However, is there a process unique to women? Is there some way that our very femaleness shapes perspectives and creates experiences in our soul-discovery? Several seminal thinkers in women's spirituality have described ways that spiritual growth is particular to women. The following draws from the work of Carol Lee Flinders (1993, 1998), Maria Harris (1991), Sherry Anderson and Patricia Hopkins (1991), Joan Borysenko (1996), and Jean Shinoda Bolen (1994) for this process of women's spiritual unfolding.

The process women undergo in their spiritual unfolding incorporates three components: *enclosure, metamorphosis,* and *emergence.* These components repeat themselves over and over in women's lives, reflected in bodily, mental-emotional, and spiritual changes. Women's bodies are intimately connected with their wisdom (Northrup, 1998). We may follow these stages as a "ritual pattern of renewal" through the inner and outer views of women's life cycles.

Enclosure

Enclosure occurs whenever life processes pull us inward, and there is need for protection. Young girls need "containment" in a safe family and community, where their wonderment, discovery, and joyful play is encouraged. When menstruating, women naturally feel inward and somewhat withdrawn. Many women have yearned for "moon lodges" where they might retreat from daily responsibilities, be

> Pallal—the Aramaic root of the word prayer—means seeing oneself as wondrously made.
>
> —Ron Roth, *Prayer and the Five Stages of Healing*

nurtured, and share quiet time with other women. During pregnancy, women enter a deep state of inner-containment, focusing on the many emotional and physical changes, and enthralled with the great mystery of life's creation. At menopause, women return to another type of enclosure, pulling inward as enormous changes take place in the body-mind that signal the next stage of spiritual evolution.

THE DARK NIGHT OR CAVE EXPERIENCE–ENCLOSURE

Women's experience of enclosure has some elements of the Dark Night stage, which can also be expressed as entering a cave. Descending into the cave symbolizes going deeply into our hidden interior, and facing our fears related to our dark side. Some consider it a "descent into hell" where we encounter all that is fearful, horrible, disgusting, and repulsive within our self-image and experiences. By facing these fearful things, and looking through them to the lessons they bring, and realizing they do not define who we truly are, we can break their spell upon our minds. This brings tremendous freedom from our "inner demons": attitudes, beliefs, fears, thoughts that have limited us from our full potential.

Metamorphosis

Metamorphosis is the transformational process that is supported by enclosure. In this process, we discover the incomparable richness of our "Interior Castle," beautifully described by Saint Teresa of Avila. Inside the cocoon of transformation, we become like the silkworm pupa which dissolves into a liquid broth. The firm walls of the cocoon are essential to protect it, and after a time of safe containment, the pupa reconfigures itself into a chrysalis. Now it cannot be contained any longer, and breaks out as a 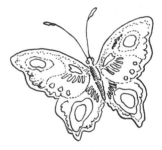 butterfly, which spreads its wings and flies away into the world. The butterfly is one of the Goddess' symbols of transformation and rebirth (Eisler, 1997). When women are in the "broth" and feeling their very identity melting away, it can be

> We have nothing to fear but fear itself.
>
> —F. D. Roosevelt, inaugural speech, March 4, 1933
>
> Love is letting go of fear.
>
> —Jerald Jampolsky, *Love Is Letting Go of Fear*

terrifying. This is a vulnerable time for women, and great damage can be done if the right support is not present. Metamorphosis is happening during prepuberty and the first few menstrual years, during the establishing of relationships, during pregnancy and childbirth, during new creative ventures, during major life events, during perimenopause and menopause, and during dying.

THE DESERT EXPERIENCE–METAMORPHOSIS

The Illumination stage of the spiritual journey can be related to women's process of metamorphosis. Once we have faced our worst fears, and overcome them, we attain a new level of empowerment. Every time we become more powerful, we are tested—will we use our new power selfishly, or for the good of others? Symbolically we "go alone into the desert" as Christ did, to be tempted by the "devil" or forces of evil (ego-pride, selfish use of power). This temptation may be subtle, more psychological than physical. We face it alone, as no one can make choices about how we use our powers except ourselves. While it may appear that choices for material world success and abundance are the right ones, it is always choices for spiritual values that bring us the greatest happiness.

Emergence

Emergence is the opening process into the woman's new state of being. She is now claiming her new self, expressing and living it fully. After menarche, the girl becomes transformed into a woman, now open physically, emotionally, and psychologically to relationships and creation of life. After each menstrual period, women open up again to sexuality or activity. After childbirth, as milk flows to nurture the baby, women expand physical boundaries to encompass the child, and enter into relationships in a new way. The mother-self emerges, identity changes, and a new stage of life is entered. After menopause, the woman is trans-

Seek ye first the Kingdom of God, and all these things shall be added unto you.

—Matthew 6:33

Before the world was I longed for thee; I long for thee and thou for Me. When two burning desires come together then is love perfected!

—Mechthild of Magdeburg, in Carol Lee Flinders,
Enduring Grace: Living Portraits of Seven Women Saints

formed again into a new identity. Ideally, the postmenopausal years are a life stage of expanded spirituality, creative self-expression, and social contribution (Flinders, 1998; Rutter, 1993).

QUIET TRANSFORMATION—EMERGENCE

Women's emergence process is similar to the spiritual journey stage of Mystical Union and Gratitude. We return from the Desert Experience transformed, as we have met and overcome its tests. Even if our outer life does not look much different, our inner essence has changed and we are vibrationally different. People around us will sense this, and feel it intuitively. Prior problems often fall away. Our sense of inner peace provides a deep anchor through life's storms. We are able to do our "life's work," whether that is on a grand scale before the public, or on a small scale with our family and friends. The Wise Woman, Creatrix, or other archetypes manifest through us, and we can bring perspective, comfort, guidance, and inspiration to others. Of our infinite abundance, we have much to give the world. Embodying archetypal powers, women often contribute to social causes and work to make the world a better place, in some way, for all.

WISDOM'S CHALLENGE: TRANSFORMING SPIRITUALLY

Menopause is the gateway to women's wisdom years. However, wisdom must be earned, developed, and grown into. The many challenges women face during the menopausal years provide lessons and opportunities to grow into wisdom. As we are challenged on many levels—physically, emotionally, socially, and spiritually—we are tempered as a steel blade by fire, refined into our pure essence, purified and cleansed of all that is not our highest expression.

Give me all that thine is, and I'll give you all that mine is.

—God to Mechthild of Magdeburg, in Carol Lee Flinders,
Enduring Grace: Living Portraits of Seven Women Saints

Everything is mine, for all that is God's seems to be wholly mine. I am mute and lost in God.

—Saint Catherine of Genoa, in Carol Lee Flinders,
Enduring Grace: Living Portraits of Seven Women Saints

So our Lady is our mother, in whom we are all enclosed and born of
her in Christ, for she who is mother of our saviour is mother of all
who are saved in our saviour; and our saviour is our true Mother, in
whom we are endlessly born and out of whom we shall never come.

—Julian of Norwich (1342–1416?), *Long Text 57*, in Carol Lee Flinders,
Enduring Grace: Living Portraits of Seven Women Mystics

As women come into the fullness of their spirituality, they also realize how
important it is to share this with others. Living in awareness of ourselves as
expressions of the Divine Feminine, we naturally transmit spirituality to others
through women's innate connectedness, relationality, and receptivity. Every stage
in the dance of Spirit is living the spiritual life, even the process of awakening and
discovering we do have a deeper self. Just being aware there is "something more"
is to have already touched it; to be searching for the Mystery is to have already
met it. Wherever we are in our spiritual journey, we have something valuable to
share with others. As our inner sense of Divine connectedness develops, and our
receptivity deepens, we may want to share spirituality in various ways.

Receptivity of the Heart

Carol Gray, a midlife woman, has been a devotee of Paramhansa Yogananda (a Hindu master who brought Kriya yoga to America) for many
years, and is a leader of the Ananda Meditation Center in Ashland. She
tells of an experience that changed her life, the way she sees the world,
others and herself.

I (was) sitting in Ananda Assissi's beautiful Temple of Light while
Swami (Kriyananda) was telling the Bible story of the woman
who touched Christ's cloak and was healed. Crowds of people
had been milling around Jesus, but only one was healed that day.
Lots of people touched his cloak, but this woman alone received
God's healing energy. Why? Because, explained Swami, she was
receptive. The crowds were intellectually open-minded, still not
truly receptive.

I started weeping because I felt like those people in the crowd.
It seemed as if I had been standing at the edge of the crowd for

(Continued on next page)

incarnations. I was open-minded but something was missing. I felt a tremendous longing for that missing piece. Then an almost indescribable blessing poured into me. At that point the tears really started to flow. . . . These tears were a mixture of sadness and joy; I felt cleansed, too, all at the same time.

After the tears stopped I gradually became aware that something in me had changed. . . . Ever since then I have felt a light, new energy in my heart; a subtle, interior shift that altered my outlook on the world. . . . I learned through this experience about the enormous spiritual power of receptivity. To be receptive, one needs an open heart as well as an open mind. I created a prayer to help remember: "Divine Mother, help me to be fully receptive to the blessings that are inherent in each moment."

—Carol Gray, *Clarity Magazine*

Creating Traditions

Creating a tradition for women's spirituality gives us ways of expressing and sharing how to live the spiritual life. Much of the feminine aspect of religion has been lost over the centuries since the Great Mother tradition was replaced by the masculine Sky Gods. Even though the image of the One God (masculine aspect) replaced the many faces of the Goddess (feminine aspect), people's yearning for the unconditional love of the Great Mother kept aspects of the Divine Feminine alive. In the Jewish tradition she is Shekhinah, the ruach (wind) that is the breath of spirit blowing through forms and bringing them life. The Christians hold a very special place in their hearts for Mary, the mother of Jesus, as the embodiment of compassion and caring through life's most difficult challenges. The Buddhists have the bodhisattvas, some male and some female, enlightened beings who return to earth again and again to help struggling people learn to live in harmony. The Hindus have a rich tradition of feminine goddesses, some who came before their major gods, representing a great diversity of Divine aspects. They see the primal creative force of the universe as feminine, and the pure vital energies which sustain life are called Shakti (a feminine energy). Native peoples maintain spiritual traditions with multiple gods and goddesses who enliven the many domains of the natural world; spirit is seen in all creatures and in the earth herself.

> Everything was sacred with our people. How sacred everything
> was. . . . The non-Indian people believe in God, but we believe in the
> universe as god. . . . Like the sun is our brother. He gives us energy;
> he gives us life . . . the moon is your grandmother. The earth is your
> mother. . . . When men begin to understand the relationships of the
> universe that women have always known, the world will begin to
> change for the better.
>
> —Cecilia Mitchell (Akwesasne), Mohawk medicine women, in Steve Wall's
> *Wisdom's Daughters: Conversations with Women Elders of Native America*

The tradition of feminine spirituality honors the earth and all her creatures. Everything in existence is seen as coming from the creative forces of the feminine spirit joining with the generative powers of the masculine spirit. The resurgence of interest in goddesses and the divine feminine reflects our understanding that the world needs to once again cherish its life forms, and the matter from which life forms emerge. This feminine force of unconditional love and healing is being called back into our consciousness, so that the planet can be brought into greater harmony.

Divine Feminine: "Made in Her Image"

Many girls and women feel the need for female images of the Deity with which they can identify. Having only male images of the Divine leaves women feeling somehow not right, perhaps imperfect or other than made in the "image of God." Having a tradition of female Divine images conveys to girls/women that the Holy One is like them. There are feminine Divine images of many colors and races, which communicates universality and teaches that Goddess is not reducible to any one image. We may honor and pray to the Divine Feminine as the Black Madonna (aspect of Mary, drawn from Astarte), Mother of Compassion (Quan Yin, Mary), Grandmother Spirit (Spider Woman, Thought Woman), Queen of Heaven and Earth (Inanna, Nana), Goddess of Fire and Transformation (Sekhmet, Kali, Pele), Source of Creative Energy (Shakti, Shekhinah), Goddess of Intelligence and Knowledge (Cerridwen), Source of Wisdom and Knowledge (Sophia, Chokmah, Athena), Creator of Life Cycles/Moon Goddess (Oya, Isis), Goddess of Intuition and Psychic Wisdom (Hecate), and many others.

The Feminine Divine, the Goddess, has innumerable forms. Find those you best relate to, and your inner prayer life may be transformed. (Chapter 6 includes many archetypal images of goddesses, focusing on those most meaningful for

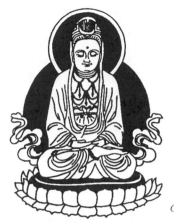

Quan Yin.
Reproduced with permission.
Copyright © Kate Cartwright.

midlife women. Also see References for books on women's spirituality and the Feminine Divine).

Rituals and Ceremonies

Many women's groups have been creating fresh, inspiring, female-focused ceremonies. These include opening a circle, honoring the four directions, equinox and solstice celebrations, puja (prayers), arati (offerings), fire ceremonies, honoring the elements, ceremonial meals, women's sweat lodges, queening/croning, and other transition ceremonies, and numerous ways women come together to pray and adore the Holy One (See Rite of Passage Ceremony in Appendix C).

Mighty, majestic and radiant
You shine brilliantly in the evening,
You brighten the day at dawn.
You stand in the heavens like the sun and the moon,
Your wonders are known both above and below,
To the greatness of the holy priestess in heaven,
To you, Inanna, I sing!

—Hymn to Inanna, Sumerian goddess, Queen of Heaven and Earth,
fourth century B.C.E., in Wolkstein & Kramer,
Inanna: Queen of Heaven and Earth

One ancient ritual practiced among women for untold centuries is opening the circle, a process now used to begin women's group gatherings. To open the circle, the leader faces each of the four directions, and ceremonially invokes the qualities that each represents, or calls forth the spirits associated with these. The directions of above and below are usually included, which creates a three-dimensional sphere. This practice actually draws from esoteric knowledge about the process of creating matter, taught in Egyptian mystery schools (Melchezidek, 2000). There are many variations on the words and ceremonial practices used. Table 5–3 offers

TABLE 5–3 Opening the Circle

The practice of opening the circle by focusing on the directions and their associated qualities has roots in the native traditions, ancient goddess religions, and Egyptian mystery schools. One woman may lead the entire ceremony or a different woman may call each direction. She begins facing east, holding an object and using a phrase or prayer to invoke the spirit and qualities of the east. This continues for south, west, and north. Often the directions of above and below are included.

EAST	SOUTH	WEST	NORTH
Air	Fire	Water	Earth
Dawn	Noon	Dusk	Midnight
Spring	Summer	Autumn	Winter
Yellow, white	Red, orange	Blue, indigo	Brown, green
Eagle	Coyote	Bear, raven	Buffalo, white owl
Feathers, wind	Candles, bonfires	Water, liquid	Soil, stones
Clarity	Passion	Fluidity	Stillness
Communication	Strong will	Renewal	Silence
Learning	Growth	Compassion	Natural cycles
Psychic work	Purification	Emotions	Nurturance
Inspiration	Senses, joy	Unconscious	Wisdom

ABOVE	BELOW
Celestial world, heavens	Underworld, hades
Infinite source of being	Dark side, shadow being
Expanded vision of cosmos	Focused vision within self
Guide to unity, connection with all beings	Guide to inner secrets, unraveling our mysteries

Here is one example of how you might invoke a direction:

Facing the north, holding a crystal, say: "Spirit of the North! Who brings all things to completion, taking us deep within to learn our own mysteries, in the silence of winter, bringer of wisdom to nurture the next cycle, I call on your presence at our circle."

a summary of the symbolism of opening the circle. (See Appendix E for more details.)

Mentoring and Modeling

The name "mentor" goes back to Greek mythology, when the goddess Athena guided and counseled the young Telemachus, preparing him to become a wise and just leader. Mentors and models abound in the workplace, medicine, academic life, the arts, and government. Spiritual mentors provide a one-on-one relationship to support another woman's quest to discover and experience the sacred in her life. Sometimes women's mentors are priestesses or ordained clergy-women, but equally valuable are wise, spiritually evolved friends. Since we are all inherently spiritual, and are in touch with different aspects of our spirituality at different times in life, women often mentor one another, sometimes simultaneously—a tribute to our relationality and adaptability.

Spiritual models may be women we may not know personally, but whose deep insights and wisdom teach, guide, and inspire us. There are more and more books, videotapes, and audiotapes by women on self-awareness, spiritual growth, and transformation. We are creating a rich contemporary network of women wisdom teachers; check your local bookstore, the Internet, or the numerous brochures offering workshops and seminars in your area.

How Women Model for Each Other

Every one of us serves as a model, at some time, for what it is to be a mature, spiritual woman. Though we may not be aware of it, we are always asking one another: "What can I learn about my life from observing your life?" We intuitively watch one another to see how things can be done. We observe public figures and celebrities, such as Oprah Winfrey, Hillary Clinton, or Jessica Tandy. We delve deeply inside the writings of Alice Walker, Betty Friedan, Linda Johnson, Merlin Stone, Carol Lee Flinders, Barbara Hand Clow, Marion Woodman, and Lynne Andrews. We find ourselves inspired by the powerful teachings of Caroline Myss, Marianne Williamson, Clarissa Pinkola Estes, Jean Shinoda-Bolen, and Christiane Northrup. These women are available to us daily as role models. By observing their actions, or ways of being in the world, we learn and make associations with how we want to be also. This becomes part of our feminine tradition of self-awareness and growth.

Isis, giver of life, residing in the Sacred Mound, Satis,
She is the one who pours out the Inundation
That makes all people live and green plants grow,
Who provides divine offerings for the gods . . .
She is the Lady of Heaven, Earth and the Netherworld
Having brought them into existence through what her heart
Conceived and her hands created . . .

—Hymn IV, hieroglyphs inscribed on the walls of Isis's Temple
of Philae in southern Egypt by Ptolemy II (284–246 B.C.E.),
originating many centuries earlier. From Harvey & Baring, 1996.

My Grandmother's Cre Dieux

As a girl, I spent most of the summer with my grandparents near the Mississippi River in rural Louisiana. My family was Catholic as far back as anyone can remember. In southern Louisiana, with its French and Spanish heritage, Catholicism is the dominant religion. Grandma's home was replete with Catholic symbols: pictures of Jesus, the Virgin Mary, and various saints, rosaries, prayer cards, and Bibles. I remember that in her bedroom there was a large picture of two children crossing a flimsy footbridge over a deep chasm. The girl, a few years older, was carefully guiding her smaller brother to find safe footing. Hovering over them was a magnificent, glowing, beautiful female angel, her wings outstretched and her hands held in open blessing for the children. I've often recalled that image of our guardian angel protecting us through life's perilous passages.

Every evening Grandma would kneel on her Cre Dieux to pray. This was a small bench on which she kneeled, with supports at elbow level on which she rested her arms while silently saying her rosary. I was glad that both the bench and elbow rests were well padded! Grandma stayed in prayer for what seemed to me a very long time; silent, absorbed, eyes closed, focused deeply inward. I wondered what Jesus, Mary, or an angel might be saying to her.

Now, when I meditate, I feel connected with that memory. In my inner awareness, Grandma's spiritual modeling flows seamlessly through time. Her communion with Spirit becomes merged with mine.

—Lennie Martin

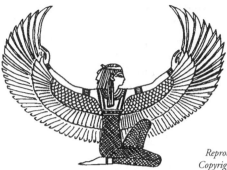

Isis with Wings.
Reproduced with permission.
Copyright © Kate Cartwright.

Transforming: Bringing Forth Our New Vision

Transforming is a mature expression of women's spirituality (Harris, 1991). We are concerned not only with our personal transforming, but also transforming our world. Mature women are birthing a new vision, brought into being through integrating all life's experiences and the spiritual growth that has come from these.

To *trans-form* is to change or shift the form, shape, configuration, or nature of something; in this case, of ourselves and the world. Every woman's life is full of transformations, some large, some small. Having gone through a transformation, we are not the same anymore. We may have shifted our attitudes, changed some beliefs (such as our unworthiness into acknowledgment of our innate value), broadened our viewpoints so we can see things differently, or stopped a habit that controlled or limited us.

People say "I don't know what it is, but you're different." We know deep within that a quantum leap was made in our consciousness; we have expanded and will never again be held down by certain limitations. Often we do not recognize our transformations until some time after they have occurred. We look back and think "Wow, I've really changed regarding that!" Of course, we sometimes know when we are in the throes of transformation, which may come in the guise of challenge, sorrow, suffering, or loss.

> Our listenings and our questionings call for a sea of change. They call for a spirituality that results from the coming together of the perspectives and the experiences of all people—and of the planet Earth too. At this point in the dance of the spirit, they also call for a spirituality that includes entering the depths and dying.
>
> —Maria Harris, *Dance of the Spirit: The Seven Steps of Women's Spirituality*

Mourning can be seen as a process of dying into life. Through this process, we discard what is no longer viable, so we can turn toward re-forming and trans-forming spiritually. For this to happen, something must be allowed to die—often spiritual or religious beliefs from the past that are too limiting—and we need to grieve the passing. This passage into grief and darkness becomes our path into light. When we can allow ourselves to mourn the passing of former ways, and then let go of the past, we free our energies for communion with Spirit, which leads to the re-birthing of the sacred within us.

The challenges in life release new potential to grow in a different direction. Suf-fering, loss, and sorrow are special doors of opportunity to contact the reality which transcends desires. Wisdom and its counterpart, compassion, emerge from encountering and integrating the lessons of obstruction and suffering. To see "negative" experiences of life as wisdom lessons is a great victory for the soul, and brings the virtues of patience, perseverance, forgiveness, and detachment. Those who master these lessons become great wisdom teachers for humanity.

One reason why we resist making internal changes is an often subconscious awareness of their impact on the structure of our lives. When we choose to be whole and integrated in body-mind-spirit, then it follows that anything in our lives not in support of our wholeness will need to go. When we release our fears and limitations, we are freed to celebrate the truth that all the good of our past remains alive within us, and what is "dead" or no longer serves growth can be allowed to drop away. We cannot fully feel the grace that connects us with our own immortality if we continue to fear and fight the passage of years. Releasing the past through greater understanding of our Divine nature is the way to rise above all that has happened to us on the physical plane.

We are drawn closer and closer to Spirit through transformation processes. Many people are writing and speaking of their experiences with beings from other dimensions. We may have awareness of spirit guides, angels, or great masters who are with us during our journey through life. Many healers and psychics provide assistance in communicating with the spirit domain, and working with energy and consciousness. In the journey to discover who we are—the mystic's quest—we find our own Divine nature and know that this essential Being is shared with all of creation and all beyond creation.

> We are not born devoid of knowledge about the working power of our spiritual nature; quite the contrary, we know instinctively that every internal change we make, every shift in perspective or belief, automatically activates an external shift in our lives.
>
> —Caroline Myss, *Why People Don't Heal and How They Can*

PURPOSE OF THE WISE WOMAN

The Wise Woman has traditionally served as a reservoir of knowledge, the container of the seeds of truth from generation to generation. She has provided counsel, advice, and guidance to others, helping them face difficulties and make choices. She draws from her many experiences in life, from the challenges she has faced and overcome, from her own lessons and transformations. She models living by higher values and spiritual principles in her daily life. Some keys of this Wisdom Tradition are:

- All advice/assistance is given from a place of inner purity, with no personal goals or agendas
- Waiting for the right timing, never imposing, always honoring
- Not being attached to any outcomes, but offering to share wisdom freely without conditions or expectations
- Living in harmony with people and nature
- Compassion for others and for one's self
- Living by inner guidance, listening to the Inner Voice of Truth
- Creative expression with or without purpose
- Personal spiritual practices, deep connection with the Divine, Source, Infinite Consciousness, Goddess or God, however you may relate to this

Elder women become the nurturers and healers of the planet. They can undertake the sacred mission of promoting the consciousness of unity—one humanity, one world with all its creatures, waters, plants, terrains, and atmospheres equally loved and valued. They can transmute planetary suffering through compassion and unconditional love. Such wise women will usher in the new millennium of higher consciousness, bringing greater peace and harmony to the world.

TAKING CHARGE OF YOUR SPIRITUAL JOURNEY

The key element for embarking on your journey of spiritual unfolding is simply the intention to do so. When that still voice deep within your soul calls for guidance, direction, instruction, or support, then the universe swings into action to provide guides, teachers, intuition, and community. Although the initiative is always yours at each step, a time comes when you realize that "you as the ego-personality" are not really in charge, but that a greater power or higher aspect of being is behind the flow of your life. At that point, follow the yogic advice to "attune your will to Divine will" and merge into the flow of grace that creates a

Wise Woman Vow

My intention is to live, this day forth, as a Wise Woman
I create sacred spaces around me, to nourish my soul.
I enter the silence of a quiet mind, to become a clear reflection
　of Divine Spirit.
I sanctify my life in the feminine waters of compassion, forgiveness,
　right thought, acceptance, and gentle guidance.
I accept and love myself as I am, and others as they are.
I reap the harvest of wisdom from each season of my life.
I care for the planet, and walk the earth with sensitive feet.
I bear the light of Divine Mother, to bless and heal, and quicken
　the vibration of the whole earth.

—Lennie Martin, March, 1998

life of inner peace, harmony, and universal love regardless of outer circumstances. These elements are helpful along the path:

- Take stock of issues or relationships that have not been brought to completion, and do the necessary clearing, healing, or releasing.
- Bring energy into your body-mind system using breathing, yoga, or other energy balancing techniques.
- Nourish your body-mind-spirit system with uplifting attitudes, harmonious behavior, and healthful nutrition.
- Develop a regular meditation or contemplation practice.
- Study and introspect to expand your awareness and connect with spiritual traditions.
- Connect with other women to share and support spiritual experiences.
- Find some way to serve or give to society or the planet.

REFERENCES

Allen, P.G. (1986). *The sacred hoop: Recovering the feminine in American Indian traditions.* Boston: Beacon Press.

Anderson, S., & Hopkins, P. (1991). *The feminine face of God: The unfolding of the sacred in women.* New York: Bantam Books.

Begley, S. (2001). Religion and the brain. *Newsweek,* May 7, 50–57.

Benson, H. (1975). *The relaxation response.* New York: William Morrow & Co.

Bolen, J.S. (1994). *Crossing to Avalon: A woman's midlife pilgrimage.* San Francisco: HarperSanFrancisco.

Borysenko, J. (1996). *A woman's book of life: The biology, psychology, and spirituality of the feminine life cycle.* New York: Riverhead Books.

Bowie, F., & Davies, O. (1990). *Hildegard of Bingen: Mystical writings.* New York: Crossroad.

Brennan, B. (1987). *Hands of light: A guide to healing through the human energy field.* New York: Bantam Books.

Burnham, S. (1997). *The ecstatic journey: The transforming power of mystical experience.* New York: Ballantine Books.

Campbell, J. (1988). *The power of myth.* New York: Doubleday Books.

Childre, D., & Martin, H. (1999). *The HeartMath solution.* San Francisco: HarperSanFrancisco.

Clow, B.H. (1996). *The liquid light of sex: Kundalini rising at midlife crisis.* Berkeley, CA: Bear and Company.

Corliss, R. (2001). The power of yoga. *Time,* April 23, 54–62.

Darras, J.C. (1989). Isotopic and cytologic assays in acupuncture. In *Energy fields in medicine.* Kalamazoo, MI: John Fetzer Foundation.

Eisler, R. (1997). *The chalice and the blade.* San Francisco: Harper & Row.

Flinders, C. (1993). *Enduring grace: Living portraits of seven women mystics.* San Francisco: HarperSanFrancisco.

Flinders, C. (1998). *At the root of this longing: Reconciling a spiritual hunger and a feminist thirst.* San Francisco: HarperSanFrancisco.

Fowler, J.W. (1981). *Stages of faith: The psychology of human development and the quest for meaning.* New York: Viking Press.

Frawley, D. (1994). *Tantric yoga and the wisdom goddesses.* Salt Lake City: Passage Press.

Gray, C. (2000). Receptivity of the heart. *Clarity Magazine.* Ananda Church of Self-Realization, Nevada City, CA, Winter, 2000, 10–11.

Greeley, A. (1987). Mysticism goes mainstream. *American Health, 6,* 47–49.

Gypson, W. (1997). Acupuncture: 5,000 years in 30 minutes. In *Complementary medicine: Integrating new & ancient therapies into your practice.* Sacramento, CA: Sutter Health and Mercy Healthcare.

Harris, M. (1991). *Dance of the spirit: The seven steps of women's spirituality.* New York: Bantam Books.

Harvey, A., & Baring, A. (1996). *The divine feminine: Exploring the feminine face of god throughout the world.* Berkeley, CA: Conari Press. Based on translation by L.B. Zabkar, *Hymns to Isis in her Temple at Philae,* Hanover, NH: University Press of New England.

Hawking, S.W. (1998). *A brief history of time.* New York: Bantam Books.

Hay, L. (1999). *You can heal your life.* Carlsbad, CA: Hay House.

Heisenberg, W. (1971). *Physics and beyond.* New York: Harper Torchbooks.

Jampolsky, G.G. (1979). *Love is letting go of fear.* Millbrae, CA: Celestial Arts.

Johari, H. (1987). *Chakras: Energy centers for transformation.* Vermont: Destiny Books.

Johnston, C. (1993). *Yoga Sutras of Patanjali.* Albuquerque, NM: Brotherhood of Life.

Kaku, M. (1994). *Hyperspace: A scientific odyssey through parallel universes, time warps, and the 10th dimension.* New York: Anchor Books Doubleday.

Kriyananda, G. (1988). *The spiritual science of Kriya Yoga.* Chicago: The Temple of Kriya Yoga.

Lesser, E. (1999). *The new American spirituality.* New York: Random House.

Lindbergh, A.M. (1991). *A gift from the sea.* New York: Vintage Books.

McWayne, W.R. (1998). *Radical reality.* Modesto, CA: RealityWorks.

Melchizadek, D. (2000). *The ancient secret of the flower of life.* Volume 2. Flagstaff, AZ: Light Technology Publishing.

Myss, C. (1996). *Anatomy of the spirit: The seven stages of power and healing.* New York: Harmony Books.

Myss, C. (1997). *Why people don't heal and how they can.* New York: Harmony Books.

Myss, C. (1997). *Spiritual madness* (Audiotape series). Boulder, CO: Sounds True.

Myss, C. (2000). *The fundamentals of spiritual alchemy.* Workshop sponsored by the Association for Humanistic Psychology, Oakland, CA, December 1–2.

Myss, C. & Shealy, N. (1998). *Vision, creativity, and intuition. The science of intuition, Part II, Sacred contracts.* St. Louis, MO: Holos Institute.

Newberg, A., D'Aquili, E., & Rause, V. (2001). *Why God won't go away: Brain science and the biology of belief.* New York: Ballantine Books.

Northrup, C. (1998). *Women's bodies, women's wisdom: Creating physical and emotional health and healing.* New York: Bantam Books.

Northrup, C. (2001). *The wisdom of menopause: Creating physical and emotional health and healing during the change.* New York: Bantam Books.

Pascal, E. (1992). *Jung to live by: A guide to the practical application of Jungian principles for everyday life.* New York: Warner Books.

Prabhavananda, S., & Isherwood, C. (1953). *How to know God: The yoga aphorisms of Patanjali.* New York: New American Library.

Roth, R. (1997). *Prayer and the five stages of healing* (Audiotape). Carlsbad, CA: Hay House.

Rutter, V.B. (1993). Woman changing woman: Feminine psychology re-conceived through myth and experience. San Francisco: HarperSanFrancisco.

Shealy, N., & Myss, C. (1993). *The creation of health: The emotional, psychological, and spiritual responses that promote health and healing.* Walpole, NH: Stillpoint Publishing.

Smith, H. (1992). *Forgotten truth: The common vision of the world's religions.* San Francisco: HarperSanFrancisco.

Smith, H. (2001). *Why religion matters: The fate of the human spirit in an age of disbelief.* San Francisco: HarperSanFrancisco.

Stein, M. (1983). *In midlife: A Jungian perspective.* Dallas: Spring Publications.

Teasdale, W. (1999). *The mystic heart: Discovering a universal spirituality in the world's religions.* Novato, CA: New World Library.

Wall, S. (1993). *Wisdom's daughters: Conversations with women elders of Native America.* New York: Harper Perennial.

Wolkstein, D., & Kramer, S.M. (1983). *Inanna: Queen of heaven and earth.* New York: HarperCollins.

Yogananda, P. (1994). *Autobiography of a Yogi* (Reprint of original 1946 edition). Nevada City, CA: Crystal Clarity Pub.

Zukov, G. (1980). *The dancing Wu Li masters: An overview of the new physics.* New York: Bantam Books.

Energizing the Energy Centers (Chakras)

Many menopausal symptoms are energetically connected to vortices of energy located near the base of the spine (first chakra), the pelvic area (second chakra) and the navel (third chakra). You can bring life force (prana, chi) into these areas by:

- Sitting upright in a comfortable position, feet flat and palms upturned resting in your lap. Sit cross-legged if you prefer.
- With closed eyes, focus on the breath moving in and out of your nostrils. Do not try to control the breath, simply watch it.
- When you feel quiet, envision a golden-white stream of light pouring onto your head and neck. With each inward breath, draw that light into your body. Feel it still present when you breathe outward.
- Focus on drawing each inward breath deeply into your lower body, between the navel and base of the spine. Feel the light flooding into the organs and tissues, filling them with energy. Push your stomach out a little with each inward breath. Do this for 10 minutes, every day if possible, but at least 5 times per week.

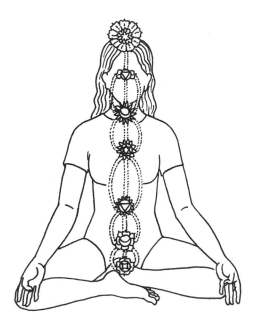

Enhancing Intuition

Intuition is a natural ability we are all born with. It is a process of broadening our attention to gather information that is not immediately obvious. It often occurs in the body first, then percolates up into consciousness. Intuition is learning to read the messages sent by our body-mind—our cells and tissues respond intuitively. All information we need is available, surrounding us in the morphogenic field (ether): the collective unconscious. Our minds can access that information, through the part that is a segment of Universal Mind.

Intuition requires that you *be in the present* by doing these steps.

- Relax: Detach from fear, stop trying, assume intuition will manifest.
- Concentrate: Focus attention by breathing, lights, sounds, exercise, crystals, and so on.
- Be patient: Wait calmly, avoid analysis, allow incubation.
- Be open: Pay attention to the unexpected, the unexplainable, the "A-HA."
- Contemplate: Play with options, alternatives, other possibilities, the outrageous.
- Write results: Write what comes as soon as possible; do not judge or screen.
- Verify: Test the results, take action, analyze-examine, and observe confirmations.

Breath and Word Meditation Technique

This simple but effective technique was developed by Dr. Herbert Benson, M.D. of the Harvard Medical School. He calls it "The Relaxation Response," and it has been taught to thousands of patients who have used it to reduce blood pressure, headaches, stomach distress, hot flashes, and many other symptoms (Benson, 1975). We have added an "expansion" phase to bring an experience of Divine connection.

Step 1: Relaxation

Sit comfortably in a quiet place. Tense muscles, then relax feet to head. Keep spine straight. Deeply relax all muscles. Close eyes, rest hands in lap. Check for places of tension.

Step 2: Concentration

Breathe deeply in and out through nose, 3 times.

Then allow breath to flow naturally.

Simply watch the breath coming in and out of your nose.

Say the word "one" silently while you exhale.

Variations: say   "peace" with inhaling,   "ful" with exhaling; or
                        "still"   "ness"
                        "one"   "world"

Step 3: Expansion

After concentrating for 10–20 minutes, stop watching breath and breathing words.

Your mind may be very still.

Feel absorbed or bathed in qualities such as:

peace   quiet

harmony   joy

love   tranquility

If thoughts come, gently release them without being disturbed.

Stay in this expanded state of mind as long as you can.

Archetypes of Midlife and Menopausal Women

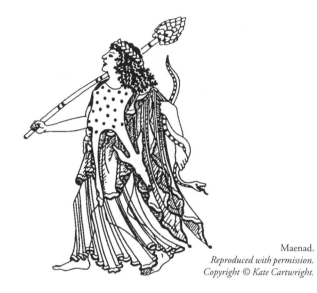

Maenad.
Reproduced with permission.
Copyright © Kate Cartwright.

Have you ever felt there are forces at work in your life that are much bigger than yourself? At times, you may have tapped into clarity or strength you never knew you had. Maybe you were tired or not feeling well, but had to teach a class or perform a concert. Fearing that you would never get through it, you found instead a mysterious energy source pouring through you to accomplish the task. Perhaps you have been surprised at your unexpected negativity or anger flashing toward someone? Cutting words may have sprung from your mouth almost before you realized you were saying them. Perhaps you have been inexplicably intimidated by a situation or person, or conversely felt comfortable and intimate with a stranger. You may wonder about the source of these reactions. They are likely coming from archetypal patterns becoming activated in you and others.

During midlife and menopause, women are naturally drawn inward as hormonal shifts alter brain biochemistry and body physiology. At some point around age fifty, women realize they are entering uncharted territory in their psyche and self-identity. Many begin having thoughts or images of mythic or historic feminine figures. They may be drawn to certain historic women or goddesses, and revisit fairy tales only to discover deeper hidden meanings in the deceptively simple stories. Having learned from many life encounters with people, we often see them fitting into categories, and find ourselves making remarks like: "Well, there's a Queen for you," or "What a warrior he is," or "She certainly is a philosopher about life."

In all these situations, we are tapping into the archetypal domain. *Archetype* means "primary pattern" or "original type." These are mental images or thought forms that have been created by the collective thoughts of millions of people through the ages. They gain their power by being held in collective consciousness and passed generation to generation. The original concepts of the archetypes of the collective unconscious were developed by Carl Jung, the Swiss psychologist, who saw them as inherent potentials in the psyche. These inherent patterns or predispositions become activated for any individual woman by a number of interconnected elements, such as family background, culture, circumstances, hormones, and stages of life (Bolen, 2001).

Jung believed that archetypal themes are expressed symbolically in myths. Joseph Campbell, renowned scholar of mythology, agreed that myths are expressions of archetypal thought forms that are basic structural components of the mind. In every human culture across time, the same mythologic motifs are found. These same structures in the mind, Campbell believed, led ancient architects to conceive the similar shapes and proportions of Sumerian ziggurats, Mayan pyramids, and

Thunder, Perfect Mind
For I am the first and the last.
I am the honored one and the scorned one.
I am the whore and the holy one.
I am the wife and the virgin.
I am the mother and the daughter.
I am the one whose wedding is great,
    and I have not taken a husband.
I am the barren one, and many are her sons.
I am the silence that is incomprehensible.
I am the utterance of my name.

—Nag Hammadi, second to third century C.E. "Voice of the Feminine Divine,"
in Shahrukh Husain, *The Goddess: Creation, Fertility, and Abundance,*
the Sovereignty of Woman, Myths, and Archetypes.

stepped Buddhist temples (Campbell, 1972). Brain researchers Newberg, D'Aquili, and Rause (2001) agree that myths are created by basic, universal brain structures and neurological processes by which people make sense of the world, and find resolution of existential tensions through flashes of transformative insight.

From the view of energy theory, archetypes are universal energy patterns that are recognized by virtually all people. These images are imprinted on our psyches, and imbedded in the unfolding patterns of consciousness evolution. Archetypal themes that appear in myths and fairy tales represent symbolic lessons for the soul's growth. Each person has a complement of archetypes to which they are magnetically connected, although different ones will be more prominent at various phases of life. Other people readily recognize archetypal traits in us, sometimes more clearly than we do. Every significant archetype creates patterns in our psyche and physical life, brings lessons for spiritual growth, and serves as a source of empowerment once we have mastered their energies. As Caroline Myss (2000) states succinctly: "An archetype is a template that everyone recognizes."

THE FUNCTIONS OF ARCHETYPES

Whether we are aware of it or not, archetypes are playing an important part in how we live our lives. The archetypal images are always hovering around in our subconscious mind, sometimes driving our behavior without our even realizing it. When we begin to see prototypes or symbolic models operating in ourselves and others, we can start to identify archetypal patterns playing out. We can learn about the qualities these archetypes are activating within ourselves and others. When we consciously tap into archetypal energies, we draw their power and wisdom to assist us on our life journey.

Seminal work on archetypes for contemporary women was done by Jean Shinoda Bolen, M.D., a Jungian analyst. Her book *Goddesses in Everywoman: A New Psychology of Women* (1984) described how women were acted upon by powerful forces of the archetypes of the collective unconscious and the stereotypes of culture. Many women recognized in themselves the patterns Bolen described in the Greek goddesses from the patriarchal Olympian world, whose struggles, powers, and limitations reflected issues in women's lives. One major effect of this book was to lay a foundation for women's spirituality, helping to bring the word "goddess" back into their vocabulary and consciousness in an acceptable way. The "goddess archetype" connected with many women's lives through dream images, a cherished object, or favorite pictures, which they came to recognize as symbols for the sacred feminine. Bolen's recent book *Goddesses in Older Women* (2001) looks at lesser known crone-aged goddesses from Greek, Hindu, and Egyptian mythology.

The Importance of Archetypes for Midlife and Menopausal Women

Knowing about our archetypal patterns gives us insight into our motives and drives. It also opens up new areas of experience, and lets us see sides of ourselves we have not yet expressed. The dark side of archetypes helps us see our fears and limitations, and the golden side shows us our potentials.

Learning about mature and elder women's archetypal patterns, and the goddesses or other figures from mythology who embody these patterns, can help women recognize and name their own inner stirrings. These archetypes represent patterns and energies in our psyches. According to Bolen (2001):

> By knowing who the goddesses are, women can become more conscious than they would otherwise be of the potentials within them that, once tapped, are sources of spirituality, wisdom, compassion, and action. When archetypes are activated, they energize us and give us a sense of meaning and authenticity.

Women naturally relate to different archetypes in various phases and circumstances of life. The maiden/young woman phase is a time of sampling life, exploring capabilities, and trying out relationships. The mother/mature woman phase involves making commitments and nourishing these, whether children, career, talent, or cause. The crone/wise woman phase is initiated around menopause as focus shifts inward to bring forth previously unexpressed aspects of self, leading to expanded consciousness and spirituality. When women move into new phases of life, this activates other archetypes bringing an infusion of energy and vitality, meaning, and authenticity. Knowing about these archetypes and drawing them into your awareness enlarges their presence within you. Their names, qualities, images, and stories are important to know, as this brings them alive in your imagination and deepens your connection with their forces.

One larger purpose of all the attention being focused on menopause is to change our personal and social views of postmenopausal women. A new cultural archetype for the midlife-and-beyond woman is being born, and we are part of it. You will find these archetypes are positive, empowering models for the postmenopausal woman. Included here are some old and new archetypal models that support a powerful, congruent, meaningful expression of the mature woman in the new millennium.

Archetypes can help women in the perimenopausal/menopausal journey as follows:

- Archetypes create images in our minds that shape our life experiences and guide our path of evolution.
- Archetypes carry lessons within their energetic domains. These lessons lead to self-knowledge and empowerment. Recognizing archetypes in ourselves

gives us insight into forces driving how we act, and makes us aware of choices leading to various outcomes.

- When we consciously draw on archetypal forces, we can access powerful energies from vast "mental forms" that exist in societal and world consciousness.

- We gain vision of the roles these archetypal patterns perform, and can see where we are heading. Most archetypes have a dark and a light side. Understanding what these encompass can help us clear out the old and open new potentials.

Roots of the Sacred Feminine

Contemporary women are rediscovering and claiming their lost tradition of sacred feminine archetypes, spiritual images, and myths. The ancient goddess-oriented cultures that flourished in Europe and the Mediterranean regions, predating the advent of Judeo-Christianity, have been unearthed by courageous and independently minded women researchers. Marija Gimbutas, a professor of archeology at UCLA who knew 20 languages, was the first scholar linking linguistic research with archeology, mythology, and comparative religion. Analyzing results of her major archeological excavations of Neolithic settlements in Italy, Greece, and Yugoslavia, Gimbutas developed a picture of goddess cultures from around 6,500–3,500 B.C.E. These peaceful, matrifocal cultures were unstratified, egalitarian societies with well-developed agriculture, medicine, architecture, metallurgy, wheeled vehicles, ceramics, textiles, government and law, and written language (Gimbutas, 1991; Stone, 1976).

Ideologically, they revered the Great Goddess in a myriad of roles connected with earth and generativity. She was the source of all life, and was worshipped as the feminine life force, an embodiment of nature. She was the creator, sustainer, and destroyer of life, and followed cycles of the moon, seasons, and phases of life. Because all living things were her children, they all shared in her divine essence. All life and the earth itself were seen as sacred. Women were the image of the goddess, and held major roles in the society's spiritual life. Women's fertility was honored, and sexuality was considered both a natural instinct and source of pleasure. Social networks and families were matrilineal (Bolen, 2001).

In old Europe, these goddess-oriented cultures were gradually overrun and destroyed by invading semi-nomadic Indo-European peoples from the distant north and east. The invaders were warlike, patrifocal, mobile, and ideologically oriented toward male sky gods. These invaders, called Kurgans by Gimbutas, viewed themselves as superior because of their ability to conquer and dominate the more culturally developed peaceful peoples who had long been settled in old Europe. The Kurgans subjugated the peoples of the goddess, diminished her power or devalued her attributes, or absorbed her qualities into their male gods (or their consorts). Far from bringing civilization to Europe, the Kurgans destroyed a highly developed civilization and imposed a warrior elite society. The social consequences of their values and language virtually eradicated the sacred feminine tradition, brought about male dominator culture based on strength, and reduced women to property. This process is eloquently described by Riane Eisler in *The Chalice and the Blade* (1997).

It took many centuries for the goddess religions and images of the sacred feminine to be suppressed. The process has never been complete, although male-dominated religions have made the sacred feminine nameless or disguised in androgenous terms, and have severely restricted her power. Classical Greece reached its apex in the fifth century B.C.E., as a male-oriented culture that granted women no legal rights. Athenian women were under the legal guardianship of men, and could not go to court, own property, sell any property worth more than a bushel of barley, or speak or appear in public except on special occasions (Keuls, 1993). However, the Greeks retained the memory of pre-Olympian mythology stretching into dim antiquity. The original divine genealogy begins with Gaia, the goddess Earth, the first parent who gave birth to the gods Uranus (Sky) and Pontus (Sea). Gaia mated with Uranus, giving birth to the Titans, the first generation of gods and goddesses. When Zeus made his power-play to take over the Greek pantheon, he first had to pursue, capture, and marry Metis, the daughter of two Titans and a pre-Olympian goddess of wisdom. Metis' heritage and counsel allowed Zeus to succeed after many battles with the Titans and establish himself as chief god on Mt. Olympus. Later Zeus "swallowed" Metis when he learned she would bear a son who would supplant him. Symbolically he took on (absorbed) her powers and qualities, including the ability to bear children as he subsequently birthed Athena out of his head.

The Judeo-Christian religions struggled to suppress the goddess cultures in the land of Canaan, the Middle East. The Canaanites worshiped Asherah, the Semitic name of the Great Goddess meaning "Mother of All Wisdom," "She Who Gives Birth to the Gods," or simply "Holiness." Asherah was married to El, and their daughter was Ashtoreth or Astarte, married to Baal. The most prominent Canaanite diety, Asherah was known for her oracles and her priestesses were addressed as Rabbatu (female form of Rabbi). This goddess culture was peaceful, with highly developed arts and agriculture.

Around 1200 B.C.E. the Israelites, after wandering for forty years in the desert, invaded Canaan. The Israelite god Yahweh was fiercely monotheistic, and would tolerate no "false gods" to be worshiped, as stated in the First Commandment given to Moses. According to Baring and Cashford (1991), the Great Father God (Yahweh) appears for the first time in the Old Testament accounts, developed from Hebrew mythology that coalesced various male deities of earlier cultures— Enlil, Ptah, Marduck, El—into a single monotheistic image.

Yahweh's Hebrew prophets undertook a relentless effort to eliminate the goddess Asherah and destroy all her symbols. Their goal was to remove even the memory that a Great Mother Goddess ever existed, and make Yahweh the first and only deity. This was an erratic process, as Asherah continued to be worshipped by Hebrew-speaking peoples for several more centuries. There were cycles ranging from 20 to 100 years in which Asherah was worshipped in Israelite temples up to the Babylonian exile in 586 B.C.E. (Davies, 1985). The Second Commandment's prohibitions against making "graven images" or likenesses of anything on earth, in heaven, or water meant it was sinful to make paintings or sculptures inspired by nature or the feminine face or body. Yahweh was a "jealous god" whose rival was a goddess of great power and antiquity.

THE GODDESS VEILED: SOPHIA

Eventually efforts to eliminate the goddess were successful, although hidden references to the feminine divine continued in both Old and New Testament scripture. In Hebrew, there is no word for goddess, producing the psychological effect of non-recognition: without a vocabulary the idea of feminine divinity is hard to imagine. In the Old Testament Book of Proverbs, however, there is a feminine force called *Chokmah* in Hebrew and *Sophia* in Greek. The English version is the neuter word *wisdom*. In the Revised Standard Version of the Bible, Sophia speaks as "wisdom" and describes herself as a feminine divine being:

> The Lord created me at the beginning of his works, before all else that he made, long ago. Alone, I was fashioned in times long past, at the beginning, long before earth itself. When there was yet no ocean, I was born . . . before the mountains had been shaped, before he made earth with its fields. . . . When he set the heavens in their place I was there . . . when he fixed the canopy of clouds overhead . . . when he prescribed its limits for the sea and knit together earth's foundations. Then I was at his side each day, like a master workman. I was his darling and delight, rejoicing with him always, rejoicing in his inhabited world and delighting in mankind.

Sophia further speaks as a wisdom goddess, saying "I have counsel and sound wisdom, I have insight, I have strength" (*The Holy Bible,* R.S.V., Proverbs 8:14, 8:22–31, 9:1).

In the *Wisdom of Solomon,* an apocryphal Hebrew text probably written about 100 B.C.E., Sophia appears as a powerful teacher and guide for King Solomon. Solomon tells that he gained his renowned wisdom from Sophia, from whom he learned everything that was both manifest in the world and hidden from view. She was clearly an inspirational, divine presence. This was difficult for a male-oriented monotheistic religion to reconcile, and therefore references to Sophia in Jewish literature are taken as merely poetic expressions (Bolen, 2001).

In contemporary Judaism, there is an unseen and unpersonified aspect of feminine divinity called the *Shekhinah*. This feminine force flows through Jewish women when they light the candles for the Sabbath meal, welcoming the sacred into their homes as the holy day begins on Friday evening. The Hebrew word *Sh'kina* means dwelling place, implying a place where God lives. The Shekhinah derives from this word, an essentially feminine energy that enters the household through its women and remains while Sabbath is observed, a time when work ceases and the house is considered a temple.

In the standard New Testament, divinity continues to be described as exclusively male and monotheistic, although God has three aspects in the Christian trinity (father, son, and holy spirit). The discovery in the mid-twentieth century of early Christian Gnostic gospels revealed a deep connection with the feminine divine among followers of Christ during the first few hundred years after his death. Thirteen papyrus codices found near the town of Nag Hammadi in upper Egypt contain 52 texts that are Coptic translations of more ancient manuscripts originally written in Greek, the language of the New Testament. Scientific dating has concluded that the original texts were written around 50–100 C.E., which means they were written as early or earlier than the New Testament gospels. Considered heretical by orthodox Christians, many such early texts were destroyed during 300–400 C.E., after Christianity became the state religion of the Roman Empire (Pagels, 1989).

The Gnostic Christians (from the Greek *gnosis,* or knowing) were autonomous groups with no hierarchy or dogma. They regarded all doctrines as only approaches to truth, which needed to be directly perceived through one's own experience. Their egalitarian practices especially offended orthodox Church fathers such as Tertullian, who criticized their willingness to listen and pray equally with anyone, even pagans, and "share the kiss of peace with all who come." Women had authority, which Tertullian considered heretical and audacious, saying the women "have no modesty; they are bold enough to teach, to engage in argument, to enact exorcisms, to undertake cures, and, it may be, even to baptize!" (Pagels, 1989). Women were as likely to lead group prayer, preach, offer sacraments, read scripture, and prophesy as were men.

In some gnostic texts, Sophia is described as a goddess, Yahweh as the son of a great mother goddess, and the Trinity as made up of father, mother, and son. According to one text, the true revelation of Christianity came through Mary Magdalene, a woman disciple of Jesus who was also his beloved. Many texts were mystical and offered a visionary perspective similar to that in Revelations. Accounts of humankinds' origins differed from the story told in Genesis, speaking of humans made "in *our* image, after *our* likeness. . . ." Some texts castigated Yahweh for his arrogance and jealousy, and chided him for his ignorance of his own mother (Bolen, 2001).

The multiple aspects of the Great Goddess can be seen in writings from the Nag Hammadi documents. One text contains a mystical, poetic female voice of divinity, referring to itself as "Thunder, Perfect Mind." Her essential quality is all-inclusiveness, as she contains within herself all opposites: creation and destruction, life and death. As the origin and completion of everything, her voice is reminiscent of St. John's recounting of his encounter with spirit, which says "I am the alpha and the omega." Every aspect of feminine being is included, merged into the mystical and unknowable.

THE FEMININE DIVINE IN ARCHETYPES

This brief excursion into the roots of the sacred feminine may have triggered nearly forgotten collective-unconscious memories for you, or, you may have felt an inner resonance with ancient truth that you know in your bones about our origins and history. Women are now reconnecting with their spiritual and multicultural heritage in many ways, calling to themselves the images and archetypes from mythology and folklore that represent women's vast powers and rich spiritual traditions. If you want to further explore the roots of the sacred feminine and its expression in mature women, you will find much fascinating and inspiring material in the works of Marija Gimbutas, Merlin Stone, Riane Eisler, Jean Shinoda Bolen, Barbara Walker, Sherry Anderson and Patricia Hopkins, Carol Flinders, Elaine Pagels, China Galland, Charlene Spretnak, Ann Bancroft, Tikva Frymer-Kensky, and many others.

There is a particular importance for women to have feminine divine images and language in our societies. Being able to personally identify with what is sacred and holy gives a deep sense of self-worth and value. Even though the Judeo-Christian tradition proposes that their God-image contains both the male and female, religious practices and common language usage communicate a different message. Until very recently, few women were ordained ministers in most Protestant denominations, and there remains overt, officially sanctioned resistance to priesthood for women by the Roman Catholic Church and in Orthodox Judaism. Use of the masculine name (God) and pronoun (He, His, Him) in scripture, preaching, and educational activities continues to support the image of a male deity. Jean Shinoda Bolen (2001) describes the impact of first seeing a woman priest:

> I remember the time that I was in an Episcopalian church and Barbara St. Andrews officiated. This was in the early eighties, and the first time I ever saw a woman priest in a clerical collar speaking from the pulpit and offering communion. It seemed strangely unfamiliar, and then it liberated something in me. It was similar to when I saw someone who is Asian like me in an honored or respected role for the first time. When I witnessed it myself, my own world grew larger.

Women in the midlife and postmenopausal stages are engaged in the process of enlarging their world. Soul and spiritual issues come to the forefront. Thoughts turn to mortality and divinity, death, transformation and continuance. Religious beliefs and personal faith often come up for review. Often at this time, a deep yearning arises to feel connected with the feminine divine and to experience the knowing (gnosis) of the sacred within. Learning about, relating to, and drawing from the archetypes of midlife and menopausal women can help fulfill this yearning.

After reading this chapter, see Worksheets on pages 281–283 for exercises on "Invoking Your Archetypes," Envisioning a New World Order," and "Contributions to a World in Balance and Harmony."

ARCHETYPES OF MIDLIFE AND MENOPAUSE

Several archetypes have special importance for women during perimenopause and menopause. Their energetic domains are inner knowledge, vision, creativity, abundance, and transformation.

The Alchemist

During perimenopause, as midlife issues arise, the Alchemist usually is activated. This archetype is portrayed in the fairy tale of the Spinner, where the heroine must learn to spin straw into gold, or else lose her life. Fearing she will be unable to perform this act of alchemy, she calls upon a fairy godmother or kind witch who comes to her aid and teaches her. The fairy godmother or witch symbolizes her own inner wise woman, the one who knows the secrets of life and mysteries of spirit magic.

All experiences, even difficult and painful ones, have value in life. They can all be spun into gold, giving gifts of understanding, compassion, forgiveness. Almost every woman has had some traumas in her life which require the power of the Alchemist to transform. Women who had abusive childhoods may undergo transformation of these wounds through acknowledging them, expressing anger, grieving loss of a happy childhood, and finally forgiving their abusers. Women who suffer serious illnesses can learn the process of regaining health or living gracefully with limitations. These women transform wounds and suffering into wisdom and strength, and can assist others through similar processes.

Despite our "broken web"—the lost feminine traditions in so many cultures—women can find images of this alchemical power in myths such as Spider Woman (Hopi), Changing Woman (Navajo), and Shakti (Hindu). These symbolize the immense creativity inherent in the feminine principle, which lies at the heart of the natural world. Feminine qualities of inclusiveness, adaptability, compassion, and honoring inner truth support both creation (bringing into being) and regeneration (renewal, healing, and reshaping).

The Alchemist energy is present in most women's menopausal transitions. We transform problems, symptoms and fears into something valuable: the precious wisdom, vision, and courage of the mature Wise Woman and the Elder Woman (see Figure 6–1).

This is the story of how this painting (Figure 6–1) came to be: Artist Alta Wertz was in her 60s, had lived through the death of two husbands and reconstructed her life, when she attended the first Crone Counsel at Jackson Hole, Wyoming. While there she felt inspired to paint a watercolor of the Crone Mother with the guidance of the spirit of the Crone—a presence who had come to her in a dream years ago. In her dream:

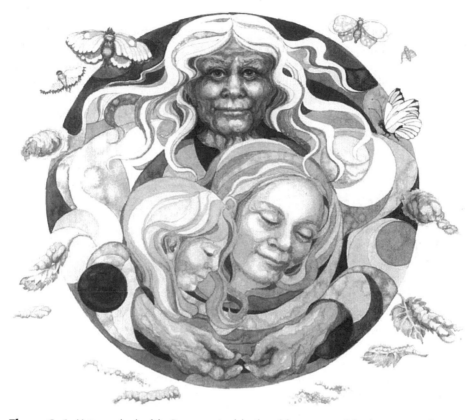

Figure 6–1 Metamorphosis of the Dreamers. A celebration of the presence of the three aspects of woman as depicted in the archetype of the Triple Goddess: maiden, lover/mother, and wise elder/crone. *Reproduced by permission of Alta Happ Wertz.*

I received a telephone call from a female with an ancient voice, who didn't identify herself, but who said she was coming over. Answering a knock at the door I found myself face to face with a very old lady, who upon entering the room immediately took my hands in hers. A powerful surge of energy flowed through me. "From now on," she said, "I will be your teacher. You are a wonderful woman." Not only that, but somewhere in the dream I was flying, wearing a red Wonder Woman cape.

Astrologically speaking, at the time I had the dream I was in my second Saturn Return, which is a time for harvesting the seed of what we have learned throughout our life and passing it on to those behind us. The Crone in my dream was making it quite clear that it was time for me to allow the "me" in the "wonderful woman" cape to make room for the "Crone-in-training" higher aspect of myself to step forward and take her rightful place.

SPIDER WOMAN

Spider Woman is the Hopi creation goddess who together with Tawa, the Sun God, brought Earth and all creatures into being. As Mother of the Earth, Spider Woman has responsibility for teaching, supporting, and transforming people, animals, and all nature. She spins the web of creation, and interweaves its intricate connections, out of her very Self, her own body. The web cannot be permanently broken, because she is constantly reweaving and respinning and because all life is also her own Self.

Spider Woman of the Hopi Indians

All the mysteries, powers, and magic of the Below are controlled by Spider Woman, the Earth Goddess. Those of the Above belong to Tawa, the Sun God. These Two had one Thought and it was a mighty Thought— that they would make Earth between the Above and the Below. The Hopi people, created by Spider Woman and Tawa, emerged through the *sipapu,* or opening, at the bottom of the Grand Canyon.

"I am Tawa," sang the Sun God, "I am Light. I am Life. I am Father of all that shall ever come."

"I am Kokyanwuhti," the Spider Woman crooned in a softer note. "I receive Light and nourish Life. I am Mother of all that shall ever come."

Spider Woman caught up clay with her slender fingers and made the Thoughts of Tawa take form. The Two sang the magic Song of Life, and all things created breathed and lived. Spider Woman continued to spin and weave the Web of Life from her own body, always teaching the people, and recreating and renewing cosmic and human harmony.

—G.M. Mullett, *Spider Woman Stories: Legends of the Hopi Indians*

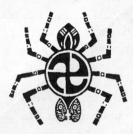

Spider.
Reproduced with permission.
Copyright © Kate Cartwright.

Touched by the Goddess: Spider Woman at Sedona

When I was 52, my husband and I vacationed in Sedona, Arizona. The week before, I had read a book on Spider Woman and the ancient Native American creation myth of how she spun the world into existence through her web. There was a dramatic electrical storm the day we arrived, with huge billowing black clouds, ear-splitting thunder and electric bolts that seemed to reach across the entire sky, down into the earth. The next morning I felt flu-like, achy and feverish. Later I discovered a small bite about an inch above my pubic hair line, and instantly recognized it as a spider bite. Physically I felt fine the next day, but the energy of unsettled things, changes, and upheavals stayed with me. A few days later my daughter called, telling me she was having a miscarriage. When at the soaring Chapel of the Holy Cross built into a sheer red cliff, I prayed to Mother Mary and lit a votive candle for my daughter's well-being. The Divine Mother's presence was tangible, with her endless compassion for our suffering. Sitting later on the edge of a vast canyon, in a circle of stones creating my sacred space, I meditated on the rose-hued cliffs on the other side, weathered and worn by centuries of rain and wind, with each layer clearly etched in gently graduated colors. Peace, unity, time-lessness, and endlessness seemed to vibrate from these ancient rocks.

My daughter lost the baby. My spider bite scabbed over and healed, leaving a faint white scar as its memento. My husband and I discussed the meaning of all this. A Sedona brochure says "The legend of The People says that the Grandmother Spirit of the world still lives in Sedona, welcoming her family home." This was all too much for coincidence. I believe that Grand-mother Spirit touched me through Spider Woman's earth-plane symbol, an initiation of sorts that began changing my consciousness. The Goddess energy, so concerned with birth, death and people's struggles in the world, graced me in the chapel and on the cliff. I knew Her presence and Her love.

—Lennie Martin

CHANGING WOMAN

The Navajo tribe's primary deity, Changing Woman is the woman who is trans-formed time and time again—she grows old and becomes young again with each change of the seasons. Changing Woman creates life and is one with all life; radiant,

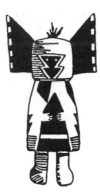

Corn Mother.
Reproduced with permission.
Copyright © Kate Cartwright.

honored, and visionary. She manifests spirit and all that is holy, while causing the ebb and flow of life by changing everything she touches. Ceremonies such as Kinaalda, the menstruation ritual initiating girls into womanhood, were established by Changing Woman.

The corn maiden, mother, and grandmother reflect the cycles of Changing Woman. Among Southwestern tribes, associations between corn and the supernatural permeated everyday life. Eastern tribes believed that women alone had the special power required to grow corn. After planting corn seeds in small hillocks, Iroquois women would circle the field at night, pulling their clothing over the earth. Through this ritual, women shared their fertility with the corn seeds.

Changing Woman Chant

There is a woman who weaves the night sky
See how she spins, see her fingers fly
She stands beside us from beginning to end
She is our mother, our lover, and friend
Our grandmother, sister, and friend
She is the weaver and we are the web
She is the needle and we are the thread
She changes everything she touches
Everything she touches changes
    Changing, holy, sacred, healing, weaving woman.
I am a woman of radiance, radiance
Buffalo woman's kin

(Continued on next page)

I am a woman of radiance, radiance
The double helix spins
Like a lightening arrow or a galloping mare
I'm pulled to the center of life
Shedding the old, I don wings of magnificence
Me and the eagle take flight.
Changing, holy, sacred, healing, weaving woman.

—Navajo song

SHAKTI

This Hindu deity represents pure, essential feminine creative power. All Hindu goddesses have Shakti-power, and when a woman expresses some aspect of a goddess, she is said to be manifesting her shakti. This feminine principle is the basis for the natural world; it is the Divine as nature. Shakti is wondrous, active, changing, growing, chaotic, free, the fuel for all activity, infinite primordial energy. In each goddess (representing various qualities) Shakti finds new expression. As people grow spiritually, Shakti-power moves upward through the body, enlivening the seven chakras (energy centers near the spine), and bringing enlightenment, Self-Realization, Divine Union, and merging with the infinite cosmic Source. Through the union of Shakti and Shiva, Lord of Bliss, Order, and Destruction, the universe is manifest in endless cycles of creation and destruction.

Shakti is the ultimate alchemist, the changer of everything, the power of transformation. When devotees have a life-altering event, such as serious illness, injury, or unexpected crises, this is often called "Shakti-pat" meaning they were hit with a great force of transformative energy.

The Guardian (Protectress-Goddess)

The Guardian archetype naturally emerges around menopause. Having completed the life phase of family care-taking or intense career commitment, postmenopausal women turn their new resources of fiery yang energy toward protection of others in many forms. They become the guardians of life: of the young and vulnerable, the environment, the animals, the values of honoring diversity, and the interrelatedness of all life. The biological pathways of empathy are well-established in emotionally healthy women, who can sense and feel from another's perspective. Their lives express tolerance of differences, appreciation of the ramifications of decisions, and cellular-level knowledge that all is interconnected.

Women manifesting the Guardian archetype have a fierce directness that cuts through to the heart of things. They will not tolerate abuses or exploitation of people, creatures, or the earth. Their creativity and relationships become more

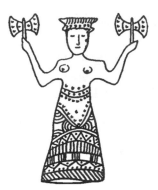

Minoan Great Mother.
Reproduced by permission.
Copyright © Kate Cartwright.

assertive, although not emulating the male oppositional qualities of domination and conquest. Women are, above all, deeply connected with others. They know the intrinsic spirituality of interrelatedness. Therefore, they work creatively for change in ways that honor the highest nature of others. The Guardian energy is seen in goddess figures such as Themis, Durga, and Demeter.

THEMIS

Themis is a Greek goddess who represents steadfastness, justice, and righteousness. She is the oracular power of the earth deity (Gaia), and carries the force that

O Ishtar, Queen of all peoples, directress of mankind!
Thou art mighty, thou hast sovereign power, exalted is thy name!
Thou art the light of heaven and earth . . .
Ruler of weapons, arbitress of the battle!
Framer of all decrees, wearer of the crown of dominion!
Thou wieldest the scepter and the decision, the control of earth and heaven!

At the thought of thy name the heaven and earth quake.
The gods tremble, and the spirits of earth falter.
Mankind payeth homage to thy mighty name,
For thou art great, thou art exalted . . .
O Lady, majestic is thy rank, over all the gods it is exalted!

—Hymn in Praise of the Goddess Ishtar of Babylonia, found on one of the "Seven Tablets of Creation," seventh century B.C.E., although the hymn is much older. From Cahill, 1996.

binds people together; the collective conscience, the social imperative, the Law. She guides the elders and unites the people in peace. As an emanation of the Great Earth Mother, the authority of Themis has prehistoric roots. In Olympian mythology, Themis is the one who must convene and dissolve the assembly of gods and goddesses at Mt. Olympus; Zeus (King of Gods) cannot summon his own assembly. Themis calls the gods and goddesses to council, presides over feasts, and ends their meetings.

At the beginning of humanity, Themis was there. She was the guardian of all people, especially the young who were to be fed and nurtured, protected, and loved. She taught people how to live together, to share, and to be family. As the people multiplied and formed clans, she showed them how to cooperate, share skills, and develop trade. From her oracles, people learned to form councils and follow the rules of order, justice, and mercy. In this way, millennia passed and Greece prospered. Later, barbarian invaders swept down and took Themis captive, proclaiming a new order of patriarchal rule using military force. Zeus was established as the King of Gods, ruling by fear and deception. Yet Themis could not be crushed, and retained her ultimate power to convene the assembly on Mt. Olympus, without which the gods could not operate. Themis would not die (Spretnak, 1984).

DURGA

Durga is the Hindu goddess of invincible power, who rides a lion (symbol of solar-yang fiery energy). She eliminates obstacles to enlightenment, and overcomes difficulties by taking us beyond disease, sorrow, darkness, and death. Wielding weapons of light, she destroys negative forces. Durga has great strength and power in battle, and was essential in the struggle of humans against demonic forces that were taking over the world, according to ancient Hindu legend. In her most fearsome expression, Durga becomes Kali, the black goddess of destruction and transformation (discussed later in this chapter).

The Nurturer and Rejuvenator

The mature mother aspect of the goddess is widely celebrated as the source of life's sustenance. She is the personified principle of renewal, the continuous regeneration of plant life and the life cycles of humans and animals. The life of humankind mirrors the circular existence of vegetation—birth, life, death, and rebirth. Death is regarded as a passageway into a new life in another realm of existence. Birth is celebrated as the re-entry of the soul into the world, after spending a time in the mysterious place of rejuvenation, often called the "underworld."

In Egypt, the mother who gives birth and destroys, who catalyzes the cyclic movements of existence, is personified in the dual faces of the goddess Hathor/ Sekhmet. In Mesopotamia, this eternal cycle was portrayed as the mythical union

She who has color of the Fire, I take refuge in her, the Goddess Durga. Fire, deliver us anew, across all difficulties to well-being. Fire, Knower of all births, as a ship across the sea, deliver us across all difficulties. Like the Sun, chanting with the mind, awaken as the protector of our being.

—Mahanarayana Upanishad, Durga Sukta 2-5,
from David Frawley, *Tantra Yoga and the Wisdom Goddesses*

of female and male, the Goddess and her lover, whose union and separation led to the seasons and agricultural cycles. The Greeks embodied this process in the pure, tender love of the mother Goddess for her daughter. They also had to undergo cycles of union and separation, as told in the myth of Demeter and Persephone.

HATHOR/SEKHMET

Deriving from an ancient Egyptian goddess who predates Isis, Hathor is represented as a cow goddess who nurtures, cares for her children, and embodies love,

I, Sekhmet, dedicate every day to love each and every one of you.
Wear My love every morning around you as a garment and it will
     protect you.
Trust My strength and it will keep you safe.
Trust My power and ask, for I will provide for all your needs
     abundantly.
Trust My knowledge and it will be yours to unfold.
Know that I am your mother, therefore I will never let go of your
     hand.
Ask Me what your heart desires and if in divine order I will comply.
Bring to me your enemies and I will fight the battles with you.
Remember, what your tiny hands cannot reach, My huge paws and
     claws can.
Remember, what your finite eyes cannot see, My timeless eyes can.
Remember, what seems impossible for you is nothing within the sea
     of possibilities contained in my womb.

—Anonymous, "Sekhmet the Lion-headed Goddess,"
in-class materials by Raven Joy

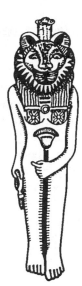

Sekhmet.
Reproduced by permission.
Copyright © Kate Cartwright.

joy and celebration of life. Sekhmet is portrayed as a lioness-headed goddess, full of solar power that destroys, purifies, transforms, regenerates, and heals. The combined force of Hathor/Sekhmet animates all creation, is the source of consciousness, and the eternal flame that keeps creation becoming. This energy is manifested on earth in all matter, most highly developed in humans through our creative abilities: we can imagine and invent, and thus bring into existence our visions.

Sekhmet has special significance for midlife women, as the teacher of fearless compassion. Through her energies we learn to turn anger to action that leads to compassion. We are able to alchemically transform fear into intuition. Sekhmet's power contains the fire that purifies sickness, as she was the patron of great healers during Egyptian times. This same power, which we call kundalini or chi, flows through contemporary healers. Remember that kundalini energy begins rising naturally in menopausal women, initiating us into a stage of greater empowerment.

When we invoke the archetypal energies of Sekhmet, this fiery power helps maintain cosmic and moral order in a very forthright and focused way. Through her, we express majesty, pride of being, and true passion. We offer a no-nonsense compassion that demands self-knowledge and discipline. Sekhmet asks us to enter our shadows, recognize and understand them, and unite the darkness-light, lunar-solar sides of our natures so we can proceed to a place of wholeness. As we become whole, we help bring the world and indeed the universe back to a state of wholeness (Sierra-Wolf, 1999).

The Myth of Hathor/Sekhmet

Ra, the Sun God who ruled the sky and all that dwelt below, grew weary and the people saw him as weak and decrepit. They no longer paid him homage and their worship grew lax. Looking with dismay on his creation, Ra called the Lion Goddess Sekhmet to set it straight. She prowled the land, saw how cosmic law was defiled and how this led to needless human suffering. She loosed her fiery wrath upon the people and the ground was littered with broken and bleeding bodies. Her taste for human blood ignited, Sekhmet's savage slaughter know no bounds. Ra grieved as he saw this carnage, but because of Sekhmet's divine powers, he knew he could not force her to cease the ravaging of earth—so, he resorted to trickery. At night while she rested, Ra called upon his priests to brew 7,000 vats of barley beer, spiked with pomegranate juice so it looked like blood. Just before dawn they poured it upon the fields where Sekhmet was sure to pass. When she awoke and resumed her feasting, she lapped up the lake of "blood" and became intoxicated. This turned her into the Cow Goddess Hathor, her other face. She resumed nurturing the world and humans were saved.

DEMETER

The power to nurture is the core quality of Demeter. Her story is one of happiness and innocence, separation and loss, and then reunion and transformation. Demeter is the ultimate caretaking mother who lives, in a way, through her daughter Persephone, selflessly nurturing her. Pluto, Lord of the Underworld, falls in love with Persephone and carries her off to Hades. When Demeter loses Persephone she is shattered. In her grief and wrath, she fails to tend the seeds and commands the plants not to grow. The earth becomes parched and barren. Demeter refuses to nurture the earth until Persephone is returned to her. Zeus orders Pluto to return Persephone to her grieving mother for part of the year. Joyfully, Demeter makes plants grow and the earth become green and full of blossoms during spring and summer. When Persephone returns to the Underworld, the earth enters late fall and winter again.

Life teaches us that to cling to something or someone is to suffer. It is essential to recognize our wholeness and be able to stand alone, yet still love and serve others, as well as be loved and served in return—to be intradependent. This is a myth of letting go of expectations (Demeter cannot have Persephone all the time), yet also learning that we can claim the power to change things, to take action, to

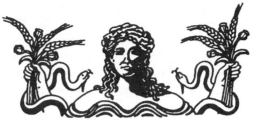

Demeter.
*Reproduced with
permission.*
Copyright ©
Kate Cartwright.

attend to our own needs and nurture ourselves. This is also the archetype of emotional depth that comes from grieving loss and surviving it. If we can survive our greatest wounds, this suffering makes us stronger. Sometimes we are happy, sometimes sad, sometimes outward, sometimes inward, sometimes moving toward the realization of a dream, sometimes moving away in defeat. Wisdom is found in understanding the duality of life, the opposite points on the great wheel. North balances south, birth balances death. In menopause, we move into the larger cycle of a woman's life—changing from mother to creatrix or matriarch, and ultimately to crone or elder.

The Queen

The Queen is a powerful but much misunderstood archetype of the midlife and older woman. We have all known such women; they have a regal air about them and seem to command attention and respect. They often radiate a sense of inner worth, of completeness in themselves, which naturally expresses generosity toward others. A certain deference seems their natural due, and we find ourselves giving it to them almost without thinking. The Queen archetype is a natural ruler, and women in whom it is fully activated will draw a loyal following, their "court" for which they set the tone. Queens also provide for their followers' well-being and want to give to them; in contemporary times this giving is more in terms of emotional support and wise advice. Some prominent American Queens include Gloria Steinem, Mary Kay, and Hillary Clinton. Oprah Winfrey is another benevolent Queen who gives opportunities to others through her abundance. Oprah provides a positive model of a woman with prestige, means, and power; through this she is helping to heal the Prostitute (selling-out of the self) archetype that plagues so many women today.

We are familiar with the Dark Queen through fairy tales and myths. A classic is the Dark Queen who pursues Snow White with intention to kill her, thus removing her as a future rival for the Queen's powers. In this mythology, the Dark Queen is driven by jealousy of the innocent maiden who signals the waning of the Queen's power as her cycle draws to a close. In the psyche, the Dark Queen represents the unknown, fearful, and dangerous parts of ourselves. As we begin to awaken (the Maiden) we must face and come to know our shadow. By examining the shadow's secrets, we dissipate fear and integrate its powers.

Hera is the prototypical Queen from Greek mythology (see Figure 6–2). It is interesting that her ancient, pre-Hellenic myth tells quite a different story from the one we are more familiar with after Zeus enters the picture as her husband.

HERA

The myths of Hera focus on the cycles of women's lives and the power of partnership. She is connected with the seasons, phases of the moon, and the life stages of maiden, mother, and elder. In pre-Hellenic times, she was especially venerated in Crete, Samos, and Argos, and her temple, the Heraion, long predates the temple of Zeus. Every spring, women gathered at the sacred spring of Kanathos as the new moon appeared to invoke the Goddess Hera for the next seasonal cycle. Hera took a ritual bath in the sacred spring, which renewed her virginity, meaning she was One-In-Herself, complete and not needing anything else. As spring colors and plants bloomed, she then presided over the Sacred Marriage, symbolized by

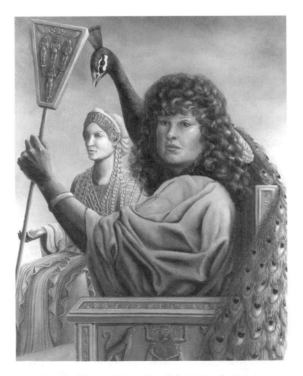

Figure 6–2 Hera. Reproduced with permission. Copyright © Sandra Stanton. *www.goddessmyths.com;* e-mail: *images@mainwest.com*

union of the lunar cow and the solar bull. These rites guaranteed fertility and fecundity for people, plants, and animals. Homage to Hera continued throughout the year. Every four years the benevolence of the Goddess was celebrated at the feast of the Heraia in Olympia. Footraces were run by girls who represented the three stages of women's life. As Hera crowned each winner, the girls said (Spretnak, 1984):

THE MAIDEN: I am the new moon, swelling with magic, pure in my maidenhood, ever growing stronger.

THE MOTHER: I am the full moon, complete in my powers, making people with my rhythms, bathing them in light.

THE ELDER: I am the waning moon, easing into peace, knowing all that went before, I am the wise one.

Hera was an indigenous goddess and ruled alone; her first consort was Herakles. After the patriarchal gods took over, Hera's story changed. As Zeus moved in from the north and took over the Greek pantheon, in the way of conquering chieftains he married Hera, a daughter of the land (Spretnak, 1984). In the myth, Zeus and Hera live a tumultuous life together, full of infidelity and jealousy, rage and lust. Hera is the Queen, regal, proud, privileged, but conflicted. She is committed to partnership but finds at the outset that it is unequal. She encounters many challenges that seem to require sacrifice. Hera has to face her powerlessness as Zeus philanders and procreates with many others. What, then, are her choices? To either accept the situation with equanimity, to become depressed and withdrawn with the humiliation of it all, to become a guerilla fighter nipping and retreating, or to take her power back and concentrate on her own growth.

This archetype demonstrates a woman's urge for union, both within and without. The continuum ranges from an unhappy partnership with another person who is on another wavelength to the ultimate spiritual union of partnership with the higher Self. It is a journey from losing oneself to gaining oneself. Only when Hera finds her independent identity can true partnership start. She withdraws from her marriage, goes on retreat to reestablish her sense of self, then is able to meet Zeus again without being the needy, wounded partner. Then begins the healthy integration of male and female without the co-dependence that fear of being alone brings forth. Marriage, therefore, can be one of the greatest teachers of our lives (Stassinopoulos, 1999).

At her best, in the fullness of her power, Hera is serene, authoritative, potent, and active. She is secure in her equality in partnership. If a partnership is not working, she takes action. This is where many women find themselves at menopause: making the decision to either stay or go, to accept things as they are or to change them. We ask the question: is a bad partnership better than no partnership? We learn ultimately that it is our partnership with ourselves that needs to be attended to first.

MARY, QUEEN OF HEAVEN

In the Christian tradition, Mary the mother of Jesus fulfills the widespread human need to relate to a loving, all-accepting, and nurturing feminine divinity. Virtually nothing is known about Mary after the death of Jesus. Mary's later life and her own death are not mentioned in the New Testament Bible, although later works in the fourth or fifth centuries C.E. became the basis for the tradition of Mary's bodily assumption into heaven. According to these texts, the saints and apostles were gathered before Mary's tomb, arguing about her status. Jesus then appeared with the archangel Michael and ordered that Mary's body be carried up to heaven. Her body was taken "to the Tree of Life," a common goddess-symbol dating from ancient Sumer, and was then reunited with her soul. Other accounts say Mary did not die at all, but was carried to heaven while still alive by Jesus, the Apostles, a host of angels, and the prophets Moses, Enoch, and Elias (Husain, 1997).

As the tradition of the Assumption was widely accepted, Mary's identity as divine was confirmed and she, like Isis, Ishtar, and others before her, became the Queen of Heaven. As a supreme goddess, she gained the appellations of "Star of the Sea" and "Mother of God." At evening services Mary is invoked with "Hail, Queen of Heaven, whence the light of the world has arisen." In her revered role as Queen of Heaven, Mary intercedes on the behalf of humankind with God and Christ. Many Catholics and other Christians find it more comforting to direct their prayers to Mary, to whom they feel closer and from whom they know will always flow unconditional love and acceptance. Mary has a long tradition of miracles and blessings. Visions of Mary in which she teaches, blesses, and encourages her faithful followers have been recorded from Europe to Mexico.

Queen Mary protects, assists, guides, and comforts those under her dominion. She is a gracious and beneficent goddess-queen archetype, the epitome of compassionate goddesses. Other great goddesses of compassion include Quan Yin (Chinese) and Tara (Buddhist).

The Wise Woman (Sage, Crone)

The Wise Woman archetype carries the seeds of knowledge for the next generation, and speaks with the voice of wisdom for society. This archetypal energy comes to women who have faced many challenges in life, and have learned the lessons inherent in these experiences. Wise Women deeply understand the multiple interconnections in the web of life. They have examined their shadow, faced their fears, and come out strong and empowered. With their clarity and insight, they become "oracles" whose advice is sought by others facing choices and challenges. They listen to their inner voice and commune with their innate Divinity, which enhances vision, intuition, and compassion.

The Wise Woman models the successful journey through life's middle and later stages. She embodies integrity and inner balance. Her expansive vision sees the symbolic meanings of things. Her commitment is to help others in self-growth, and to relate ever more closely to Spirit. Her methods may at times appear extreme, for she knows the ephemeral quality of material things, and exhorts others toward their own higher awareness, often through causing them to cast aside their illusions. This is the transformative aspect of the Wise Woman, for part of her purpose is to initiate us into the closing of cycles, the finishing of natural processes, and the mysteries of death and regeneration.

At menopause the woman rests in the "pregnant void" and creates an energetic opening for a new state of consciousness. Once established in wisdom-mystery, mature women embody the processes of transformation, death, and regeneration. They know the fullness of cycles, from beginning to ending. The shadow self, darkness, underworld, and the unknown are their domains. Women draw from powerful archetypes of the Wisdom or Transformation Goddesses, who have numerous forms such as Hecate, Kali, The Black Madonna, and Oya.

The Blood Mysteries

There is an ancient tradition called women's *blood mysteries*. The "water" that flowed through women as menstrual blood was seen as the "fountain of life." People observed that women's monthly bleeding stopped during pregnancy—they retained the blood to make a baby. This was a magical thing, a special power women possessed. Then when women became older and stopped menstruating, they retained the blood to make wisdom. This was an even greater power, commanding respect and awe. This "wise blood" enabled postmenopausal women to become trusted advisors, visionaries, healers, oracles, and keepers of knowledge for the group.

HECATE (HEKATE)

Hecate is a Greek goddess who represents the crone (wise woman) aspect of the ancient Triple Goddess (maiden, mother, crone). She is the goddess of death and regeneration, who stands at the crossroads where the three roads come together. Her vision encompasses the road behind, which we have already traveled, and the roads ahead which we can now choose. Her understanding of the consequences of choice is deep and profound, for she knows the secrets of life, death, creation, and immortality. As one who has gleaned wisdom from experiences in many dimensions, Hecate provides wise counsel and guidance to those who would deepen their understanding of life's mysteries.

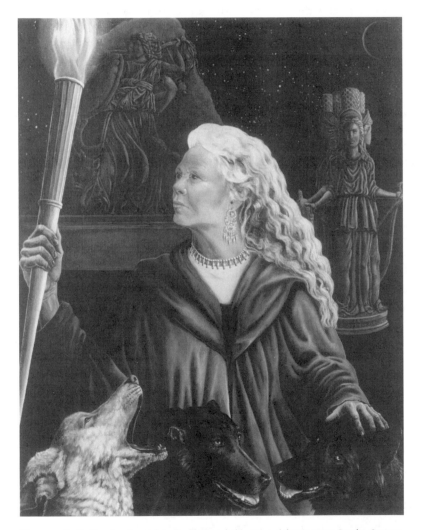

Figure 6–3 Hecate. *Reproduced with permission.* Copyright © 1998 Sandra Stanton. *www.goddessmyths.com;* e-mail: *images@mainwest.com*

Hecate

But when the moon slipped away, shrinking gracefully into its own death . . . the mortals guarded themselves against visiting spirits from the underworld. Hordes of ghosts led by Hecate and Her baying hounds roamed the earth on moonless nights. Yet She protected those mortals who purified themselves in Her name. . . . When Hecate's rites were observed, the black nights passed silently one into another. But if the Goddess was defiled, She unleashed the power of Her wrath and swept over the earth, bringing storms and destruction.

Until the new moon slit the sky, Hecate shared clues to Her secrets. Those who believed understood. They saw that form was not fixed, watched human become animal become tree become human. . . . Awesome were Her skills but always Hecate taught the same lesson: *Without death there is no life.*

—Charlene Spretnak, *Lost Goddesses of Early Greece*

Associated with the waning moon, Hecate's energy brings us into the darkness. In spiritual terms, darkness is the unknown, the abyss, the uncharted territory, the mystery. We each carry within ourselves a personal pattern of darkness and light. Light means a place of illumination where we access personal power and truth through the freeing effects of expanded awareness and consciousness. However, to expand our light we must expand our personal power, requiring us to leave the safety of the known. Venturing into the unknown means exploring the mystery of ourselves and revealing our secrets and fears, so they may be resolved. To do this, we must enter the darkness. Fearsome forces may dwell in the darkness. Hecate's myth represents these forces as howling demons and baying hounds, ghosts stalking the earth, and terrible storms and destructions (see Figure 6–3).

KALI

The Hindu goddess of creation and destruction, Kali is portrayed as dark blue or black wearing a garland of skulls and dancing on the chest of Shiva (her male consort—pure Beingness, origin of life force) with her fangs or long tongue protruding. For the ignorant, Kali represents the terrible force of death; for the wise it is the power of transformation. Kali grants eternal life—when we are willing to surrender our mortal, transient, material nature. When her force awakens within

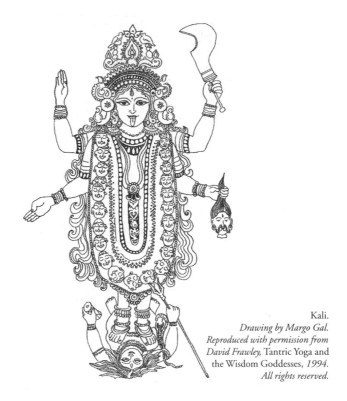

Kali.
Drawing by Margo Gal.
Reproduced with permission from
David Frawley, Tantric Yoga and
the Wisdom Goddesses, *1994.*
All rights reserved.

us she works to break down all limitations and attachments, so we can transcend the known and enter the Great Mystery.

Kali is an intoxicating personification of primal energy, an incarnation of the essential feminine force with overwhelming intensity and legendary strength. In the myth of Kali, demonic forces had been dominating and oppressing the world for a long time. Humans appealed to the gods, but the gods were defeated by the powerful demons and fled in humiliation. In desperation, the people prayed to the Daughter of the Himalayas to save gods and humankind alike. The gods sent

Kali is time or eternity. . . . To see death or decay inherent in all things is part of her recognition. Those who know the truth of Kali see the old person in the child, and the child in the old man. They see the flower in the decayed stump, and the decayed plant in the flower. They grasp time from both ends and embrace eternity.

—David Frawley, *Tantric Yoga and the Wisdom Goddesses:*
Spiritual Secrets of Ayurveda

forth their energies as a stream of fire, and from this emerged the Great Goddess Durga. In a pivotal battle against the demons, the Goddess Kali sprang from the brow of Durga, and attained victory through her fierce and merciless fighting. Kali manifested herself to annihilate the demonic power and to restore peace and equilibrium.

In order to defeat the demonic forces, Kali had to eliminate everything that brings dualism or separation into the world. The splitting of reality by judgments about good-evil, pure-corrupt, mine-yours, right-wrong is the source of separation. Kali had to destroy the very source of this dualism within the psyche of people and gods. She wiped out everything, so existence could be restored to its natural state, and gods and people could return to an undivided view of life. The good-terrible mother, the creator-destroyer, Kali personifies the eternal flux of life, from which all things arise and into which they disappear. Her energies compel us to accept darkness and light, death and life as the two sides of the coin of existence (Mascetti, 1998).

BLACK MADONNA

The Black Madonna is an enigmatic archetype whose origins reach back to the Great Mother-Earth Goddess of prehistoric times. Great Mother worship flourished throughout Europe from 7,000 to 3,500 B.C.E., and goddess figures over 30,000 years old have been found from Yugoslavia to France (Gimbutas, 1989). As many as 450 Black Madonna images existed in Europe at one time, about half of these in France. Some have been destroyed, lost, or tucked away in private collections. There are also statues or icons in South America, England, Mexico, and the United States (Krymow, 1998).

Black Madonna may be a statue, painting, or icon, representing Mary and Jesus with dark brown or black faces. Darkness has a wide range of symbolic meanings, such as deep space, the womb, the earth, the unknown, ancient wisdom, death, sorrow, the unconscious, the descent, mysteries, and the shadow side. For Tibetan Buddhists black signifies the stage just before enlightenment; the Sufi tradition holds that darkness is the final stage of the soul's journey to beatitude. Black means mourning in the West; fertility in Old European cultures; purity in Turkish tradition; and black is the first step in the medieval alchemical process (the *nigredo*) (Galland, 1990).

Darkness has significance for how our universe operates. Dark matter may comprise as much as 90 percent of the entire universe, according to recent research in theoretical physics. The world and universe we can see, called the "luminous world," is believed to be only a fraction of what exists. Dark matter cannot be seen, but it can be observed indirectly through its gravitational effects on galaxies. Though we cannot see or measure dark matter, we feel it through the movements of stars, planets, and galaxies. It is a most intriguing idea that much of what exists is invisible, undetectable by the five physical senses, and operating by cosmic laws we do not yet comprehend. There is indeed great mystery in darkness.

Midlife women going through the dark night, and delving into their shadow self, will find resonance with the Black Madonna. When this connection occurs for us, the coming of the Black Madonna into our consciousness symbolizes the growth of the psyche in the direction of merging spirituality with every-day life, the body, and the earth. Spirituality is not separate from earthly life, and we do not have to reject involvement with life in order to expand spiritually. This is the feminine way, the dawning of Feminine Divine awareness within. To long for darkness is to long for transformation, for integration, for healing, for balance.

Black Madonna of Czestochowa, Poland

Located in the Jasna Gora Monastery is a fifteenth century copy of the original icon, whose origin is still debated. Most art historians believe it was painted from a fifth century Byzantine prototype called the *Hodegetria,* "The One Who Leads the Way." This famous image of the Madonna and Child was worshipped in Constantinople and revered by ships' pilots for its guidance. But legend has it that the original Black Madonna was painted by St. Luke, the disciple of Jesus Christ, using wooden planks of the table from the household of the Holy Family in Nazareth. While Luke was painting the picture, Mary told him about the life of Jesus, which he later retold in his gospel.

Many miraculous events and healings connected with this Black Madonna have occurred over the centuries. In the fifteenth century the monastery was invaded and a looter struck the icon twice with his sword. Before he could strike a third time, he fell to the ground in agony and died. In the mid-seventeenth century, a small force of Polish soldiers defeated a huge army from Sweden that was plundering the country at Jasna Gora. The Madonna is credited for the Polish victory against the Bolshevik Army in 1920. While the Russians were invading Poland, they saw an image of the Black Madonna in the clouds, and withdrew.

The archetypal roots of the Black Madonna (and of Mary) extend to Mesopotamia and connect with Ishtar, a Sumerian/Babylonian goddess called the Queen of Heaven. She was a moon goddess associated with

(Continued on next page)

vegetation, fertility, and love prior to the third millennium B.C.E. Her worship spread to Greece and Turkey, and was carried by the Hittites into Europe. Ishtar was also associated with the underworld, and her face is black. Other names for Ishtar have been Astarte and Asherah (Hebrew), and Cybele and Artemis (Greek).

In the mother aspect, the Black Madonna (Mary) is connected with the Egyptian goddess Isis. Like Mary, Isis was a virgin who brought her son Horus forth "of herself." Isis often is depicted suckling her son Horus. Being Egyptian, Isis has brown-black skin. The worship of Isis persisted in various forms of the Mother Goddess across the Mediterranean countries and into France, Central Europe, and Russia. Thus, the Black Madonna is the most contemporary form of a very old goddess, having different names, forms and functions in various cultures.

OYA

Out of the Africa comes Oya, the powerful Yoruba goddess of change and transformation, who is the Primeval Mother of Chaos. She is called Queen of the Nine (tributaries of the Niger River) and Goddess of the Winds of Change. Oya represents the wild, turbulent forces of nature and is depicted surrounded by lightning, fire, storms, earthquakes, and tornadoes. Although she can bring destruction, Oya's power is also cleansing and rejuvenating. With her machete (sword of truth) she cuts through everything that is stagnant, stuck, degenerating, and unfit, and which no longer serves our growth. By pruning away the old, dying, and unnecessary parts of ourselves, Oya's energy clears the way for new growth and expression. Oya does what is necessary, what must be done for movement, progress, growth, and renewal.

In her manifestation as the wind, Oya carries souls into and out of the world. She becomes the energy of our first and last breath. Through her functions surrounding death she is connected in popular legend with cemeteries, and her pictures often show her wearing a necklace of skulls. Her great powers may be represented by bulls or horses—animals which can be domesticated and made to serve humankind, but which also may revert to wild behavior and unbridled passions.

Oya is also Queen of the Marketplace, an unusual title for a goddess. The realm of business is capable of creating wealth or ruin, and unless one is shrewd and astute, marketplace forces can get out of control. In all these symbols, we feel the immense uncontrollable power of Oya, a dark goddess of earth and the underworld who can destroy or transform us.

And thou who thinkest to seek for me, know thy seeking and yearning shall avail thee not unless thou knowest the mystery: That if that which thou seekest thou findest not within thee, thou will never find it without thee. For behold, I have been with thee from the beginning, and I am that which is attained at the end of desire.

—Wiccan Charge of the Goddess, *Panegyria,* No. 75, 1998, in Lady Brita, *The Seduction of the Dark Side*

Descent of the Goddess Archetype

For about two years, I'd been yearning for some way to relate to a Divine Feminine. My spiritual tradition, based on Paramhansa Yogananda's teachings, drew primarily from a male line of Indian gurus and Christ. Many prayers and chants were done to Divine Mother, but I felt the need to experience this feminine deity in other forms. In my meditations, I began tentatively saying prayers to the Goddess, and inviting Her presence. It was not easy at first, having related conceptually to male deities for so long. Different images floated through my mental field: goddesses, saints, and priestesses from Greece, Egypt, Celtic lands, Catholic traditions, middle Europe, Asia, and China. I began to study and learn more about these female forms of Spirit.

One evening in meditation, an astonishing event happened. I actually "felt" both physically and through inner awareness, that a huge Goddess energy was descending upon me. It was like an enormous umbrella, slowly lowering onto my field of consciousness, gently pressing upon my aura. I had no clear image of the Goddess, no particular face or shape; but instead felt Her as unfathomable power, infinite awareness, total beingness in everything. My form was completely permeated with this awesome energy, vibrant and radiant with its ecstatic expansiveness.

I have no doubt that what occurred was an invoking of the Goddess Archetype. I had prepared my mental-consciousness field for Her, and had actively invited Her to appear. So She did—and with aplomb. In this experience, I also realized She was calling me into Her service. As the Goddess Archetype became part of my energy field, I took on the sacred mission of this archetype, to bring wisdom-compassion into the world, especially to women for their spiritual empowerment.

—Lennie Martin

> Nothing—the nameless
>   Is the beginning;
> While Heaven, the mother
>   Is the Creatrix of all things.
> All mysteries are Tao,
>   And Heaven is their mother;
> She is the gateway
>   And the womb-door.
>
> —*Tao Te Ching* by Lao Tsu

FORMING A NEW ARCHETYPE: THE CREATRIX

Drawing from models of the mature, midlife and elder woman so richly expressed in other cultures, such as Greek, Native American, Hindu, Buddhist, Old European, and Ancient Egyptian, may be helpful, but there may not be a perfect fit unless you have experience with those cultural backgrounds. The Triple Goddess (maiden-mother-crone) found so universally among cultures provides a good model, but once we have moved past mother by completing the menopausal journey, the crone does not quite express where most Western woman find themselves. Crone seems more fitting for an elder woman, well advanced in years. With women living longer, the mid-age time has also expanded and the phase of advanced age has receded.

Women in their 50s to 70s need a ncw model.

The Fourth Face of the Goddess

We are proposing that women add a fourth face to the Triple Goddess: the Creatrix. Some are already calling this face the Queen and having Queening Ceremonies instead of Croning Ceremonies. The Queen does present a regal, noble, and powerful image. These are qualities that mature women would do well to cultivate. However, the Queen archetype has a number of other particular qualities that may not really apply to many women: expecting deference, needing lavish surroundings, naturally "ruling" others, drawing loyal followers, creating a "queendom" to rule over, generosity and largesse, and providing for those under their "rule."

The Creatrix has a more universal and broad image (see Figure 6–4). She is noble and powerful, in the sense of inner knowledge and self-worth, and deep understanding of the innate value of all others. Hers is a creative force born of maturity, much broader than the capacity for reproduction. Through her flow innumerable possibilities for creating, bringing into manifestation, and taking processes into their fullness and completion.

From the viewpoint of cycles and seasons, the Creatrix would be autumn, the time of harvest, grasses and stalks browning and drying, ripened grain, fruit heavy on vines. She can be in the fullness of her sexuality, with increased capacity for sensuality. She knows how to enjoy life's bounties. In this context we might see the Triple Goddess and a Fourth Face as:

- the Maiden is spring
- the Mother is summer
- the Creatrix is autumn
- the Crone is winter

In the moon cycle, so fundamental to women's rhythms and so ignored by contemporary western society, this quartet would appear as:

- the Maiden as the new and waxing moon
- the Mother as the full moon
- the Creatrix as the waning moon
- the Crone as the dark of the moon

Qualities of the Creatrix Archetype

The Creatrix blends many qualities of the other mature women archetypes described in this chapter. Here is an ideal image of the Creatrix archetype, the highest we might aspire to were we to follow Christ's admonition to "Be ye therefore perfect . . .": The Creatrix has the *Alchemist's* capacity to transform painful, difficult experiences into strength, courage, and wisdom. Drawing from the *Guardian,* she is assertive, outspoken, empathetic, deeply connected with others and the earth, and willing to challenge actions that damage herself or others. As the *Wise Woman,* she offers insight, clarity, and support to others in their journey of self-discovery, carries the seeds of wisdom for future generations, and expresses the transforming power of spirit within. As the *Nurturer-Rejuvenator* she has experienced the darkness, knows the shadow self, and comes into wholeness by integrating her own dark and light patterns. Her wholeness flows through the endless cycles of life, bringing balance into the world.

Perhaps the greatest perfection we can attain, after all, is simply being truly ourselves. If this archetypal image resonates with you, we are happy to have connected. If it does not seem to fit, remember there are many archetypal expressions and all have worth. Archetypes are symbolic concepts, mental field-forms, that capture sets of qualities through images. Their immense power derives from the global collective mental forms that we have infused with meaning over the centuries. Each women resonates with the symbolism most meaningful to her. Whatever it takes to be fully you, then that is the best pattern. We are all unique, so let us celebrate our diversity.

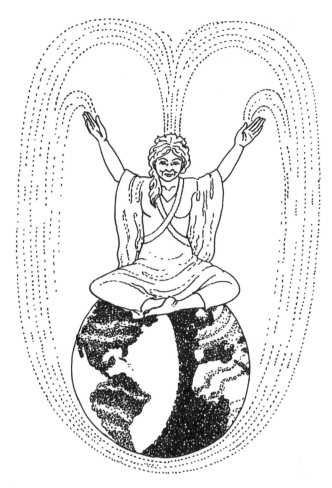

Figure 6–4 The Creatrix. Pouring love, protection, and abundance upon the entire world, the Creatrix archetype lives in the hearts of menopausal women.

Creatrix Blessing

From the mind of infinity   (*hands in prayer, touch forehead*)
With the heart of compassion   (*hands in prayer, touch heart*)
Through the power of creativity   (*hands in prayer, touch navel*)
I pour blessings of peace, love,
    abundance and harmony   (*making arc with hands above head to sides*)
Upon the Earth and all its beings.   (*bring hands in prayer back to heart*)

ENVISIONING THE FUTURE

Join women all around the planet now to envision a whole new world order. We can imagine, create an image, of a world where women are listened to and respected, and where feminine values prevail. It is important to hold these images in your mind, because if you can envision it, you can create it.

What follows draws from broad feminist principles, which some women respond to, but others resist or dismiss. Whether you connect with these feminist principles or not, probably you can still agree that some changes are needed in society and the world. Just try these on "for size" and see if they make sense to you.

What Feminism Really Means

Feminism means humanism. It means deeply honoring the feminine aspects of the self—in both women and men. It means envisioning a society where sexism no longer exists, where opportunities and self-expression are not limited by one's gender. Such a society would support the special needs of girls as they grow up. Girls would be of equal value as boys, and given equal treatment and opportunity in all areas of education and career.

Feminine values are life-enhancing for all people, creatures, and the earth's environment. Life is seen as precious and sacred, to be treated with utmost respect. Everyone is valuable, regardless of position in society, wealth, physical attributes, or intelligence. Cycles are acknowledged in all life processes. Being is more important than doing or having. These values promote peace, harmony, freedom, joyousness, kindness, connectedness, and relations.

Healing the Broken Web

It seems that midlife women, in fulfilling our potential as "New Millennium Women," are being called to heal the broken web of our feminine matrix, torn asunder in many areas by 5,000–6,000 years of patriarchal dominance. Looking around, we see a world that is inhospitable to women, children, and most living

> Yes, and I long for one thing more: to learn how to listen to the delicate vibrations of my soul, to be incorruptibly true to myself and fair to others, to find in this way the right measure of my own worth.
>
> —Karen Horney, in Peg Streep (Ed.), *An Awakening Spirit*

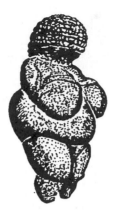

Venus of Willendorf.
Reproduced with permission.
Copyright © Kate Cartwright.

things—including Gaia, the planet herself. This is the result of male-dominated power structures, and of value systems that view the world as a collection of resources to be mined, used, and developed to promote material wealth for a select few. Let us ask this question of ourselves and everyone else who will listen: What will it take to create a society that:

- Cherishes all children
- Respects all adults
- Honors its elders
- Is kind to all creatures
- Sees the Earth as sacred?

Patriarchy: From Silence to Violence

To begin answering this question, we need to take a look at patriarchy as a power system. Please note: This does not mean blaming men as being wrong. Although they appear to benefit from this, most men are as damaged and limited by patriarchal values as are women. It is the system of beliefs and values that is the problem. Here are the main ways patriarchal systems control and suppress women, and others who do not fit the dominant male profile, which in the West means being white, physical, materialistic, rational, non-emotional, and reasonably wealthy:

- *Androcentric language* that expresses and organizes things in terms of the experience of men. This results in male-centeredness, even if it is not consciously intended.
- *Privilege accorded to men.* Women have cooperated with male privilege because they have received certain benefits by aligning themselves with

> It is time now, however, for the pendulum to swing back toward the feminine so that a physically healthy earth and an emotionally healthy world population can be preserved and encouraged.
>
> —Joan Borysenko, *A Woman's Book of Life*

men. In supporting privileges for their men, women could then identify with their more powerful positions. This is a process of identifying with another in order to gain some of his power.

- *Silencing women's voices* has been necessary to keep them subjugated. This did not happen easily; the history of the patriarchy is also the largely unwritten history of women's resistance to it. It took over 2,500 years for women to be fully disempowered. Many measures were needed: laws, edicts, and reinterpreted scriptures. Brute force was necessary, and we have legends of heroic women warriors, such as the Amazons, who resisted fiercely. The outcome was a system in which only male voices had legitimacy.

- *Commodifying women's sexuality* in thousands of ways. Using sexualized images of women and girls deeply dishonors our sexuality. It turns females into objects, things used for purposes of selling something, enhancing male self-image, and creating female images that reinforce our roles. This keeps women confused about our real sexual nature. One of the worst things about this "soft core pornography" is that it eroticizes status and power differences between men and women. Some types even eroticize violence.

- *Separating woman from each other* builds walls of suspicion and distrust. Society defines "good" women as distinctly different from "bad" women. This is the basis for the madonna/whore image that has haunted women for centuries. We can be cruel to each other, with labels like "slut" and "bitch." We lose the ability to listen, dialogue, and connect with each other. Girls learn to distrust women and fear what will happen to them. The strong trend for women's circles is beginning to overcome this separation.

- *Violence* is the ultimate weapon of the patriarchy in keeping women suppressed. Men are generally larger and stronger than women, so physical force is a "bottom-line" way to exert control. Even knowing that force can be used keeps women fearful. We see daily acts of violence against women and girls, often by complete strangers. Women no longer feel safe in streets and parking lots, or even in their homes. The vast majority of men would never use such force, and abhor this rampant violence in our society. However, it just takes a few men capable of carrying out brutality, rape, and murder against women to help maintain the power of the patriarchy.

> Every piece of misogynist scripture or liturgy represents a place where women were still thought to be resisting. . . . For it isn't merely that women have been gagged and muffled all these millennia. . . . It is also that in the domain of patriarchy only one sort of voice has any legitimacy; only one (men's) counts as a real voice.
>
> —Carol Lee Flinders, *At the Root of This Longing*

- *Dethroning the goddesses* and demonizing women's religious practices were key in disempowering women. Images of the sacred were shifted from feminine to masculine, goddess/earth mother religious myths were retold, rituals and symbols were cannibalized. Male sky and warrior gods emerged who were angry, judgmental, harsh, controlling, and often violent. These gods formed covenants with men to give them power and to subjugate women. The feminine became the source of evil, temptation, and sabotage of men's spiritual aspirations. Women were excluded from holy community and many religious rites. Gradually women took these attitudes inside, with devastating effects on their self-worth. The wellsprings of women's spirituality were closed off, but are now flowing upward like released geysers—the Goddess has returned.

Sacred Serpents—Prophecy and Wisdom

The symbol of entwined serpents was found in ancient times throughout the Mediterranean and Middle East, associated with revelation, prophecy, and vision. The earliest accounts are of the Sumerian Goddesses Nidaba, the Learned

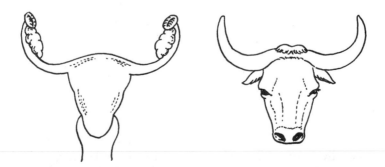

The bull and the uterus: The bull is a mystical life-source, an earthly manifestation of the cosmogonic primordial waters. . . . Why such close association with the Goddess? (Because of) the extraordinary likeness of the female uterus and fallopian tubes to the head and horns of a bull. –Marija Gimbutas, *The Language of the Goddess*

One of the Holy Chambers, often depicted as a serpent; and Ninlil, Great Mother Serpent of Heaven. All existence was thought to begin with serpent-creative power. Inanna (Nina) was a serpent goddess, oracle, and dream interpreter. Ishtar of Babylon was depicted sitting upon the royal throne of heaven, holding a staff with two snakes coiled around it.

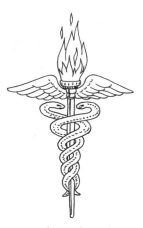

The Cobra Goddess religion was well established by predynastic times in Egypt. Cobra symbols were worn on the foreheads of Egyptian royalty. Called Ua Zit (Au Set, Auset), the Cobra Goddess was the source of creation, and existed before anything else. This symbol is associated with Isis, whose name derives from Auset or Aset. The cobra, represented by an eye, symbolized mystic insight and wisdom. Snakes were found in prophetic goddess temples throughout Egypt.

On the island of Crete, the snake was more often associated with the female deity than in any other Mediterranean area. The Cretan Serpent Goddess was depicted holding snakes in her hands, or with snakes coiled about her body. It is thought that her worship was brought to Crete from Egypt around 3,000 B.C.E. Similar serpent goddess temples were found in Canaan (Palestine) and Cyprus.

The sacred serpent appeared in Greece connected with the Oracle Goddess at Delphi. The priestess who gave divine revelations was Pythia, and a snake called Python was coiled about the tripod stool upon which she sat. The Oracle's advice was sought on many matters, as the priestesses were understood to have direct communication with the deity who possessed the wisdom of the universe. The earliest temples at Delphi were built by women; at this holiest of shrines the Goddess was worshipped as the Primeval Prophetess (Stone, 1976).

In later times the priests of Apollo took over the shrines and killed Python. There are many legends of male warrior-gods slaying snakes and dragons, the mythic symbols of the creation goddesses, and thus subjugating or taking on their power. Around that time, the early Greek physician Aesculapius became associated with the symbol of two serpents coiled around a staff—the caduceus, now a symbol for the medical profession.

Our Daughters, Society, and Ourselves

The web of feminine existence is being healed and made whole by women changing their lives and inner reality. We need to include the girl-children and adolescents of society in this healing process for it to be complete. For many women, our own wounds have been so great that we have not been able to focus on our daughters, whether our own children or all girls in Western culture. The gulf separating women and girls has seemed so large, and the forces maintaining it so tremendous, that many women have felt powerless to make any changes.

The research and writings of many women have raised consciousness about the strong impact of our "girl-poisoning culture." Around puberty, girls lose their voice, face the wall of negative cultural stereotypes of women, have a drop in self-esteem, and their math and science scores plummet. Girls who are gifted, creative, intelligent, and outspoken seem to turn off and shut down. They are overwhelmed by the constricting images of what a teenage girl should be, and the fearsome realization that by becoming women they are losing their unique selfhood (Pipher, 1994).

Many women have written about the processes by which girls and women become disempowered and alienated, and how they reconstruct their self-image and regain their voices. For more about this, see Suggested Reading at the end of this chapter.

We are beginning to reweave the web for girls by creating new traditions for menarche rites, and providing a wealth of written material supporting their value and self-image. Teachers are becoming aware that girls need support to maintain their voices and sense of self after puberty. One example is the "Power and Promise of Girls" program for sixth-graders launched by Tim Flinders and co-teachers in Petaluma, California. The program has three main purposes:

- Making the classroom more welcoming to girls by having images of women scientists, explorers, artists, and political leaders on the walls, and by inviting women speakers doing a wide variety of work.
- Providing girls opportunity to speak out and express themselves through public speaking and performance.
- Creating a way for girls to share and connect with each other, through regular meetings in which girls share personal stories about courage, challenges, issues, and solutions (Flinders, 1998).

What Girls and Women Need

These elements have been identified by many women writers as the keys to helping girls grow up whole, healthy, and self-confident. They can certainly apply to grown women at any age, and women going through the menopausal transition.

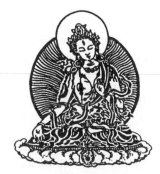

Tara.
Reproduced with permission.
Copyright © Kate Cartwright.

- *Retreats in a female space.* A regular opportunity to be sequestered, alone and in silence, to go within and revel in the mysteries of the female body is essential. The natural tendency of women to seek quiet, contemplative time during menstruation must be supported in some way.

- *Special songs and dances.* Music and movement communicate with the body-mind in ways that go far beyond words. Singing, chanting, dancing, and moving rhythmically in ways that celebrate femininity will create a deep inner sense of being special and precious. This also helps create community among girls and women.

- *Learning life skills and self-mastery.* Girls and women must be prepared to handle their lives in practical ways. Skills that assist us to know our emotional nature and learn positive ways of self-expression are essential. Effective communication is a critical foundation.

- *Touch and laying on of hands.* Humans need to be touched. Most rites of passage include ritual cleansing, symbolizing the metamorphosis that is occurring. This is like massaging the girl/woman into a new form, the likeness of her next stage and the goddess.

- *Physical and athletic expression.* The image of women as weak is reinforced by keeping them physically under-developed. How important physical activity is to health is well known. Girls and women need encouragement to pursue sports and exercise, and social structures that support this. We are seeing a phenomenal response to professional women's sports, such as soccer and basketball, that are drawing thousands of enthusiastic spectators.

- *Adornment.* Girls and women love to wear beautiful jewelry and clothing. Special types of adornment are part of most rites of passage. If we find the deeper symbolism in dressing up, we can honor and celebrate our feminine traditions.

- *Communion with divinity.* The importance of connecting with spiritual forms that reflect back women's images cannot be overstated. By communing with feminine divine forms, girls and women can find those holy expressions within.

- *Deference and support by men.* What would the world be like if men showed respect for women and acknowledged their special needs without labeling them as weaknesses? Mutual support between the sexes would help men and women develop to their fullest expression, and not be limited by artificial definitions imposed to keep the power balance tipped toward one group.

- *Opportunity to serve the community.* Everyone expands by giving to others. Recreating the web of interconnectedness requires that girls and women learn the importance of serving their community and the world in some way.

> People generally speak of women as the weaker sex . . . now (we) recognize that women cannot be considered as weak. From ancient times woman has been held in high esteem. . . . By and large, they uphold truth and righteous conduct. . . . Women are the torch-bearers of refinement . . . and emancipation . . . given due recognition and encouragement, they will shine with brilliance in all fields and will serve the home, nation and entire world gloriously, contributing to the welfare of entire humanity.
>
> —Sathya Sai Baba, *Sai Echoes from Kodai Hills*

WISE WOMAN VISION FOR A NEW WORLD ORDER

Postmenopausal women and those on the threshold of this phase are entrusted by millennia of tradition to carry their culture's highest vision for the future. Knowing the rich history of women's spirituality and social leadership provides a foundation for this responsibility. Becoming familiar with and activating the archetypes that are strongest in you brings an additional level of consciousness and empowerment. As women come into their wisdom years, they can see the purpose and meaning of their own lives more clearly, as well as the values most worth supporting in their societies. For those with children, becoming a grandmother offers

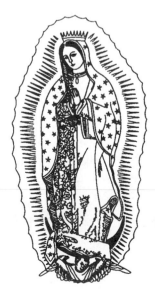

Our Lady of Guadalupe.
Reproduced with permission.
Copyright © Kate Cartwright.

the opportunity to enrich the lives of three generations. In the Seneca Native American tradition, women were taught to think and act in terms of seven generations. As Jill, the 21-year-old daughter of clan mother Janice Sundown Hallett, states: "We are taught that we are to look out for the welfare of the seventh generation. I am the seventh generation of my elders from the past. What I'm doing today is I'm looking at the seventh generation, the faces that are yet unborn" (Wall, 1993).

In her three-book series on women turning 50, 60, and 70, Cathleen Roundtree (1993, 1997, 1999) interviewed mature women from all walks of life, some well-known and others not known at all. She asked them about what kind of lives they led and what they have learned. Many women speak about how they came to realize that service, to their community or the world, was vitally important. Tabra Tunoa built a jewelry-making business into a multimillion-dollar corporation, and then joined Social Venture Network, an organization of socially responsible businesses making $5 million a year or more. Poet and activist Mitsuye Yamada helps people who are involved in struggles, whether political or cultural or within family and self. In her mid-70s Yamada was working with Amnesty International and the Multicultural Women Writers, a group she founded in 1980. With her help, women have written and published on such themes as the impact of strong women in their lives, the invisibility of Asian American women in American culture, and the plight of aging women in a youth-oriented culture.

Native American women are helping to shift their cultures from pessimism to optimism, and from despair to hope. Recovering from the devaluation of women that resulted from the influence of Western culture on women-centered tribes, numerous writers are telling the true story of the powerful influence of women in both traditional and contemporary American Indian life. All aspects of life are being affected, from the secular to the sacred. Paula Allen, a Keres Pueblo Indian of the Southwest, gives many examples of women's involvement in spiritual traditions. She relates the story of the late Essie Parrish, who was the Dreamer of the Kashia Pomo:

Look at us, hear us! . . . Heart of Heaven, Heart of Earth! Give us our descendants, our succession, as long as the sun shall move . . . May the people have peace . . . may they be happy . . . give us good life . . . grandmother of the sun, grandmother of the light, let there be dawn . . . let the light come!

—Mayan prayer to Huracan, Heart of Heaven, Grandmother Sun and Light, in P. G. Allen, *The Sacred Hoop: Recovering the Feminine in American Indian Traditions*

The dreamer is the person responsible for the continued existence of the people as a psychic (tribal) entity. It is through her dreams that the people have being; it is through her dreams that they find ways to function in whatever reality they find. It is through her dreams that the women keep children safe in war, that healings are made possible, and that children are assured a safe passage through life . . . The Dreamer, then, is the center of psychic/spiritual unity of the people. (Allen, 1986)

Modeling Joyful Expansion

The photograph is arresting: a joyful woman with an arm outstretched, who is smiling at the sun, standing on stilts, with one breast removed. This is Californian Terry Sendgraff, a woman in her sixties, a lesbian who developed and now teaches a low-flying trapeze dance form she calls Motivity. Another project she developed is Women Walking Tall, in which she teaches women as old as 75 to walk and dance on stilts. She says what she is really teaching by using this medium of fascinating movement is authentic self-presentation. Ebullient and irrepressible, Sendgraff describes her sixties as "filling up and spilling over . . . full and present, what could feel better?" Through her imaginative work she is helping many others feel better as well.

—From Cathleen Roundtree (1997), *On Women Turning 60*

Taking Charge of Your Archetypes: Women Making a Difference

Fulfilling the archetypal patterns of mature and elder women, we can make a difference in our families, society, and world. As related by an unnamed Native American elder woman:

This is the time of the woman . . . Spiritual communications come through the feminine side . . . Everyone comes into this world with a work to do, and there are special forces to guide in accomplishing that work. To truly do this work with the purest expression, you must be with the spirit, mentally and physically. (Wall, 1993)

Women in the wisdom years can fulfill their potential and embody spirit by:

- Healing ourselves, bringing ourselves to the greatest wholeness and integration of which we are capable.

One and the same rhythm and tune pulsates within all of creation. Once we realize this truth, all the contradictions and differences will dissolve and disappear. Then we will hear the eternal music of the Self, both within and without. The divine flower of peace, love, and tranquility will blossom, and its fragrance will spread all over the world.

—Mata Amritanandamayi Devi (Ammachi), Address
at the United Nations, 1995

- Fulfilling the promise of the rich harvest of fall, the Creatrix archetype, with an abundance of gifts for others.
- Activating other midlife and mature archetypes with which we connect, so their power and attributes can express through our bodies, minds, and lives.
- Supporting other women in their healing of themselves and their attainment of wholeness, completion, and integration.
- Assisting girls through menarche and into womanhood, so they retain their bright gifts, abilities, self-confidence, and belief in their potential as women.
- Putting energy into making changes in our society, to continue to reduce the impact of patriarchal values, and to bring feminine values into the world.
- Cultivating global consciousness that recognizes how everything is connected in an intricate web.
- Making personal choices that support the environment, human rights, animals, peace, and nonexploitation of third world peoples.
- Respecting our differences. Each woman's life has its own unique tapestry. We can never fully know the deeper purposes of another's journey. Each of us chooses to enjoy our life in our own way, some not feeling drawn to community or social action. We would only ask that you be fully aware of the impact of your choices for material comfort, entertainment, recreation, food, and health. That is because everything each one of us does affects the web of existence.

Blessed be! To each and every one of our dear sisters.

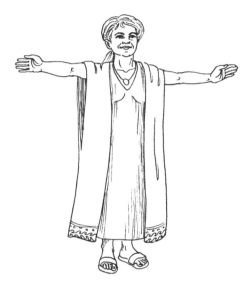

Sisters

Sisters
Such sweetness of soul streams through your spiritual veins that
Your laughter, like a medicine man's rattle, breaks man's web of
    sorrow into showers of blessings;
One million little blessings like butterfly kisses and soft snowflake
    forests
Touch our hearts and fire love in our souls;
Your laughter makes the roses open to the morning sun
And the ice melt that we may drink.
Sisters
Whose courage mutes my voice and freezes my being into a reverent
    stillness;
I am without breath, without a pulse.
I break apart into a thousand sorrows
Floating like lotuses on a mirrored pond, each held afloat by one of
    the millions of your small prayers.
Your prayers, like so many dolphins swimming silently with babies
    on their backs, carry the burdens of humanity
To the soul of the Buddha's compassion
And a tear drops from his eye.

—Judy Kenny, Nevada City, CA

REFERENCES

Allen, P.G. (1986). *The sacred hoop: Recovering the feminine in American Indian traditions.* Boston: Beacon Press.

Anderson, S., & Hopkins, P. (1991). *The feminine face of God: The unfolding of the sacred in women.* New York: Bantam Books.

Baring, A., & Cashford, J. (1991). The hidden goddess in the Old Testament. In *The myth of the goddess: Evolution of an image.* London: Viking.

Bolen, J.S. (1984). *Goddesses in everywoman: A new psychology of women.* San Francisco: Harper & Row.

Bolen, J.S. (1991). *The wise woman archetype: Menopause as initiation* (Audiotape). Boulder: Sounds True.

Bolen, J.S. (2001). *Goddesses in older women: Archetypes in women over fifty.* New York: HarperCollins.

Borysenko, J. (1996). *A woman's book of life: The biology, psychology, and spirituality of the feminine life cycle.* New York: Riverhead Books.

Brita, L. (1998). The seduction of the dark side. *Panegyria, 75,* 3–6.

Cahill, S. (ed.). (1996). *Wise women: Over two thousand years of spiritual writing by women.* New York: W.W. Norton and Company.

Campbell, J. (1972). *Myths to live by.* New York: Viking Press.

Davies, S. (1985). The Canaanite-Hebrew Goddess. In Olson, C. (Ed.). *The book of the goddess past and present.* New York: Crossroad.

Eisler, Riane. (1997). *The chalice and the blade.* San Francisco: Harper & Row.

Flinders, C.L. (1998). *At the root of this longing: Reconciling a spiritual hunger and a feminist thirst.* San Francisco: HarperSanFrancisco.

Frawley, D. (1994). *Tantric yoga and the wisdom goddesses: Spiritual secrets of Ayurveda.* Twin Lakes, WI: Lotus Press.

Frymer-Kensky, T. (1992). *In the wake of the goddesses: Women, culture and the Biblical transformation of pagan myth.* New York: Fawcett Columbine.

Galland, C. (1990). *Longing for darkness: Tara and the Black Madonna.* New York: Penguin Putnam.

Gimbutas, M. (1989). *The language of the goddess.* San Francisco: HarperSanFrancisco.

Gimbutas, M. (1991). *The civilization of the goddess.* San Francisco: HarperSanFrancisco.

Husain, S. (1997). *The Goddess: Creation, fertility, and abundance, the sovereignty of woman, myths, and archetypes.* Boston: Little, Brown & Co.

Joy, Raven. (1999). Sekmet, the lion-headed goddess. Unpublished class material.

Kenny, J. (1998). Sisters. Unpublished poem. Nevada City, CA.

Keuls, E.C. (1993). *The reign of the phallus: Sexual politics in ancient Athens.* Berkeley, CA: University of California Press.

Krymow, V. (1998). Black madonnas: Still black and still venerated. Accessed 12/00: *http://www.udayton.edu/mary/resources/blackm/blackm.html*

Mascetti, M.D. (1998). *Goddesses: Mythology and symbols of the goddess.* New York: Barnes & Noble.

Mata Amritanandamayi Devi. (1996). *Unity is peace.* Address at the Interfaith Celebration in honor of the 50th Anniversary of the United Nations. New York, October 21, 1995. Amritaprui, Kollam, India: Mata Amritanandamayi Mission Trust.

Mullett, G.M. (1979). *Spider Woman stories: Legends of the Hopi Indians.* Tucson: University of Arizona Press.

Myss, C. (2000). *The Fundamentals of Spiritual Alchemy.* Workshop sponsored by The Association for Humanistic Psychology, Oakland, CA, December 1–2.

Newberg, A., D'Aquili, E., & Rause, V. (2001). *Why God won't go away: Brain science and the biology of belief.* New York: Ballantine Books.

Pagels, E. (1989). *The Gnostic gospels.* New York: Vintage Books.

Pipher, M. (1994). *Reviving Ophelia: Saving the selves of adolescent girls.* New York: Ballantine Books.

Roosevelt, F.D. (1933). Inaugural speech, March 4, 1933. Accessed 8/01: *www.viothia.org*

Roundtree, C. (1993). *On women turning fifty: Celebrating midlife discoveries.* San Francisco: HarperSanFrancisco.

Roundtree, C. (1997). *On women turning sixty: Embracing the age of fulfillment.* New York: Three Rivers Press.

Roundtree, C. (1999). *On women turning seventy: Honoring the voices of wisdom.* San Francisco: Jossey-Bass Publishers.

Sathya Sai Baba. (1998). Sai manifesto for women. *Sai echoes from Kodai hills.* Prashaanthi Nilayam, Anatapur District, India: Sri Sai Books and Publications Trust.

Sierra-Wolf, S. (1999). Awakening the solar fire. *Nicki Scully's News from the Cauldron* (Spring), *1,* 19.

Spretnak, C. (1984). *Lost goddesses of early Greece: A collection of pre-Hellenic myths.* Boston: Beacon Press.

Stassinopoulos, A. (1999). *Conversations with the goddesses.* New York: Stewart, Tabori & Chang.

Stone, M. (1976). *When God was a woman.* New York: Harcourt Brace & Co.

Streep, P. (1993). *An awakening spirit: Meditations by women for women.* New York: Viking Study Books.

Tao te Ching by Lao Tsu. (1997). Translated by Gia-Fu Feng and Jane English. New York: Vintage Books.

Wall, S. (1993). *Wisdom's daughters: Conversations with women elders of Native America.* New York: Harper Perennial.

SUGGESTED READING

AAUW. (1991). *Shortchanging girls, shortchanging America.* Washington, D.C.: American Association of University Women Educational Research.

Belenky, M., Clinchy, B., Goldberger, N., & Tarule, J. (1986). *Women's ways of knowing: The development of self, voice, and mind.* New York: Basic Books.

Debold, E., Wilson, M., & Malave, I. (1993). *Mother-daughter revolution: From good girls to great women.* New York: Bantam Books.

Gilligan, C. (1993). *In a different voice.* Cambridge, MA: Harvard University Press.

Johnson, L. (1994). *Daughters of the goddess: The women saints of India.* St. Paul: Yes International Publishers.

Lerner, G. (1986). *The creation of patriarchy.* Oxford: University Press.

MacKinnon, C. (1987). *Feminism unmodified.* Cambridge: Harvard University Press.

Rutter, V.B. (1993). *Woman changing woman: Feminine psychology re-conceived through myth and experience.* San Francisco: HarperSanFrancisco.

Worksheet 6–1

Invoking Your Archetypes

Archetypes are all around you in the domain of thought and consciousness, the mental or mind field. You can follow these steps to increase awareness of their presence, draw these powerful thought forms into your mind, and invoke their powers into your life.

- Read and learn about various midlife and menopausal women's archetypes. Knowing their stories and qualities will bring them alive in your mind.

- Discover an archetype to which you feel drawn. Listen to your inner responses as you read or think about this archetype. If you are inclined, use intuitive methods such as a pendulum or Tarot cards to confirm that this is an active archetype in your consciousness field.

- Enter a quiet, meditative space. Open your awareness to receive, then invite or call the archetype to be present.

- Allow images, thoughts, or ideas to flow into your mind without judging or evaluating them. Simply observe and experience. Listen inwardly for any type of communication from the archetype.

- When the connection with your archetype seems complete, thank it for coming and ask it to remain present in your consciousness field if it is an archetype from which you want to draw power.

- You may want to write your experiences in your journal shortly afterward, while they are fresh in your memory.

- Repeat this process for other archetypes you want to invoke.

Worksheet 6–2

Envisioning a New World Order

If you could help co-create the world to make changes for healing the Earth, and for the health and well-being of all its inhabitants, what would you like to see? Let the sky be your limit. Imagine wildly the best of all possible worlds. My vision for the World, its people, creatures, the Earth:

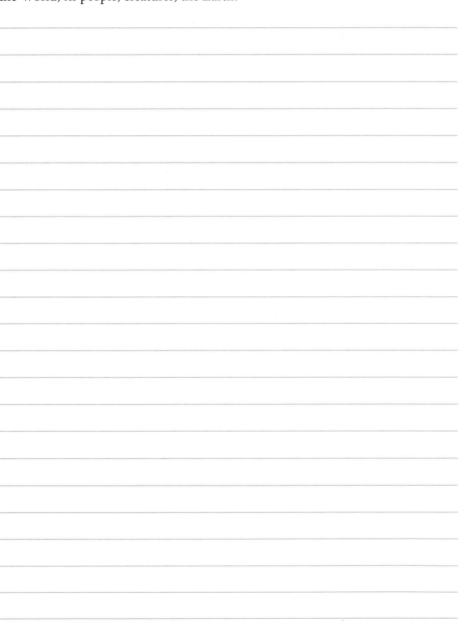

My Contributions to a World in Balance and Harmony

List some ways you personally can begin to make a difference. Remember, peace, love, and harmony begin at home, within yourself and your family. Here are just a few areas where we can make contributions:

- Food banks, soup kitchens
- Humane societies, especially ones that save animals' lives
- Protecting whales, dolphins, sea turtles
- Protecting old-growth forests
- Protecting wild, scenic rivers and lakes
- Women and children's shelters, safe houses, domestic violence services
- Buying from ecologically responsible businesses
- Choosing plant-based diets and organic foods
- Not watching violent, sexually exploitive movies and television
- Praying regularly for world peace

Here is what I am able to do:

Yoga Postures for Menopause

Posture	Physiological Effects	Menopause Benefits
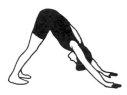 Downward-Facing Dog (Mountain Pose)	shifts blood flow to head balances endocrines strengthens arms, stretches legs	decreases hot flashes builds bone in arms, wrists limbers leg muscles, joints
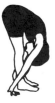 Jackknife (Standing Forward Bend)	stimulates circulation, digestion releases tensions in legs shifts blood flow to head massages abdominal, pelvic organs	supports calm emotions releases emotional tensions improves digestion improves pelvic congestion
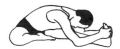 Head-to-Knee	limbers legs, lower back massages abdominal, pelvic organs stimulates peristalsis stimulates adrenals, liver, spleen	promotes peace, tranquility releases fear, insecurity aids anxiety, depression aids constipation and pelvic congestion

Posture	Physiological Effects	Menopause Benefits
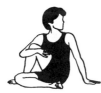 Simple Inverted Pose (milder) Shoulder Stand (more intense)	draws blood to brain, eyes, ears, nose stimulates thyroid, parathyroid improves circulation, rests heart drains blood from legs, pelvic area	decreases hot flashes aids thyroid, parathyroid relieves varicose veins and hemorrhoids benefits skin, complexion creates peace, balance
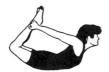 Half Spinal Twist	strengthens, limbers spine and neck stimulates adrenals, kidneys expands shoulders, opens chest	aids estrogen production balances heart qualities (joy, compassion, love)
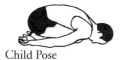 Bow Pose	stimulates, balances circulation tones digestive, pelvic organs, adrenals and limbers spine, hips	balances hormones aids estrogen production increases energy in spine
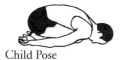 Child Pose	stimulates leg circulation relaxes, tones abdominal organs brings blood flow to brain stimulates pelvic organs	relieves fatigue in lower body, mental fatigue relieves low abdomen, back muscle tension may help irregular periods

Posture	Physiological Effects	Menopause Benefits
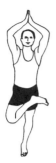 Tree Pose (and other standing poses)	tones leg, feet muscles balances spinal column, muscles coordinates muscle activity	builds and strengthens bone develops good posture reduces stress, promotes calmness
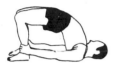 Bridge Pose	strengthens low back stimulates pelvic organs stretches leg, abdominal muscles	energizes pelvic organs balances hormones aids estrogen production calms moods, anxiety
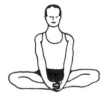 Butterfly Pose (supported)	opens, stretches thighs and pelvis removes constriction of uterus ovaries, vagina	balances hormones relieves pelvic congestion calms moods, anxiety, fears
  Legs Up Wall (supported inversion)	increases circulation to chest, head	reduces stress, anxiety reduces varicose veins relieves hot flashes

Yoga postures reproduced with permission from Ananda Yoga Teacher Training Program and the Ananda Expanding Light Retreat, Nevada City, CA 95959.

APPENDIX B

How to Start a Women's Group

Many of the ideas and suggestions presented here are from the experience author Pam Jung had as a member of a women's group for eight years.

Women getting together to talk about their lives, their relationships, what brings them joy, and what brings them sadness is as old as time. Unfortunately, with the busyness of our lives today, it does not usually happen unless a formal group is formed. The rewards of such a group, if the chemistry is right, can be anything from pleasant to life-transforming. The challenges may be great as well.

Because the effectiveness of a group and its longevity depend entirely on its members, much depends on who participates. Often groups start when a couple of friends think it is a good idea to try and agree to invite others to join them. Unless members are psychotherapists, the group is not considered a therapy group; rather, it is an opportunity to share sisterhood.

Some elements that help a group succeed are:

Honesty

A feeling of emotional safety (no hurtful words or actions accepted)

Equality (no permanent leader; rotating facilitators are best; consensus required)

Kindness

Acceptance (people's rates of growth are different)

Nonadvice giving (keeping one's own counsel unless specifically asked to give advice; women want to be heard, not fixed)

Patience and commitment (when the road is bumpy, stick with it; the outcome might surprise you)

Some elements that will sabotage a group:

Insecure, controlling egos

People who do not feel "heard"

Feelings of being unsafe (rules arrived at by consensus being broken instead of renegotiated; feeling under "attack" by another)

A group has a mind/will of its own—while you can take another group's experience as a guide, the group you form will reveal its own direction. The following are some guidelines to consider:

> A women's group usually does best when all members are treated equally. But that doesn't mean that there cannot be a facilitator's position that is rotated either by time served, or by whose home you are at that week/month. A facilitator is not necessarily a leader. She can be simply a timekeeper, or she can suggest topics, books, or experiences to explore.
>
> A small group usually is better than a large one. Five to seven members is good—large enough so that absenteeism will not diminish the group experience, yet small enough that each woman has an opportunity to share during the evening.
>
> If you are meeting in homes, rather than a neutral space, many groups have found that it helps to rotate the home setting among the members (very egalitarian).
>
> Groups that want to have both a social connection as well as a "sharing life's issues" connection find that having a social hour first (such as dining together and sharing light conversation) allows for a concentrated discussion or processing session later.
>
> Try some ground rules, such as: (a) no advice given unless the person sharing asks for it; (b) what to do if a major conflict between two members arises; (c) each person holds a "talking stick" while sharing (this means no interruptions until she has finished); (d) strict confidentiality (this means no talking about issues with your spouse later); (e) no gossiping—it's deadly (this means not talking behind anyone's back in a mean-spirited manner, especially about absent members).
>
> You might want to have re-evaluation points when your group decides major issues, such as whether to continue meeting, whether to change the rules, or whether to open it up to new members. A re-evaluation point at six months, then a year, can unearth unbalances that need redressing. It can also relieve any feelings of entrapment.
>
> To establish trust, commit to each other. If you meet once a week, you might want to set a guideline that members be present at least three out of four times. Expect shadow sides to emerge as buttons are pushed. If you feel committed to the group and stick with it, and do not give in to the all-too-human desire to quit when there is discomfort, you will find rewards. With this commitment you may find yourself more able to process life's issues more honestly and in more depth.

What makes for a good mix of women in a group? The issue of chemistry has a magical, ineffable quality to it—"you either have it or you do not." Another variable—age range—is important. The closer you are in age, the more interests you may share. Your group probably will not last as long (or may become purely social) if it comprises young women who are dating, on the one hand, and "old marrieds" with grandchildren on the other.

Allow members to have their emotions. There is no need to "rescue" someone from the unpleasant. Tears and expressions of pain are to be heard, not "made better." Nonverbal tenderness, as in getting the crying woman to lie down in the center of your circle and simply be touched or massaged gently by the members, can be a real gift to someone who is hurting. You might talk as a group about how to handle emotions, such as anger, if/when they come up.

Everything has a life cycle, and so does a group. The group may last any length of time, from a couple of months to many years. Good luck with your group!

APPENDIX C

Rite-of-Passage Ceremony

Marilyn was turning sixty and she wanted something very different from a normal birthday party. She wanted to celebrate her sixty years and acknowledge all the people and experiences that had gone into making her what she was now.

So Marilyn called together her friends to help her make this birthday special. The ceremony took place in her large comfortable yurt (a tentlike structure), which was resplendent with candles and sweet-smelling with incense. About twenty people were present to witness Marilyn's rite of passage into the seventh decade of her life:

> The guest of honor—Marilyn—seats herself at the head of the circle of her friends. The mistress of ceremonies (MC), dressed in robes of white and gold, welcomes everyone to this celebration and starts the first of the rites.

> Marilyn meditates briefly on each of the six decades of her life, giving special emphasis to the gifts of each decade and what they signified to her. "What do you want to take forward with you into the next decade?" asks the MC. (An alternative to this has more chance involved: the honoree picks at random from a pot a stone for each decade, inscribed with a word [courage, patience, determination] that defines at least one of the lessons of that decade and drops it into a body of water [pond, stream, water pot], which symbolizes her subconscious and how that shaped her future.)

> Marilyn's time for taking vows is announced. The MC begins intoning each vow, as previously written by Marilyn, and Marilyn answers "I will" to each one. She promises to develop her intuition, to serve the community, to dedicate time to self-study, and much more. At the conclusion the MC says "May God/Goddess, who has given you the will, support you in the performance of these responsibilities."

> A blessing comes next. The MC (this doesn't have to be one person; several can take turns) puts her hands on Marilyn's bowed head and offers a prayer of thanksgiving for Marilyn, for her gifts, for her wisdom, and for her importance to all those assembled.

> Time for gift giving. Marilyn receives a bracelet made of links, symbolizing how she "links up" people to one another. It is passed around so that every

person can put her or his special energy into it. All the while beautiful, soft, angelic music plays in the background.

Sharing time begins as all the assembled friends take turns offering something about Marilyn that they particularly cherish about her or wish for her. Sweet memories are shared. One friends says that she wishes for Marilyn peace and increasing wisdom. Another thanks Marilyn for her special brand of friendship.

Now, the MC says a benediction and invites everyone to hug Marilyn. The ceremony is complete, and the socializing begins.

When asked what she thought of her ceremony, Marilyn said, "Experiencing group energy focused totally on me was like going to my own funeral, only I was there in the flesh to witness what others think, say, and feel about me. It was very powerful."

Following are suggestions of other creative things you can do:

- Invite everyone to dance, drum, and chant.

- Change clothing at an appropriate point in the ceremony, to symbolize taking off the old and putting on the new

- Draw a line in the dirt (this is great for a fiftieth party) and invite the honoree to cross over it, symbolizing her entering the second part of her life—the wisdom years. This also may be used for later birthdays (seventy, eighty), to symbolize entry into cronehood.

- Do a reading: medicine cards, tarot, or the I Ching

- Make beautiful altars of personal, symbolic, spiritual items (read *Creating Women's Circles or Sacred Altars* by Sadena Cahill)

- Guests make pieces of art featuring words or images that have been offered by the honoree. The pieces are then made into a mobile, using string and twigs.

- An outside gathering can include a ceremonial fire. Write on a piece of paper either (or both): (1) what you want to purify or burn up in the sacred flame—for yourself and for the honoree (procrastination, greed, emotional volatility, and so on), or (2) what blessing or attribute you want to bring to yourself and to the honoree. Consign these papers to the flames, which in turn take the messages to the universe. This can be a great way to witness, release, and affirm. Dance around the fire either in cadence or wildly, maybe with face painted, or sway while holding hands around the fire

- Humor is always welcome, if it is kind. A friend kneels before the honoree and takes from a basket a mixer, strainer, wooden spoon, wine opener, or other such thing and says "you have been like a —— in my life, causing ——." For example, "you have been like a mixer in my life, mixing up my preconceived notions about what life should be all about and opening up to me new vistas about how to live more completely."

- The honoree closes her eyes and feels the love from special moments in her life. Then she extends her hands and offers this loving energy to all participants as in a benediction.

APPENDIX
D

Seclusion

Seclusion usually has a spiritual connotation, although it is also used for personal growth. It is, nonetheless, time alone. Time to think, to meditate, or pray, and to feel connected with your deeper self.

Seclusion can be like taking the vacation of vacations. The difference is that in a normal vacation you are exploring the outer world; in a seclusion it is the inner world that beckons and intrigues. In seclusion you "knit up the raveled sleeve of care." The result is refreshment and renewal in your body, mind, and soul.

Here we describe a simple seclusion, which can be done over a long weekend, just to get your feet wet. Total immersion might be a week or longer—very worthwhile if you can do it.

- Choose a quiet place where you will really be alone—a friend's cabin, preferably in nature, would be great. Camp only if you are totally comfortable with this, otherwise you will spend too much psychic energy processing the newness of your experience—energy that better is spent going within.

- Spend three nights or more, so you can truly relax and feel as though you are away from it all.

- Take with you only inspirational reading, one to two books at most. Do not bring popular writing such as *People* or the latest murder mystery; during this time you want to feed your mind "good food."

- Sleep until you are completely rested.

- Monitor your thoughts. If you find yourself obsessing about a current problem at work, stop. Replace those thoughts with an uplifting song, or mantra, or inspiring words, such as "all good things come to me; they bring me peace." Think about God, or goodness, or love.

- Take long walks.

- Meditate during your walks; in the morning before breakfast, an hour before retiring, and any time during the day; as much as you like.

- Think about the blessings in your life and be grateful. When a negative thought arises, try gently turning it around to a positive.

- Eat lightly (smaller portions) and also eat lighter foods; this will give your body a rest and will help you feel lighter.
- Pray for others throughout the day. Pray for yourself.
- Do some yoga stretches; breathe deeply and slowly.
- Lie on your back, looking up at the clouds, and wool-gather, letting your thoughts float here and there.
- Think of yourself as your best friend—that you are spending enjoyable time alone with your best friend.
- Take a long soak in a bath, perhaps with candles and soft music.
- Maintain a quiet environment; no music for most of the time might be best, but soft music such as harp and chanting may be uplifting. Absolutely no television or videos.

The purpose of all the above is to quiet the mind. This takes practice and might seem impossible at first, but persistence pays off. As the mind takes a holiday from its fretful, busy thoughts, peace descends. This leads to calm balance, a sense that you are whole rather than fragmented. It helps you to learn to trust yourself and to like yourself more.

How to Create Your Own Circle

Whenever you are doing a ceremony of any kind, it adds special focus and brings a sacred atmosphere to gather in a circle and call up the Four Directions. This is an ancient rite that dates back at least to 5,000 B.C.E. in the old European (pagan) and Mediterranean goddess religions.

According to many ancient and native cultures, such as Native Americans (Indians), old European cultures (Celts, Druids) and indigenous peoples in Asia, Africa, and Australia, each direction (east, south, west, and north) has an element of nature associated with it, in a pairing that brings out mystical and spiritual qualities. Thus, East is paired with the element Air, South with Fire, West with Water, and North with Earth.

Instructions for circling:

Calling Up a Circle

Everyone gather around into a circle and hold hands.

The mistress of ceremonies says a prayer.

Drop hands and turn to face the starting direction—East.

The mistress of ceremonies intones the greeting to the East (see description below), usually holding up an eagle feather or some other item that symbolizes the element Air.

When she finishes speaking, everyone can join in, acknowledging their approval, with "aho."

She and the group then turn to the next direction (South) and follow the same format with the content specific to the south.

And so on, until all four directions have been addressed. This is enough for many. However, some traditions call in three more directions: down (Mother Earth), up (Father Sky), and around (Great Spirit).

Releasing a circle

As you call up a circle at the beginning of your event or ceremony, so do you release the circle at the end of it. This is a perfect ending that helps people feel complete.

As you spiraled from East to North in calling a circle, so you unspiral by starting with the North and ending with the East.

Again everyone stands in a circle, facing North.

The mistress of ceremonies (or someone else) thanks the spirits, elements, and powers of the North for giving their special gifts to the circle.

She continues through the last direction (East), and can end either with a prayer or with "And so it is."

The event or ceremony is now over.

Qualities of the Directions and Elements

East/Air

Time of day: Dawn

Season: Spring

Scents: Basil, bergamot, mint, dill, parsley

Colors: Yellow, white

Animal: Eagle

Objects: Feathers, wind chimes

Minerals: Amber, topaz, citrine

Qualities: Clarity, communication, the mind, learning, psychic work, inspiration.

The returning magic of sunrise brings new hope, reawakening of nature, and anticipation of clarity and illumination. New understandings are given of our relationship to the Earth and the universe, and new skills are learned to live in greater harmony. We learn to understand our experiences and gain new perspectives and knowledge. When we seem lost, exhausted, or disillusioned, the gift of the East is new awareness, new ways of seeing things, that help us find our way out of the maze. The lessons of Air are lightness of being, freedom, hope, and discovery.

Invocations

In calling the circle: "Powers of the East! Bring your morning song to my heart, and in return, I will take flight into the air of your dawn."

In releasing the circle: "Thank you, powers of the Eastern gate, for bringing us new awareness, freedom, and hope. We release you with gratitude."

South/Fire

Time of day: Noon

Season: Summer

Scents: Frankincense, black pepper, clove, lime, rosemary, ginger

Colors: Red, orange

Animals: Coyote, mouse

Objects: Candles, bonfires, hot peppers

Minerals: Ruby, garnet, carnelian, bloodstone

Qualities: Passion, strong will, growth, purification, sensuality, joy.

The vital life force of warmth and fire rushes forth, bringing full bloom to our passions and purposes. We feel the pulsating power of the universe within our bodies, a heat like the sun at midday. We express our full creative force, to manifest our dreams and visions, to act on our desires and achieve our goals. Emotions are intense under the influence of fire; we protect our dreams, rage at limits or pain, fight back, hold on to what is ours. Bonds are created with others, and we rejoice together in our victories.

Invocations

In calling the circle: "Powers of the South! From my fingertips I cast forward my fire, lighting the peaks of my creation, dancing the fullness of life."

In releasing the circle: "We release you, oh powers of the South, with thanks for stimulating our creative force and helping us onward to victory."

West/Water

Time of day: Dusk

Season: Autumn

Scents: Sandalwood, chamomile, jasmine, iris, rose, vanilla, ylang-ylang

Colors: Blue, green, turquoise, indigo

Animals: Bear, raven

Objects: Glass, cup, bowl, ocean, river, lake, stream, juice, wine

Minerals: Pearl, moonstone, obsidian, amethyst, opal

Qualities: Fluidity, renewal, emotions, compassion, feminine, unconscious.

All nature teaches us the path of change when we face the West. Watching the fiery sunset slowly fading away, the trees release their leaves, the fruit ripen and fall, the bear prepares for hibernation, and we know the time is coming to go within. We may cling with fear to what we know we must release. The flowing water, ever moving, ever changing, tells us to let go, to accept and flow with change. With the serenity of the sea's tides and the enthusiasm of the river's currents, we find courage to look inward, to heal, to follow inner guidance, and to have faith. We harmonize with the rhythms of our lives.

Invocations

In calling the circle: "Powers of the West! As the sun sets, and waves break to return again as moontides, I will flow as the river's currents to the place of courage, daring to look within and receive the healing waters of change."

In releasing the circle: "Powers of the West, we offer thanks for our healing and release you now."

North/Earth

Time of day: Midnight

Season: Winter

Scents: Pine, cedar, honeysuckle, lilac, spikenard, vertevert

Colors: Brown, green

Animals: Buffalo, white owl

Objects: Plants, flowers, dirt, salt, grains, bread

Minerals: Emerald, turquoise, malachite

Qualities: Stillness, silence, natural cycles, nurturance, wisdom, unity.

In the North—darkness, winter, midnight skies, stillness, silence—we learn to be still ourselves and to be one with the Earth and the Universe. Deep within, like the dark, warm womb, is where the human spirit evolves safely and securely. In the darkness, we come to know ourselves, to hear the rhythm of our lives, the thread of spirit that weaves consciousness beyond and before time. From our deepest center, a shining form unfolds, alive and powerful, growing and evolving in vision and wisdom. This is our true self, our essence of being which needs its passage through the Earth to refine and expand its potentials. Each cycle through the dark womb of Earth helps us gather wisdom, learn the power of darkness, and rejoice in the gift of light.

Invocations

In calling the circle: "Powers of the North! Where the mountain carves her silhouette across the midnight sky, where the frozen silence takes me deep into my own mysteries, I open my heart to the wisdom of unity with Earth and Universe."

In releasing the circle: "Oh, powers of the Northern gate, we are grateful for Mother Earth's wisdom and your gifts of introspection. We release you with thanks."

RESOURCES

Artists

Kate Cartwright
Website: *www.katecartwright.com*
E-mail: *katecartwright.com*

Sandra Stanton
Website: *www.goddessmyths.com*
E-mail: *images@mainwest.com*

Laboratories

Aeron LifeCycles Laboratory
1933 Davis St., Ste. 310
San Leandro, CA 94577
1-800-631-7900
Websites: *www.aeron.com; www.hrtdoctor.com*

Saliva tests for estrogens, progesterone, testoterone, DHEA, cortisol, melatonin. Urine test for calcium loss (Pyrilinks-D). Available to health care providers.

DiagnosTechs Laboratory
206-251-0596

Wisdom Hormone Support Program
1-800-705-5559

Salivary hormone test kit offered by Dr. Christiane Northrup in partnership with Aeron Life-Cycles Laboratory.

ZRT Laboratory
1815 N.W. 169th Place, Ste. 3090
Beaverton, OR 97006
503-466-2445
Website: *www.salivatest.com*

Human Identical Hormone Therapy

Compounding or Formulatory Pharmacies

Pharmacies that provide human identical hormone products are listed below. Prescriptions must be ordered by a health care provider.

College Pharmacy
833 N. Tejon St.
Colorado Springs, CO 80903
1-800-888-9358

Madison Pharmacy Associates
429 Gammon Place
Madison, WI 53719
1-608-833-7046

Women First Pharmacy Services
1-877-296-6361 (toll-free)

Women's International Pharmacy
at two locations

13925 W. Meeker Blvd., Ste. 13
Sun City West, AZ 85375
1-800-279-5708

5708 Monona Drive
Madison, WI 53716
1-800-279-5708

Website: *www.wipws.com*
E-mail: *info@wipws.com*

Health practitioners who use human identical hormone therapy are listed by the following:

Aeron LifeCycles Laboratory
1-800-631-7900

Natural Woman Institute
Los Angeles, CA
1-530-477-8080
Website: *www.naturalwoman.org*
E-mail: *info@naturalwoman.org*

Professionals and Patients for Customized Care
1-800-927-4227

Newsletters, Websites, Organizations, and Suppliers

Women at the Gateway
Website: *www.women-at-the-gateway.bigstep.com*
E-mail: *pfjung@jps.net*

Dr. Christiane Northrup's Health Wisdom for Women
(monthly newsletter)
Phillips Publishing, Inc.
7811 Montrose Road
Potomac, MD 20854
1-800-211-8561
Website: *www.drnorthrup.com*

Dr. Andrew Weil's Self Healing: Creating Natural Health for Your Body and Mind
(monthly newsletter)
Thorne Communications, Inc.
42 Pleasant St.
Watertown, MA 02472
1-800-523-3296

A Better Way to Midlife Health (Website)
Women First HealthCare, Inc.
Website: *www.womenfirst.com*
E-mail: *contactus@womenfirst.com*

The North American Menopause Society (NAMS)
P.O. Box 94527
Cleveland, OH 44101-4527
1-530-477-8080
Website: *www.menopause.org*

Websites on Breast Cancer

oncolkink.com
cancernet.nih.gov
webmd.com
cancer.org

National Alliance of Breast Cancer Organizations
Website: *www.nabco.org*
E-mail: *nabco@aol.com*

Website on Bladder Control

Let's Talk about Bladder Control for Women
National Institute of Diabetes and Digestive and Kidney Disease
1-800-891-5388
Website: *www.niddk.nih.gov*

Websites on Depression and Obesity

nimh.nih.gov
intelihealth.com
webmd.com
cbshealthwatch.com

Government Initiative on Obesity and Overweight

U.S. Department of Agriculture
Website: *www.nutrition.org*

SADD

Full-spectrum lights may be purchased through the following companies.

American Environmental Products
Fort Collins, CO
1-800-981-7157

Apollo Light Systems, Inc.
1-800-545-9667

Environmental Lighting Concepts, Inc.
Tampa, FL
1-800-842-8848

Medic-Lite
(Ultra-Bright Medic-Lite 10,000)
Lake Hopatcong, NJ
1-210-663-1214

Ott Lights System, Inc.
(Ott lights)
Santa Barbara, CA
1-800-234-3724

Pacific Spirit
Forest Grove, OR
1-800-634-9057

The SunBox Company
1-800-548-3968

Alternative Health Information

Alternative Therapies in Health and Medicine
(peer-reviewed journal)
Website: *www.alternative-therapies.com*

Alternative Medicine Foundation
5411 West Cedar Lane, Ste. 205-A
Bethesda, MD 20814
1-301-581-0116
Websites: *www.amfoundation.org; www.herbmed.org*
E-mail: *amfi@amfoundation.org*

Herb World News Online
by the Herb Research Foundation
Website: *www.herbs.org*

The National Center for Complementary and Alternative Medicine (NCCAM)
National Institutes of Health
P.O. Box 8218
Silver Spring, MD 20907-8218
1-888-644-6226
Website: *http://altmed.od.nih.gov/nccam*

The Review of Natural Products
Facts and Comparisons
(source of drug, herbal, patient and disease management information)
111 West Port Plaza, Ste. 300
St. Louis, MO 63146
1-800-223-0554
Website: *www.drugfacts.com*

UCB Wellness Letter
by the School of Public Health, University of California, Berkeley
Website: *www.wellnessletter.com*

Therapeutic Touch

To locate a practitioner of therapeutic touch, contact:

Nurse Healers-Professional Associates International
1-801-273-3399
Website: *www.therapeutic-touch.org*

INDEX

Figures in the text are indicated by *italic* page numbers.